Language Competence Across Populations

Toward a Definition
of Specific Language Impairment

Language Competence Across Populations

Toward a Definition
of Specific Language Impairment

Edited by

Yonata Levy
The Hebrew University

Jeannette Schaeffer
Ben-Gurion University of the Negev

LEA LAWRENCE ERLBAUM ASSOCIATES, PUBLISHERS
2003 Mahwah, New Jersey   London

Lawrence Erlbaum Associates, Inc., Publishers
10 Industrial Avenue
Mahwah, NJ 07430

Cover design by Kathryn Houghtaling Lacey

Cover drawing of children communicating
by six-year-old Shirel Libersat.

Library of Congress Cataloging-in-Publication Data

Language competence across populations : toward a definition of Specific
    Language Impairment / edited by Yonata Levy, Jeannette Schaeffer.
        p. cm.
Papers of a workshop held in the spring of 2000 in Jerusalem, hosted by the
    Institute for Advanced Studies of the Hebrew University of Jerusalem.
Includes bibliographical references and index.
ISBN 0-8058-3999-2 (cloth : alk. paper)
1. Specific language impairment in children—Congresses.   2. Learning
    disabled children—Congresses.   3. Chidren—Language—Congresses.
    I. Levy, Yonata.   II. Schaeffer, Jeannette.
RJ496.L35 L355   2002
618.92'855—dc21   2002069204
                                                                    CIP

Books published by Lawrence Erlbaum Associates are printed on acid-free
paper, and their bindings are chosen for strength and durability.

Printed in the United States of America
10 9 8 7 6 5 4 3 2 1

Contents

v

Preface

In spring 2000, the people whose work appears in this volume gathered in the majestic city of Jerusalem for a workshop on language development across populations. The title of the volume is indicative of the approach that characterized the meeting. Our main concern was the variability seen in human linguistic competence across populations of children, yet a major focus of our discussion was the phenomenon of specific language impairment (SLI). Although we acknowledge the challenges posed by SLI to our understanding of the structure and function of human linguistic competence, we also pay close attention to data concerning other populations of children that suggest points of similarities with the classical SLI profile. The composition of the chapters in this volume attests to this dual focus: More than half the chapters are concerned with SLI, but the remainder (a little less than half, yet still quite close in number) concentrates on language in other nonstandard populations of children.

This volume brings to the fore intriguing findings concerning language development in the populations studied. It discusses criteria for the definition of SLI, compares and contrasts SLI with profiles of children with other disorders and dialects, and offers a comprehensive look on human language, which ties together spoken and sign languages. Methodological concerns that affect the credibility and generalizibility of the findings are discussed and controversies between opposing linguistic approaches to acquisition are presented. The common thread that gradually reveals itself is a theoretical issue of central importance to cognitive theory, as well as to our understanding of the biological correlates of language—the question of how much variability linguistic competence can take in children as they develop.

The workshop was made possible through the generosity of a number of scientific institutions in Israel. The Israeli Science Foundation (ISF) provided major funding for the project. Without ISF funding, the meeting could not have taken place. The Institute for Advanced Studies of the Hebrew University in Jerusalem gave us financial help and, most importantly, hosted the meeting. The Institute was an island of tranquility and intellectual creativity amidst the bustling life of this uniquely beautiful, highly inspiring and, at that time, hopeful and peace-seeking city. We are grateful to the staff and management of the Institute for their hospitality and professional help before and during the days of the workshop. We were fortunate to receive financial help from the Abrahams-Curiel Department of Foreign Literatures and Linguistics at Ben-Gurion University of the Negev, and from the Authority for Research and Development of the Hebrew University of Jerusalem. We hope that this book proves itself worthy of their generous support. Lastly, we thank Izchak Schlesinger, whose profound wisdom and gentle manners enriched us all during the days of the workshop.

Yonata Levy
Jeannette Schaeffer
Jerusalem, September, 2001

LANGUAGE COMPETENCE
ACROSS POPULATIONS

I

THE CHARACTERIZATION
OF SPECIFIC LANGUAGE IMPAIRMENT

AN INTRODUCTION

Jeannette Schaeffer
Ben-Gurion University of the Negev

Within the general theme of the present volume, language competence across populations, this first section takes a special focus. It concentrates on one particular population, namely, children with specific language impairment (SLI). Specific language impairment has been studied for several decades, and is viewed by many researchers as a disorder distinct from other (language) disorders. However, as several contributions in this volume show, it is not always clear in what sense the language characteristics of children with SLI are different from those of children with other disorders. Thus, it is important to investigate the differences and similarities in linguistic behavior between the various populations. This provides more insight into the possible specificity of the disorders, as well as into the general constraints on language development. In order to maintain the hypothesis that SLI is a distinct disorder, it is necessary to create a set of exclusionary and inclusionary criteria on the basis of which the disorder can be isolated. The chapters in this section contribute to this goal.

Another focus concerns the crosslinguistic aspects of SLI. Originally, descriptions and theories of SLI were based mostly on data from English SLI. However, a recent wave of crosslinguistic research has challenged certain traditional characterizations of SLI. Several chapters in this section add in an important way to the recharacterization of SLI because languages other than English (e.g., Dutch, French, Hebrew, and Inuktitut) come under investigation.

A few questions help in organizing thoughts on the characterization of SLI: How can anyone know if a child is specifically language impaired? And what does specific language impairment mean exactly? Despite decades of research on language impairment, there is still no consensus on a definition of SLI.

A first step is to decide in what kind of terms to define SLI. Would it be useful to formulate a definition on the basis of theoretical models of linguistics and/or cognition? Should there be a list of symptoms (description)? Or should the definition have some explanatory value as well? Should the aim be for one general, crosslinguistic definition, or should the definition be customized according to (groups of) target languages? Are there subtypes of SLI? If yes, on the basis of which factors should these subtypes be distinguished?: Comprehension versus production? The different components of language, for example, the lexicon, syntax, semantics, morphology, phonology, pragmatics?

Leonard (1998) listed several inclusionary and exclusionary criteria for the diagnosis of SLI. Although diagnostic criteria are not the same as a definition, they could help in formulating a definition. The inclusionary criterion of a significant deficit in language ability is the most straightforward. A diagnosis of a language problem can usually be made with confidence. The trick is to distinguish SLI from other disabling conditions of which language problems are a part. Furthermore, a "language problem" can manifest itself in many different ways (recall the different language components: lexicon, syntax, etc., and the specifics of the target language). The exclusionary criteria require normal behavior in areas other than language, such as nonverbal IQ, hearing, brain structure, speech organs, and physical and social interactions.

Although the exclusionary criteria narrow down the number of candidates for SLI considerably, and are therefore very useful, the one single inclusionary criterion remains vague, and brings things back to the main question: Which parts/forms of language must be impaired in order to be diagnosed with SLI? When there are answers to these questions, then an adequate set of test batteries can be developed to serve as selectional criteria. The chapters in this section show that by keeping alive the interaction and exchange of information between models of linguistic theory and crosslinguistic data studies on SLI, it is possible to refine the inclusionary criterion and therefore come closer to a more detailed definition of SLI.

First consider linguistic theoretical models that distinguish different components within language. At least three major components of language can be identified: the lexicon, the computational system (Chomsky, 1993), and the pragmatic system. The computational system can in turn be subdivided into syntax, semantics, morphology, phonology (grammar), and the mechanism that processes their information (parser). Approaching SLI from this angle, then, a limitation in language ability can be lexical, syntactic, semantic, morphological, phonological, or pragmatic in nature, or a combination of two or more of these components.

The studies presented in this section all concern the question of whether these linguistic components are the exact ones that can help in an understanding and investigation of SLI, or whether the pie should be cut slightly differently. Whereas Wexler, Crago & Paradis, Van der Lely, and Schaeffer approach the problem from a (generative) linguistic theoretical angle, Rice, de Jong, and Ravid and colleagues are more concerned with the description of the symptoms of SLI. Furthermore, several authors propose to divide SLI up into subgroups, either according to the target language (Ravid et al. and Crago & Paradis) or to homogeneity (Van der Lely).

In addition, there is the crosslinguistic issue. Some authors in this section focus on English, the traditional language of investigation—namely, Wexler, Rice, Van der Lely. On the other hand, other chapters discuss other languages: Schaeffer and de Jong investigate Dutch; Crago and Paradis deal with French and Inuktitut; and Ravid and colleagues look at Hebrew. This provides for an interesting comparison between the manifestations of SLI in different languages.

The progress made in this section concerns the original inclusionary criterion of "language deficit." It is an attempt to formulate in much more detail what kind of language deficit characterizes children and adults with SLI, both in terms of symptoms and linguistic theory. A closer look at the individual chapters illustrates these issues.

Wexler (chap. 1) concentrates on the relation between linguistic theory and SLI. He argues that, in principle, the study of linguistic theory and the study of language development (including disordered language development) could and should mutually influence each other. If something goes wrong with language development (different from "normal"), then it should reveal something about the nature of normal language development, which in turn tells something about linguistic theory. Conversely, without a description of normal linguistic abilities given by linguistic theory it would be difficult to ask the question of what goes wrong.

The empirical issues that Wexler discusses include the rates of finiteness (optional infinitives, or OIs), properties of agreement and case, and the development of object clitic pronouns. He shows that errors concerning these phenomena occur both in normal child language, and in the language of children with SLI, with one difference—namely, the error stages last much longer for children with SLI. Wexler suggests a syntactic constraint of a specific type that is genetically determined and is accountable for the observed delays. The upshot of his account with respect to the search for a definition of SLI is linguistic-theoretical: SLI is caused by a maturational delay of a specific syntactic constraint.

From a more bird's-eye point of view, Rice (chap. 2) also emphasizes the importance of the mutual influence between the study of (impaired) language development and linguistic theory. In most children, the emergence of morphology and syntax occurs at the same time as other advances in social and cognitive development. The co-occurrence of multiple developmental dimensions complicates the determination of the extent to which these dimensions are truly distinct or codependent. Children who display unexpected discrepancies in their acquisition of language provide valuable insights into the ways in which language can be spared or affected, relative to other developmental dimensions. The exact nature of the discrepancies can further an understanding of the linguistic system, and how it emerges in young children.

The two types of discrepancies Rice discusses are timing in the emergence of language acquisition and the trajectory of change over time, and expected and unexpected variation across children. On the basis of data with English-speaking children (normal and SLI), she concludes that children with SLI are delayed in the onset of speech and their (morphosyntactic) developmental stages are protracted (timing), and they show high variability on linguistic measures that do not detect variation for unaffected children (variation). Thus, Rice suggests that the definition of SLI should include the terms *timing* and *variation*.

Crago and Paradis (chap. 3) illustrate the interaction between linguistic theory, acquisition theory, and the characterization of SLI by comparing varying language learners (L1, L2, and SLI) acquiring a variety of languages (French, English, Inuktitut) on a variety of grammatical topics. They address the following questions: Does the type of language learned affect the pattern of impairment seen in children with SLI? Are impaired learners different from all other learners of L1 and L2? Conversely, are L2 learners distinct from L1, both normal and impaired? Or, do commonalities exist across all learners at certain stages of development? What can account for the shared characteristics?

Crago and Paradis show that just as data from children learning structurally different languages continue to reshape language acquisition theories and linguistic theory, a broader range of cross-learner data (e.g., SLI in languages other than English and normal L2 development) leads to further refinements of these theories. This chapter underscores the significance of testing acquisition theories over a wider set of learners in order to develop such theories, as well as to better understand the groups of children on which they are based. Furthermore, comparing the end state grammars of the SLI population to the grammars of adults learning a second language helps elucidate both maturational claims regarding language development as well as certain recent claims in the L2 literature that second language learning adults are "impaired" speakers. Specifically, Crago and Paradis show that nonimpaired second language learners of French produce OI during a period of around 3 years, after age 7. This is not predicted by Wexler's claim that the protracted period of OI in SLI speech (extended optional infinitives, EOI) is accounted for by the delayed maturation of certain UG principles, as maturation of these principles is not supposed to take place after age 7 in normally developing populations.

They also show that SLI in a morphologically rich language such as Inuktitut cannot be explained by Leonard's processing account, because the Inuktitut child with SLI studied by Crago and Paradis fails to produce systematically even stressed morphemes and those that have a CVC structure. Thus, Crago and Paradis' study is a major example of the importance of testing hypotheses that emerged from studies on English SLI in other languages.

As Van der Lely (chap. 4) points out, current research on SLI shows that the language deficits found are rather heterogeneous, even if only one language—English—is considered. She examines the relation between SLI in English-speaking children who show relatively pure language impairments with those who evince coexisting (subtle) cognitive deficits. In addition, she considers the linguistic differences in children with SLI. At the broader level, the distinction between different SLI forms appears clear; for example, children with pragmatic SLI show little overlap in linguistic characteristics with those children with grammatical impairment (cf. Bishop, 1997, who argued that pragmatic disorders may also coexist with grammatical impairment). At a narrower level, the distinction between different forms of SLI become less clear, that is, with respect to the relation between variable deficits within grammar (e.g., syntax, semantics, morphology, or phonology). Although there appear to be some children with primary phonological impairment, thorough investigation of all these areas within grammar are not typically carried out with the same rigor in the same population of children. Even at the narrowest level of characterization, that is, within syntax or morphology, differences between studies are also apparent with respect to impairments in tense, agreement, or more general core aspects of the human syntactic faculty that involve movement. These differences are subsequently reflected in the resulting hypotheses characterizing or accounting for the SLI performance. Whereas some differences between studies may reflect the focus of the investigations in different labs, or the interpretation of data rather than the data themselves, there do appear to be some genuine, qualitative differences that call for theoretical discussion.

Van der Lely formulates the heterogeneity problem as follows: What is the relation between the different forms of SLI? Are there multiple disorders that result in different impairments that can variably coexist? Or is there a single disorder that, for some unexplained reason, variably manifests itself in children? As she notes, there is some empirical and theoretical justification for considering that deficits in phonology versus morphosyntax have a different origin—particularly if consideration is given to the adult language disorder literature. However, it is by no means clear that this model is appropriate when considering development, as Van der Lely sensibly points out.

By studying highly selected subgroups with clearly defined linguistic characteristics, Van der Lely addresses some of the problems mentioned here. She argues that the core deficit responsible for the grammar of children with grammatical-SLI (G-SLI) is in the syntactic mechanism of "Move," the movement of syntactic constituents from their base-generated position to their surface position. More specifically, whereas this basic grammatical operation is obligatory in normal grammar, it is optional in the grammar of children with G-SLI. This would account for the broad range of language deficits and a core feature of G-SLI grammar—the inconsistent use of certain syntactic operations. Thus, although acknowledging the heterogeneity of SLI, Van der Lely emphasizes the importance of studying subgroups that are as homogeneous as possible, in her case children with a specific syntactic deficit. This suggests that different (homogeneous) subgroups of SLI should each receive their own definition.

Schaeffer's (chap. 5) contribution draws on the distinctive language components already mentioned and concentrates on the question of whether and how the pragmatic system is distinct from the grammar, and whether this is reflected in the speech of children with SLI. She uses the Dutch language.

A survey of the literature on the pragmatic abilities (to be specified later) of children with SLI reveals a variety of results. In some studies, children with SLI perform below the level of MLU controls. In other instances, no differences are found, and in still others, the children with SLI perform at higher levels. Furthermore, a few studies report no differences between children with SLI and normally developing children of the same age. For the studies reporting poorer performance on pragmatic skills by children with SLI than control children, there remains the question of whether the weaker morphosyntactic abilities of the children with SLI get in these children's way, restricting their ability to exhibit pragmatic knowledge that they possess or whether they really lack certain pragmatic principles.

Most of these studies concern pragmatic abilities such as speech acts, conversational participation and discourse regulation (initiations, replies, topic maintenance, turn taking, utterance repair, etc.), and code switching. As Schaeffer argues, it is feasible that these (extra-linguistic) pragmatic skills are shaped by morphosyntactic abilities. If children have problems with their grammar, then this might discourage them, possibly resulting in nonassertiveness and lack of initiative. However, on the other hand, none of the pragmatic skills previously mentioned directly influences the realization of the morphosyntax.

Schaeffer points out that there is another part of the pragmatic system that seems to have a more immediate impact on the grammar. This part is concerned with speaker and hearer knowledge. Speakers need to take into account what their interlocutor, the hearer knows. Schaeffer refers to this pragmatic requirement as the "concept of nonshared knowledge." The application of this pragmatic concept affects several syntactic phenomena.

In earlier work, Schaeffer argues that normally developing Dutch-speaking children under age 3 perform poorly on scrambling, due to the lack of the pragmatic concept of nonshared knowledge. On the basis of her studies of Dutch children, Schaeffer is able to show that syntactic structures that are dependent on this pragmatic notion are preserved in children with SLI. In addition, Schaeffer's results provide support for the theoretical hypothesis that the pragmatic system is a component separate from the grammar, developing at its own pace. Thus, as for the definition of SLI, Schaeffer's contribution suggests that it should include the exclusionary criterion that the pragmatic system is not impaired in its own right.

De Jong (chap. 6) points out that linguistic theory is not always a straightforward guide for research on SLI. It is often difficult to decide on theoretical issues on the basis of data from normal, adult linguistic data. One of the critical roles of data from SLI research is to help to evaluate the adequacy of these theories. However, as de Jong wonders, what counts as evidence to the contrary? What if there is an alternative explanation? In other words, what is the explanatory value of linguistic theories for SLI?

These questions are explored by investigating (verbal) inflectional morphology and topicalization in the speech of Dutch children with SLI. De Jong argues that, although guidance by linguistic theory in the investigation of SLI is potentially helpful, the focus should remain on the profiling of SLI (namely, listing patterns of symptoms), which may vary depending on the language, and characterizing of SLI in its own right, adopting linguistic terminology.

Another example of the relevance of language typology for the definition of SLI is provided by Ravid, Levie, and Ben-Zvi (chap. 7). They point out that the domain of inflectional morphology has been studied extensively in English in comparison with more morphologically rich languages such as Italian and Hebrew, where language impaired children fared on the whole better than English-speaking children with SLI (Dromi et al., 1993). It seems that children growing up in synthetic languages featuring a variety of morphemes find inflectional morphology tasks easier than children growing up in languages with impoverished inflections. Note that Crago and Paradis's work is very important in this regard because it shows that an Inuit child with SLI omits inflectional morphology, despite the fact that Inuktitut is morphologically very rich. Such findings are not compatible with one general definition of SLI, which includes, for instance, the claim that children with SLI omit tense morphemes. Ravid and colleagues make an interesting proposal that addresses this concern.

The chapters in this section all contribute to a refinement of the characterization of the inclusionary criterion "language deficit," making use of both linguistic theory and language typology. The continuation of this path of research, together with the exclusionary criteria listed in Leonard (1998), should ultimately lead to a comprehensive definition of specific language impairment.

REFERENCES

Bishop, D. V. M. (1997). *Uncommon understanding: Comprehension in specific language impairment.* Hove, England: Psychology Press.

Chomsky, N. (1993). A minimalist program for linguistic theory. In K. Hale & S. J. Keyser (Eds.), *The view from building 20* (pp. 1–52). Cambridge, MA: MIT Press.

Dromi, E., Leonard, L. B., & Shteiman, M. (1993). The grammatical morphology of Hebrew-speaking children with specific language impairment: Some competing hypotheses. *Journal of Speech and Hearing Research, 36,* 760–771.

Leonard, L. (1998). *Children with specific language impairment.* Cambridge, MA: MIT Press.

1

Lenneberg's Dream: Learning, Normal Language Development, and Specific Language Impairment

Ken Wexler
Massachusetts Institute of Technology

The field of language acquisition has made remarkable progress in recent years. There is no area of cognitive science that has advanced at a quicker pace. The field is full of reliable and nonobvious generalizations, relations to other fields are understood, a good deal about the relation between normal and impaired development is understood, and the relative contributions of learning and development have begun to be sorted out in a coherent manner. This chapter sketches out some of these results and attempts to give an overall view of the central questions and the answers that current research suggests. For the domain of phenomena I will pick one important case, the development of central properties of sentence structure. I have sacrificed breadth of coverage in phenomena and precision of technical development in order to have space to discuss the central questions and to make the results available to nonspecialists. A major purpose of this chapter is to show how important discoveries concerning impaired linguistic development (SLI), one of the foci of this book, flow naturally from and contribute to the advances in the study of normal language acquisition.

THE COMPUTATIONAL SYSTEM OF LANGUAGE

The area of language considered here is a central one—what Chomsky (1995) called the *computational system* of language. This is the part of language internalized by the mind/brain that is responsible for basic properties of sentence construction, that is, the part of language central to the conveying of compli-cated and noncontext-bound ideas, the part that seems bound up with spe-cies-specific biological properties. A more traditional term for this part of lan-guage is *grammar*. This chapter concentrates on sentence grammar, mostly ignoring phonology, the lexicon, and pragmatics.

The properties of the computational system (grammar) that I will dis-cuss include properties of syntax and semantics. There is more known about the development of syntax, and I will concentrate on that area, al-though semantics is discussed at different points.

The computational system of sentence grammar has two parts. First, there are *principles* that hold of all languages; by hypothesis, they are com-puted by the brain as the result of genetically guided mechanisms. Second, there are *parameters*, which are set differently by different languages. The parameters are set by an individual as the result of experience. The idea is that they can be set simply from experience, so that children can easily hone in on the correct grammar given that they have the principles.[1]

This framework poses the following questions for the study of the devel-opment of language:

(1) a. How does the computational system of language develop?
b. What is learned?
c. What is genetically guided?
d. What develops late under genetic guidance?
e. What kind of variation in development is there across lan-guages?
f. What kind of impairment occurs in development and learning?
g. What does variation across languages and individuals tell about the genetic structure of language?

These questions are among the most central for any biological system, such as language, that is influenced both by genetics and the environment. It is hard to see how progress can be made on other developmental ques-tions in the cognitive (neuro-)science of language without finding reason-able answers to these questions.

One way to begin to think about the above questions is to ask: What ac-counts for child errors, for nonadult language? In particular, are errors

---

[1]A long series of works shows that the problem of parameter setting is not so obviously sim-ple as the theory postulates. See Wexler and Hamburger (1973), Wexler and Culicover (1980), Manzini and Wexler (1987), Wexler and Manzini (1987), Clark and Roberts (1993), Gibson and Wexler (1994), Dresher (1999), Fodor (1998), Bertolo, Broihier, Gibson, and Wexler (1997), and many other works. Nevertheless, because children set their parameters so well and quickly, as we will see there should be a simple solution.

caused by the missetting of parameters, or by the growth of mature forms of principles? That is, we would like to know the answers to (2):

(2) a. Are parameters sometimes misset by children?
   b. Do some principles take time to develop in their mature adult form?

It is quite natural to suppose that parameters are sometimes misset by a child and that this missetting leads to observed child errors. After all, parameter settings are at least partially the result of experience—different languages have different parameter settings and the only possible way these parameter settings could be attained is via learning. As far as I know, there is no evidence that variation in normal language development is genetically linked, that is, that children from a long genetic background of Italian speakers find learning Italian easier and that children from a genetic background of Chinese speakers find learning Chinese easier. The fundamental empirical result is that any normal child can easily learn any natural language.[2]

We could thus understand child errors as the result of difficulties in the process of parameter setting. Such a hypothesis has often been made. In fact, many developmental psycholinguists have assumed that errors in setting parameters were the only errors that children made in developing syntax, outside of errors in learning the lexicon (see Wexler, 1998, for discussion).

It is also quite natural to suppose that principles take time to develop in their mature adult form (2b). After all, biological organisms generally develop over time; their mature forms are different from their immature forms. This development is in central cases taken to be genetically guided, although influenced by the environment, but not so much as to alter the central character of the development. In fact, the problem of development has often been taken to be the central problem of biology.

The answer to (2b) can tell us much about the developmental structure of the genetic system of language. We will have to answer this question at least partially before we can understand, for example, how genetics is involved in the common observation that children do make errors in language at an early age and that their systems are at least to some extent nonadult.

The structure of very early child sentences (up to about age 3;0) tells us a great deal about the answers to the previous questions. A useful tool (in

---

[2]There has been almost no formal empirical study of this question, and it would not be totally inconceivable that in fact there is some genetic linkage to linguistic variation. Given the common experience that a child brought up in a language easily learns that language, any genetic linkage would be expected to be extremely subtle.

addition to empirical investigations) is the simple confrontation of different possible answers to these questions, asking whether these answers can or cannot predict the empirical results. Commonsensical as this tool is, it has only occasionally been used in past understanding of linguistic development, where a priori hypotheses have often been taken for granted, without consideration of the empirical facts or the alternative possibilities. For example, it has often been assumed without empirical argument that all errors in child language are due to errors in learning. My strategy here is to keep all reasonable general answers open, arguing for one or the other on the basis of confrontation with evidence.

INFLECTION AND TENSE

This section describes some very simple properties of simple sentences. One central property of sentences is that they often have *tense*. Tense is the category that encodes certain time relations. For example, in English there are two tenses, *present* and *past*:

(3) a. Mary likes candy (*present* tense)
    b. Mary liked candy (*past* tense)

In many languages, tense is indicated by an "inflection" on the verb, for example, the *s* on *like* in (3a) and the *ed* on *like* in (3b). Tense is a grammatical category; it is not the same as *time*. For example, in (4) the time of leaving is taken to be next week, the future, but the tense in English does not distinguish a future tense. (It does in some languages.) Tensed verbs are often called *finite* verbs. Untensed or nonfinite verbs also exist, as in *go* in (5).

(4) Mary leaves next week

(5) Mary wants Bill to go

There is much more to the finite–nonfinite distinction than the encoding of tense and form of the verb. Finite and nonfinite verbs behave very differently in many languages.

Consider one example of this central role of tense, an example that will soon be of use in describing children's behavior. Many languages are what is called *verb-second* (V2) languages. This means that in simple clauses, or the main clauses of more complex sentences, the verb always appears in second position, although it does not appear there in most clauses. For example, in Dutch (Dutch examples are from Wexler, Schaeffer, and Bol, in press), verbs usually appear at the ends of sentences; Dutch is what is called a *verb-final language*. But in main clauses, the finite verb appears in second position.

(6) morgen   gaat Saskia een boek kopen
     tomorrow   goes Saskia a   book buy
     ADV V_{fin} SUBJ   OBJ V_{nonfin}
     'Saskia is going to buy a book tomorrow'

V_{fin} indicates a finite verb; V_{nonfin} indicates a nonfinite verb. Nonfinite verbs occur at the end of a clause in Dutch. This is why *kopen/buy* appears at the end of the clause. On the other hand, *gaat/goes* is a finite verb; it is marked for present tense, and it appears in second position in the sentence. Either the subject *Saskia* (a name) or the object *een book/a book* could have appeared in first position instead of the adverb. But the verb could not have appeared there.

In most cases, it is possible in Dutch to tell if a verb is finite or nonfinite by its inflection or ending. The verb *kopen* is nonfinite because the verb is the root *koop* plus the nonfinite (or infinitival) ending *en*. *Gaat*, on the other hand, shows the typical *t* ending of the third person singular present tense (the subject *Saskia* is third person singular).

Syntacticians understand that the finite verb of main clauses *moves* (from final position) to second position, but it is not necessary to go into the technical discussion of verb movement here. Finite verbs in subclauses remain in final position; they do not move.

The verb-second parameter asks whether or not a language is a V2 language; there is a yes–no answer. (Much of this discussion ignores complexities; hopefully, linguists will understand). Dutch is a verb-second language, as are many other languages around the world. English and French are not verb-second languages. Thus, in order to answer whether children sometimes set parameters incorrectly, (2a) it is necessary to know whether or not, for example, they set the verb-second parameter correctly. The remarkable difference in grammatical structure that is related to the choice of finite or nonfinite verbs has been a major tool in our ability to answer this and many other questions.

OPTIONAL INFINITIVES IN CHILDREN

One of the major discoveries of the last decade in early linguistic development was the discovery of the *Optional Infinitive (OI) Stage* (Wexler 1990, 1992, 1994), which lasts in normal children from birth (so far as we can tell) to around age 3;0.

(7) The properties of the OI stage are the following:
   a. Root infinitives (nonfinite verbs) are possible grammatical sentences for children in this stage.
   b. These infinitives coexist with finite forms.
   c. The children nevertheless know the relevant grammatical principles and have set their parameters correctly.

(7a) tells us that young children often appear to leave tense out of verbs that require it. For example, here are two examples from a young child (less than 3;0) speaking Dutch:

(8) pappa schoenen wassen
    daddy shoes wash-INF
    'Daddy wash (non-finite) shoes'

(9) ik pak 't op
    I pick it up
    'I pick (fin) it up'

The form of the verb in (8) (ending in *en*) indicates that it is a nonfinite verb. Examples like (8) confirm (7a). But (8) is *finite*; it has a first person singular present tense, confirming (7b). Wexler (1990, 1992, 1994) and many others analyzed individual subject data to show that at a particular age, the child produced both kinds of verbs, finite and nonfinite.[3]

But there is a crucial difference in the examples in (8) and (9). In (8) the verb (nonfinite) appears in final position, where nonfinite verbs go in Dutch. In (9), the verb (finite) appears in *second* position.[4] These examples are thus in accord with (7c). The children are putting the finite verbs in second position, where they go, and they are putting the nonfinite verbs in final position, where *they* go.

To show that these examples are not chosen arbitrarily it is necessary to count all the relevant verbs from children. Table 1.1 shows is some data from a study of the development of 47 normally developing Dutch children (Wexler, Schaeffer, & Bol, in press).

For the youngest group, 83% of their main clause verbs (i.e., 126 nonfinite verbs out of a total of 152 verbs) are OIs, basically ungrammatical in the

---

[3]Wexler (1994) suggested that the increasing proportions of finiteness with age made it natural to think that at extremely young ages children produce 100% nonfinite forms. Wijnen (1998), de Jong (chap. 6 in this volume) have produced evidence that this is so.

[4]Example 6 is ambiguous between second and final position, of course. It has been included to make the point that in counts of the finiteness/word order correlation, research on the OI stage has not counted the ambiguous forms like Example 6 in deciding where the verb appeared. See Poeppel and Wexler (1993).

TABLE 1.1
Proportions of Optional Infinitives by Age

Age Group	% OIs
1;07–2;00	83% (126/152)
2;01–2;06	64% (126/198)
2;07–3;00	23% (57/253)
3;01–3;07	7% (29/415)

adult language. For the oldest group (3;1–3;7), the OI rate is only 7%. This is a well-documented trend in the study of OIs; the OI rate decreases over time. The same result holds in individual children; a child produces fewer and fewer OIs over time. Developing adult finiteness behavior (essentially 100% finite utterances) is thus not a question of learning at one time.

So it is quite clear that (7a) and (7b) hold of this population. To see that children produce both finite and nonfinite utterances at a given age, individual children have to be studied. That in fact is the typical method of studying the OI stage, which for reasons of space are not illustrated here. The point is to show what OI rates look like over a broad sample of children, so that the reader understands the great prevalence of OIs; there is no reason to think that any child in Dutch escapes the OI stage at the relevant age.

In order to test (7c), it is necessary to see whether finite verbs appear in second position and nonfinite verbs appear in final position. Wexler, Schaeffer, and Bol did this calculation, following the usual procedure of only counting root (main) verbs, so as not to make the results look better by counting nonfinite verbs that should be infinitival. The results are shown in Table 1.2, for the same set of 47 normal children, where only nonambiguous order is counted.

Almost 2,000 (99%) of the verbs in second position are finite, and only 20 are nonfinite. More than 600 (98%) of the verbs in final position are nonfinite, but only 11 are finite. Finite and nonfinite verbs could hardly be behaving more differently in terms of word order. Because most of the children are producing both finite and nonfinite verbs, this lack of error also means that individual children are placing essentially all their finite verbs in second position and nonfinite verbs in final position.

TABLE 1.2
Finiteness/Position Contingency Normally Developing Children

All Normal Children	V2	V_{final}
Finite	1953 (99%)	11 (2%)
Nonfinite	20 (1%)	606 (98%)

(7c) is supported in this data as strongly as anything in child development (or almost all of the cognitive sciences, in fact) ever is. Very little leeway has to be given to measurement error or noise, even at the youngest ages. This is the kind of data that psychologists studying cognitive development almost never see, close to categorical data. It seems quite reasonable to consider the small number of exceptions to the finiteness/word order correlation to be performance errors or some other kind of error of measurement.

VERY EARLY PARAMETER SETTING, LEARNING, AND IMITATION

From the earliest investigations of the OI stage (Wexler 1990, 1992, 1994), data like this were taken to show that children set parameters correctly very early. In particular, this data shows that children set the V2 parameter correctly. From their earliest utterances, Dutch children place finite verbs in second position and they place nonfinite verbs in final position. This is what would be expected if they knew that Dutch were a verb-second, verbal-final language and they produced OIs.

Children speaking V2 languages like Dutch and German not only place the finite verb in second position during the OI stage, but they place any major constituent in first position in a finite sentence, as is expected in a V2 language. Poeppel and Wexler (1993) showed data confirming this point in German, and there is a great deal of evidence that it is true.

On the other hand, children learning non-V2 languages do not show the verb-second properties. They do not put finite verbs in second position (this can be seen, e.g., in verb-final languages like Japanese and Korean), nor do they put any constituent into first position (e.g., English-speaking children do not do this). In other words, whereas Dutch children show the behavior discussed here, children developing non-V2 languages do not show this behavior.

Wexler (1990, 1994) argued on the basis of these kinds of phenomena that children set their verb-second parameter (*yes* or *no*, depending on the input language) correctly from the moment that the question could be asked, that is, from the moment that children entered the two-word stage, producing a verb and another constituent in the same utterance. (Before this stage, the question of correct parameter setting cannot be settled by production data because utterances of one word do not give word order information.) He argued further that the same thing was true of all central parameters concerning clause structure and inflection (see Wexler, 1998, for a discussion of several parameters). These parameters included the V2 parameter, the verb-to-tense (verb raising) parameter, word order parameters like VO or OV, and the null subject parameter. There is no evidence that any parameter is misset by young children.

(10) *Very Early Parameter Setting* (VEPS): From the earliest observable ages (around 18 months), children have set their parameters correctly.

It will take an advance in experimental techniques to determine whether VEPS is true at even younger ages. See Soderstrom, Wexler, and Juczyk (2000, 2002) for some evidence in English that infant techniques might help to settle that question of earlier ages.

One might question whether the strict correlation between word order and finiteness that has been shown actually does constitute evidence for correct parameter setting. Perhaps children are only good imitators, perhaps they are a kind of imitating automaton that reproduces the input. Children hear finite verbs in second position (in main clauses) and nonfinite verbs in final position, so perhaps they are simply repeating these verbs in the word order in which they hear them. Call this the *automaton* view (to distinguish it from a more sophisticated view of imitation discussed shortly). There seems to be no way to maintain the automaton view, however.

First, the automaton view suggests that children do not actually understand sentences, they do not understand verbs and nouns and how to put these together, for example. This contradicts the experience of not only developmental psycholinguists, but also of parents. The evidence cannot possibly be reviewed here, but it is a distinctly surprising view.

Second, the automaton view does not explain why children always place finite verbs in second position, because they hear finite verbs at the end of clauses when these clauses are not main clauses. Somehow children would have to ignore these subordinate clauses. But how would an automaton that did not analyze sentences know that a verb was part of a subordinate clause?

Third, the automaton view does not have a learning theory. Note that it is not enough for a child to be able to learn that one form follows another form. To capture even simple V2 facts, the child will have to associate the finite verb (presumably a verb with a certain phonology for this view) with "second" position, and the nonfinite verb with "final" position. In addition, the child will have to know what counts as a constituent, and any constituent (including adverbs) can appear in first position. That is, second position is not defined as "second word in a sentence." (The child produces utterances in line with this knowledge.)

Fourth, the automaton view does not explain why children produce OIs at all. Basically, all simple sentences in the input are tensed, so why does an imitating child go out of the way to produce untensed sentences that are quite at odds with what has been produced?

Fifth, why does the child in many languages produce such a large percentage of OIs at an early age? Notice in Table 1.1 the 83% OI rate for the 1;7 to 2;0 age group. Wijnen (1999) argued that at the very earliest ages in Dutch, there are actually 100% OIs. If the child is imitating the input, even if some kind of stray input or misanalysis led to the occasional utterance of an OI, why should almost all the child's early utterance be OIs, which are not attested in the input (see, e.g., Poeppel and Wexler, 1993, who found no input OIs)? Even if parents actually use a few OIs, for whatever reason, why should a young child's productions be overwhelming OIs? This behavior is quite the opposite of imitative behavior.

Sixth, and quite strikingly, there are a number of systematic errors that children make that have no basis at all in the input, but that relate to their understanding of OIs as nonfinite. A major example is the errors on subject case in English that do not show up in Dutch or German. Another section discusses these errors and why they are so difficult for an automaton model to handle.

This is just the beginning of a set of questions that the automaton view cannot explain. Recently, there has been an attempt to make the imitating view more sophisticated, to continue to think of the child as having no linguistic knowledge, but of having a richer set of learning mechanisms than the simplest behaviorist views would have allowed. A prime example of such a theory is that of Tomasello (2000) (see also Conti-Ramsden, sect. II in this volume, for more discussion).

Tomasello argued that young children have essentially no knowledge of linguistic categories, principles, or processes. He posited "that in the beginning children make virtually no linguistic abstractions at all (beyond something like 'concrete nominal')" and "at younger ages children simply do not possess the abstract syntactic competence characteristic of older children and adults" (pp. 241, 247). Although he did not specify ages exactly clearly, the surrounding discussion suggests that he was claiming that children, until about age 3;0, do not have linguistic categories. Tomasello concentrated for the most part on the category of "transitive verb." He claimed that children, until about age 3, do not have the category of transitive verb.[5] Although he did not discuss these processes, his theory would assert that

---

[5]Critiquing Tomasello's' supposed evidence for his view that 2-year-olds do not even know the category of transitive verb is beyond the purpose of this chapter. Tomasello's experiments showing that children do not much generalize from inchoative novel verbs (*the ball is meeking*) to transitive novel verbs (*the boy is meeking the ball*) in no way establishes that children do not have the concept of transitive verb, contrary to Tomasello's claims. For this is not a systematic syntactic pattern in English (*the book fell/*the boy fell the book*), and it would not be a good generalization for the child to draw; it is not a generalization supported by universal grammar at all. As for the experiments that show that young children who are taught novel verbs in passive

young children do not have such processes as verb movement or noun phrase movement until (if ever[6]) much later.

Tomasello claimed that the classic learnability arguments have been made against learning theories that are only "straw men"—"simple association and blind induction" (p. 247).[7] He believed these arguments do not hold if these straw men are replaced by "the more cognitively sophisticated learning and abstraction processes involved in intention reading, cultural learning, analogy making, and structure combining" (p. 247).

Tomasello's description of these "more sophisticated" learning processes was not clear enough to see how they would actually work; there was no attempt at formalization, and nothing in the way he described them makes them look new or sophisticated in any particular way.

But it is worth considering the most important process that Tomasello discussed, namely, "intention reading." Tomasello agreed with generative-based critiques that classical imitation "very likely plays only a minor role

---

form do not reproduce them in active form, the result is no surprise to those generative accounts (Babyonyshev et al., 2001; Borer & Wexler, 1987, 1992), which say that children at this young age do not have the syntactic basis for verbal passives; the linguistic system has not sufficiently matured, that is, the A-chain deficit theory. A more telling experiment (on the assumption that the novel verb technique is tapping children's linguistic abilities at all) would be to teach the children the novel verb in passive form (*the dog was meeked by the cat.*), and then ask a passive-inducing question (*what is happening to the dog*)? Especially if the verb were *nonactional* (Maratsos, Fox, Becker, & Chalkley, 1983) (and thus had no homophonous adjectival passive), the A-chain deficit theory would predict that the child could not answer with a passive form despite the passive introduction of the verb (see Babyonyshev et al., 2001; Borer & Wexler, 1987; Fox & Grodzinsky, 1998). But this experimental type was not done by Tomasello.

[6]I write "if ever" because Tomasello would really like to argue that even adults do not have such processes; the subtext (often explicit) of his work is that linguistic theory is not describing psychologically true phenomena. There is no space here to illuminate Tomasello's misunderstandings. He somehow thinks that linguistic theory is concerned with mathematical rather than psychological properties; he seems to not understand that mathematics is a tool used scientifically to describe scientific theories, as in, for example, physics. On Tomasello's reasoning, the theory of physics would not be "physical," because it uses mathematics. The reader is urged to read Tomasello's work in order to see that this seems to be his reasoning. There seems to be a kind of tradition in parts of psychology that says to attempt to understand language and its development in precise, scientific terms is somehow wrong, that language cannot be studied like other fields of science, it just is not precise enough. Tomasello's attempts seem to fall into this category. It is difficult to square the incredible regularity and interaction of phenomena that I have reported in the text with the anti-precise notions of language and its development that Tomasello seems to be urging.

[7]This claim is false. The classic learnability arguments were made assuming any mechanically specifiable (i.e., actually computable in a well-grounded, accepted sense in the cognitive sciences) learning theory. See, for example, Wexler and Hamburger (1973) and Wexler and Culicover (1980). It was shown that for certain classes of linguistically motivated processes, no specifiable learning theory (that did not assume specific linguistic knowledge) could learn all the possibilities. Nothing special had to be assumed about "simple association." As for the denial of "blind induction," this is exactly what the theories that he is attacking do.

in language acquisition." Tomasello saved the imitation theory by renaming imitation; he called it "mimicking" (p. 218). Then Tomasello used the name "imitation" for a completely different process, one in which the learner understands the intention of an actor, tries to reproduce the intention: "In cultural (imitative) learning, as opposed to simple mimicking, the learner understands the purpose or function of the behavior she is reproducing" (p. 238): Tomasello went on,

> Thus, a child might hear her father exclaim, "Look! A clown!" To fully understand his linguistic behavior (with an eye toward reproducing it) she must understand that her father intends that she share attention with him to a particular object; that is to say, understanding a communicative intention means understanding precisely how another person intends to manipulate your attention. (p. 238)

And, finally, Tomasello claimed that "to comprehend the totality of an adult's utterance, the child must understand his overall communicative intention and also the communicative role being played by the various constituents of the utterance" (p. 239).

According to this theory, therefore, the child can somehow (unspecified) figure out what the adult intends to say, and the child can then map the string of sounds to this intention; furthermore, in some more complicated (unspecified) way, the child can figure out what the *constituents* of the intention are and how these are mapped to the constituents of the sentence (see Tomasello, 2000, p. 239).

This suggestion appears to be the major theoretical proposal that Tomasello made concerning how language learning takes place. Interestingly, the basic assumption—that children need to be able to figure out something about the intended meaning of an utterance in order for language learning to proceed—is a staple of generative acquisition theories, at least since Wexler and Hamburger (1973), Hamburger and Wexler (1973), and Wexler and Culicover (1980). Those authors argued that "semantic information" had to be available to the language learner, and they gave an explicit discussion of this assumption, and what had to be assumed to make it work. (See Wexler, 1982, for particular attention to this point.) Essentially, the semantic information helped the learner to construct the "deep structure" of the sentence.

The argument was mathematical and empirical, in the tradition of scientific reasoning. Namely, certain linguistic variation possibilities could not be learned if only "surface information" (Wexler and Hamburger's term) were available to the learner; the learner had to supplement this with information concerning the intended meaning.

In more modern learning theories, changed as the result of more recent discoveries concerning the form of syntactic parameters, the same basic assumption about the necessity for semantic information helping the learner is made. Thus, Gibson and Wexler (1994), for example, assumed that semantic information helps the learner to figure out which noun phrase is the subject of the sentence and which is the object.

The essential point is that Wexler and Hamburger and Wexler and Culicover showed that even with the semantic information, there were unlearnable linguistic processes unless it were assumed that the learner had access to grammatical universals. In the case of Wexler and Culicover, they were very concerned with showing that learners could learn their language from fairly simple sentences, because very young children cannot handle very long sentences. They demonstrated that transformational grammar (in a specified sense) could be learned from sentences with no more than two degrees of embedding, so long as children had access to semantic information and universals of grammar. Both were necessary. And this was formally, mathematically demonstrated.

Although particular theories have changed, this is the essence of theories of language learning in the generative tradition—both semantic information and grammatical universals are necessary for language learning. Tomasello posited that semantic information (what he relabeled "intention reading") is necessary and helpful for language learning. I agree completely and am glad that he has accepted these arguments from generative learning theory. But without making any arguments, Tomasello also claimed that semantic information (intention reading) is sufficient for language learning. There are good arguments otherwise, and Tomasello made no counterarguments.

Tomasello's theory can be called the *intention learning theory* (with its most singular characteristic being that the child has no grammatical categories). How does the intention learning theory do on the six problems I mentioned earlier for the automaton view? It seems to overcome the first problem, because, unlike the automaton view, the intention learning theory does assume that children attempt to understand sentences. But, nothing in the intention learning theory can solve the rest of these problems. If the child does not have access to grammatical categories or to the setting of parameters, then there is no way to explain the patterns of OI behavior.

In fact, Tomasello did explicitly try to explain OI behavior via the intention learning theory. He wrote that "a major part of the explanation is very likely the large number of non-finite verbs that children hear in various constructions in the language addressed to them, especially in questions such as *Should he open it?* and *Does she eat grapes?* The child might then later say, in partially imitative fashion: *He open it* and *She eat grapes*" (p. 240).

This seems to be an attempt to deal with one of the problems raised earlier, namely, problem 4: why does the child use OIs at all? Tomasello here retreated from the intention learning theory and moved back to the mimicking theory, which he earlier rejected. For the input was in the form of a question, on his account, and yet the child uses the forms in a statement. Surely the difference between question and statement is one of the most simple and basic aspects of communicative intention. Any intention-reading learner would and should pay attention to the major difference between the intentions of questions and statements, and would not associate a form that goes with one intention (the question) with another intention (the statement). And there is good evidence that the child does pay attention to this difference; young children do not use auxiliary-first (inverted) order to make a statement; they would do that if they imitated question word order when they were making a statement. What does intention-reading theory have to say about why word order is not mislearned and verb form is mislearned?

So Tomasello seemingly rejected intention reading here, and went back to mimicking. But then we have all the problems associated with mimicking, which Tomasello explicitly acknowledged, even though he rejected mimicking.

But putting aside the fact that Tomasello's suggestion about why OIs exist contradicts his theory (being more allied with the automaton view), there are still many problems. In most of the other OI languages discussed in the literature (e.g., all the Germanic languages except English), questions are not typically asked by using a finite inverted auxiliary, plus a nonfinite verb; they only are asked this way when there is a modal or other type of auxiliary in the meaning of the sentence. But for a main verb, the verb itself is used: *isst sie Ei/eats she eggs/'does she eat eggs'?* (German). Children tend to use 100% (or almost 100%) OIs in their youngest ages. On Tomasello's proposal, this means that children use the (auxiliary) question model for the form of the verb almost 100% of the time, for some unspecified reason ignoring the declarative input. But then children should produce the finite verb before the subject almost 100% of the time, when they are using only a finite verb, because in (non-subject) questions the main finite verb always precedes the subject. But children very rarely do this, and certainly nowhere close to 100% of the time.

The questions, thus, are not answered by Tomasello's suggestion. For example, consider question 2; why don't children use the input that has finite verbs at the end of the clause (any sentence with a finite verb in an embedded clause) to imitate and thus put finite verbs in sentence final position instead of verb second position? They essentially never do this. So children use misleading input to lead to an almost 100% error rate but they do not use other misleading input at all, i.e., they get a 0% error rate. The theoretical and technical tools do not seem to be available in intention reading learning theory (or in the mimicking theory to which Tomasello retreats) to explain substantial empirical properties of development.

It is very important to reiterate that this is not a criticism of the notion of intention reading/leaning; although a very difficult concept to work out explicitly, I have long argued that it is part of language learning and the generative field mostly accepts this proposal. So it is useful for Tomasello to update the multipurpose learning school of language learning so as to help it to become more cognitive, at least recognizing the need for the child to attempt to understand what is being said. This is an advance beyond automaton theories. What is wrong in Tomasello's theory, and other antigenerative, antinativist theories of its type, is the claim that genetically guided knowledge is not part of the child's endowment. Tomasello's recognition that traditional learning theory approaches were too limited is welcome, and as he attempts to add concepts to the theory it would be useful if he kept adding the ones that have been proposed in generative-based theories. If he and others attempt to actually work out process models of learning, as has been carried out in detail in generative learning theories, he might discover that intention learning is not sufficient.

I will return to intention learning when case errors are considered (problem 6). Meanwhile, it is safe to conclude that the strict patterns of morphology and word order correlations that children produce in the OI stage is good evidence for their having set parameters correctly.

OI'S IN ENGLISH

One reason it took so long to discover the OI stage is that so much modern work (since roughly Brown, 1973, on language acquisition) has been carried out in English or influenced by research on English. Unlike other Germanic languages, Romance languages and many/most other languages that have nonfinite forms, the English infinitival verb has no audible inflection. The infinitival form of the verb sounds just like the stem of the verb, *to go, to walk, to eat.* Compare the infinitival form of *speak*:

(11) French: parl   + er
     German: sprech + en
     English: speak + Ø

The English infinitival suffix is phonetically zero, it is unpronounced. Therefore OIs were not discovered because there was no obvious "extra" morpheme that had been added to the verb while the tensed/agreement morpheme was omitted. In Dutch, *en* is added to the stem when children produce an OI, and this form is extremely noticeable, it is clearly not a stem, and it does not belong there. So it is just an accident of English that OIs are a less obvious phenomenon.

But OIs clearly exist in English, as Wexler (1992, 1994) showed. As was well-known since Brown (1973), children often produce what sounds like the stem form instead of the third person singular form, for example, *push* instead of *pushes*. Similarly, they produce what sounds like the stem form instead of the past tense form, for example, *push* instead of *pushed*. Wexler argued that these forms were expected if tense was omitted from the structure and a nonfinite form was therefore the appropriate form. The analysis of the form would be as in (12), where the phonetically empty morpheme Ø is the spell-out of the nonfinite/infinitival morpheme in English:

(12) a. pushes → push + Ø
      b. pushed → push + Ø

These nonfinite forms in English showed all the properties of OIs. For example, the proportion of nonfinite English forms decreased in a child as the child aged, just as OIs do. Wexler also showed that children understood the grammatical properties of the tense morphemes in English, just as they understand the properties of the finiteness morphemes in other languages. For example, they appeared only in the correct positions; children, for example, do not say, *Mary not pushes the chair* (see also Harris and Wexler, 1996). If they omit the auxiliary, then they say *Mary not push the chair*. Furthermore, children understand the semantic properties of the tense morphemes; they do not use the present tense morpheme when past is appropriate (**pushed* → *pushes*) or the past tense morpheme when present is appropriate[8] (*pushes* → *pushed*) (see Rice, Wexler, & Cleave, 1995, and Rice & Wexler, 1996, for children age 3 and above; Schütze & Wexler, 2000, for age 2;6 and older). In either case, children in the OI stage might use the "stem" (nonfinite) form instead of the correct tense form, but they will not substitute the wrong tense form. All these predictions and many others follow from the assumption that young English-speaking children are in the OI stage even though there is no obvious "infinitival" morpheme.

The relevant stage is called the *Optional Infinitive stage*, because of its most prominent characteristic in the original languages in which it was discovered. But as Wexler (1990) argued, the stage is in no way limited to what are traditionally called infinitival forms. Rather, the prediction is that nonfinite forms occur; often these do not take the form of infinitives. For example, in many sentences in English, finiteness is marked only by an auxil-

---

[8]These experiments were done in ordinary discourse contexts, and the prediction of course is just for these contexts. Children might have somewhat different properties of tensing in special contexts, for example, children even at older ages sometimes use present tense in narratives more than adults. But these differences involve conventions of discourse; children clearly are not making mistakes on whether to use a particular morpheme as a present tense or past tense morpheme.

iary. These auxiliaries have no semantic function other than to mark the inflectional properties of finiteness (tense and agreement). The OI stage predicts that these morphemes are omitted for the same reasons (which have not been discussed yet), as are the inflectional finiteness morphemes on the main verb. This prediction is strongly confirmed, in English and in many other languages. An English example is that auxiliary *be* is quite often omitted by children: *Mary going.*

The prediction is quite strong. Namely, when measured by rate of use in obligatory context, the finiteness morphemes in English should pattern together in development, taking a very similar course, showing relatively minor fluctuations from each other. This was shown to hold by a detailed analysis of longitudinal data from a large group of children using structural equation modeling in Rice, Wexler, and Hershberger (1998).

At the same time, other morphemes that share identical surface (phonological) patterns do not behave similarly to the finiteness morphemes. As Rice and Wexler (1996) showed, plural *s* in no way patterns like third person singular *s*. The latter is a finiteness (tense) morpheme, and thus part of the OI stage predictions, and the former is not. Plural *s* develops much faster than third person singular *s*; there is hardly any delay. It does not pattern with the finiteness morphemes as expected. For this and many other reasons, we know that the use of these morphemes is not delayed because of their particular surface or phonological properties; rather, there is a deeper grammatical factor that underlies the OI stage.

SUBJECT CASE

One of the most important features of the OI stage analysis is that it makes it possible to bring together in the same system a myriad of phenomena that have been known to some degree but have previously had to be understood in completely different terms. It has been known for a very long time that children in English often substitute ACCusative case pronouns for NOMinative case pronouns. They often produce forms like those in Example 9:

(13) a. her going
     b. me here
     c. him like candy

In English, subjects of root clauses are NOM, *she, I, he* instead of the ACC forms used in (13). Schütze and Wexler (1996) showed that the case errors that children made were always substitutions of the ACC form for the NOM form; they essentially never substituted NOM for ACC. That is, in object po-

TABLE 1.3
Nina's Third Person Singular Subject Pronouns: Finiteness vs. Case

Subject	Finite Verb	Nonfinite Verb
he + she	255	139
him + her	14	120
Percent non-NOM	5%	46%

Note. From "Subject Case Liscensing and English Root Infinitives," in *BUCLD 20* (p.), by C. T. Schütze and K. Wexler, 1996, Somerville, MA: Cascadilla Press. Copyright by Reprinted by permission.

sitions, for example, children always used ACC forms; children do not produce utterances like *Mary likes he.*

So one of the major facts that has to be explained is this asymmetry. It cannot follow from any kind of standard "frequency" argument. As Schütze and Wexler pointed out, Colin Philips showed that in the input NOM forms are much more likely to appear than are ACC forms. So the children are going out of their way to substitute the form that is far less frequent in the input.

Another major fact is that the incorrect ACC subject forms like (13) essentially never appear when the verb is finite. They only appear when the subject is an OI. Here, for example, is Table 1.3 from Schütze and Wexler (1996) analyzing the CHILDES data of Nina (McWhinney & Snow, 1985). (See also Loeb & Leonard, 1991.)

There is an extremely small possibility of using ACC subject pronouns with finite verbs.[9] Schütze and Wexler provided statistical arguments that this effect is not one simply of correct case and correct finiteness developing simultaneously; rather, a child at a given age shows a strong correlation between finiteness and case marking such that the child will alternate finite and nonfinite verbs, and NOM and ACC subject case for pronouns, but will never use ACC case with a finite verb: *her is going now.*

The empirical linkage of ACC subjects to OIs suggests that in fact ACC subjects are only possible because OIs exist. Bromberg and Wexler (1995) suggested that ACC pronouns were default pronouns, used because TENSE was missing in OIs, on the assumption that NOM was only possible with tensed subjects. Schütze and Wexler provided a more detailed model, arguing that it was the AGREEMENT part of the finite verb that licensed NOM case. Because OIs lacked agreement, they could not license NOM case on

---

[9]The counterexamples are actually smaller than 5% because for independent reasons Schutze and Wexler developed a more complicated model, the AGR–TNS Omission Model (ATOM), which is a better description of the OI stage than the Tense Omission model that is essentially being discussed here. Under ATOM, some of the 5% counterexamples are not counterexamples. ATOM is briefly described later in the text.

the subject, and the default pronoun was used. There is good reason to believe that, in fact, agreement is responsible for NOM, but these arguments are not rehashed here; see Schütze and Wexler (1996).

Schütze and Wexler (1996) proposed the AGR–TNS omission model (ATOM), which says that in the OI stage either AGR or TNS is optionally omitted by the child. The nonfinite form of the verb is used whenever either AGR or TNS is missing. When AGR is present, whether or not TNS is missing, the NOM subject pronoun is selected. When AGR is missing, even though TNS is present, the default case form of the pronoun is selected.

What is a default form of case? It is the case form that is used when there is no structural case position. For example, in English, people say *it's him*, not **it's he*. Or they answer the question *who wants candy?* with *me*, but not with **I*. In these positions of the pronoun, nothing in the structure of the sentence dictates whether the case should be NOM or ACC, so the default form takes over, and this is ACC in English. Schütze and Wexler in fact showed that English-speaking children in the OI stage always correctly used the ACC form of the pronoun in true (adult) default positions.

As Schütze and Wexler discussed, in German and Dutch, the default case of noun phrases is NOM, not ACC. And they consider the literature, which shows that the English subject case error is not replicated in German or Dutch. This is exactly as predicted. When the verb is an OI in German or Dutch, the child will use the default form, just as in English. But the German/Dutch default form is NOM, so the child will use the NOM form. And this is exactly what happens. In contrast to the 46% ACC rate for Nina discussed previously, German or Dutch children in the OI stage use essentially no ACC subjects, even of OIs. The rate is almost 0%.

So children in the OI age range know what the default form of case is in their language. The default form varies from language to language: ACC in English, NOM in German/Dutch. This means that it must be learned from experience. Given the previous results, it is known that children in the OI stage have correctly learned the default form in their language, even when these have opposite values (e.g., ACC in English, NOM in German/Dutch). So just as in the case of parameters (and default case could be looked at as a kind of parameter, although it does not have to be), children learn the language specific aspects of simple clause and inflectional structure very early and very well.

It is no mystery how children learn the default forms. Although nobody knows the answer, because nothing is directly known about learning in language (because of the difficulty in observing an act of learning), it seems pretty reasonable to infer that children choose as the default form just that form that appears in "default" contexts, that is, contexts where there is no structural case position. Given their knowledge of the Principles of UG, children can calculate which contexts these are, and it remains only to learn

which form appears in these contexts. This learning is done by simple observation, given the calculations that children perform.

So the Principles and Parameters framework, together with the theory of
Optional Infinitives, understands why children behave as they do—why they
give these complicated and specific interactions between tense and case,
for example. Furthermore, this theory understands how children could easily learn default case.

How would an imitating/automaton model attempt to deal with these
facts? Because ACC forms do not occur in subject positions for the most
part, why does the child produce such? For the intention learning version
of an imitation model, Tomasello (2000, p. 240) suggested that children in
English imitate the kind of pronoun they hear in constructions like *let her
open it*; "they may just imitatively learn the end part of the sentence." These
are small clause constructions, which take ACC subjects. This means that
children have to ignore the fact that these forms never occur as the first
word (subject) of the main sentence. So how could they ignore this fact and
at the same time learn, say, the verb-second property of German or Dutch,
which they know so exquisitely? Learning theorists would be delighted to
see a learning mechanism that could have both those properties.

Tomasello indicated that children "basically **never**" use NOM pronouns
for ACC pronouns[10] (**Mary hit I*) because "they never hear adults say anything like this in any linguistic construction" (p. XX). He must have meant
that NOM pronouns never follow verbs, that is, he assumed that sequences
of words occurring next to each other are crucial for imitation, although he
did not state his assumptions explicitly. At any rate, his claim is false: Consider sentences like *Mary knows I like candy*, or *who did Mary tell I like
candy?* In the first sentence, the NOM pronoun *I* follows the verb *knows*; of
course, *I* is not the object of *knows*. In the second sentence, the NOM pronoun *I* follows the verb *tell*. Of course, the pronoun is not the *object* of *tell*; in
syntactic terms there is a trace of the object between *tell* and *I*. But Tomasello was assuming that children have no knowledge of such syntactic categories, of relations like subject and object, of traces; presumably, they are
only paying attention to sequences of words. So there is evidence in the input for NOM pronouns following verbs, in the sense of input evidence relevant to Tomasello's model.

But the situation is far worse. In German or Dutch, children do not use
ACC subject pronouns. Yet, the German or Dutch equivalents of *Mary saw
him go* exist, with ACC NPs as the subjects of the small clauses. So the input

---

[10]Tomasello did not reference any works on the pronoun facts in children, but the patterns
he was assuming are some of those argued for in Schutze and Wexler (1996). He treated the pronoun facts in the same paragraph as the use of OIs, suggesting that he implicitly recognized that
it has been argued that the phenomena go together in the OI stage.

situation in German or Dutch is similar to the input situation in English, with respect to the juxtaposition of ACC case and nonfinite verbs (*him go*). On the imitation learning model, Dutch and German children should produce as many ACC pronoun subjects as English-speaking children. But they do not produce any.

The methodological problem with the imitation learning view is that its mechanisms are not well-specified; each time a phenomenon in children is discovered, the model can make up a reason why there is evidence in the input for it. This is what Tomasello (p. 232) called a "fudge factor" when he discussed maturation. But maturational theories (Babyonyshev, Ganger, Pesetsky, & Wexler, 2001; Borer & Wexler, 1987, 1992, among others) make crosslinguistic predictions about differences in development, which could easily invalidate the model. Tomasello did not test his ideas against cross-linguistically different predictions—so far as I know the observations just made are the first such tests of the imitation learning ideas, tests with a negative outcome. In contrast to formal maturational ideas that have been proposed, it is harder to make such predictions for the imitation learning view, because what counts as an adult model and what counts as imitation and what counts as an intention have not been specified sufficiently. Nevertheless, the arguments just made show that the imitation learning view is wrong for the cases discussed.

The theory proposed—linking principles, parameters, and OIs—explains and clearly predicts this result. Children learn the default case form of their language. They cannot learn this from the subjects of OIs, because these sentences do not exist in the adult input. But they learn the default form, as already suggested, from sentences with NPs that are not in a structural case position. Once they learn the default case form, they use it for the subject of OIs.

But the imitation learning view has no recourse to a notion like default case. Such a notion presupposes a notion of structural case. The default case is the case used when the NP is not in a structural case position. The imitation learning view, by definition, asserts that the child has no implicit notion of structural case. Thus, it can have no implicit notion of default case, in the relevant sense.[11]

Note that what an imitation learning view—like all such views denying that young children have any kind of computational linguistic system—would like to assert is that the notion of *default* defined here can be replaced with a notion based on frequency in the input. That is, the default form should be the most frequent form in the input. But this is just false; consider that the NOM form in English, which is not the default form, is by far the most frequent in the input. In Dutch and German, the default form is NOM; although there is no data, presumably NOM is the most frequent form in the input in these languages also. So the sense of default that is needed is orthogonal to frequency in the input. What is needed is a computational notion of default, part of the child's system of language. Children, it turns out, and not surprisingly, have a computational system of language.[12]

VARIATION ACROSS LANGUAGES
IN THE OI STAGE: THE NS/OI CORRELATION

Although many languages go through an OI stage, many do not. For example, Italian, Spanish, and Catalan do not go through the OI stage. The percentage of OIs in these languages, even at very early ages, is extremely small. More than 20 languages have been studied at this point, and there is a generalization that fits the data perfectly so far (Wexler, 1998, also see Sano & Hyams, 1994):

(14) The Null-Subject/Optional Infinitive Generalization (NS/OI): A child learning a language goes through the OI stage only if the language is not an INFL-licensed null subject language.

NS/OI says that Italian, Spanish, and Catalan do not go through the OI stage because they are null subject languages. German, Dutch, English, and French, on the other hand, are not null subject languages, and they do go through the OI stage. See Wexler (1998) for a discussion of more languages and more data.

So, why should NS/OI hold? Wexler (1998) derived the existence of the OI stage as well as NS/OI from the assumption that what characterizes young children is a particular limitation on their computational systems called the *Unique Checking Constraint* (UCC).

---

[11]Tomasello's work appears to not understand the relation between finiteness and subject case, a classic fact about languages that any theory would have to take account of. He made a point of discussing what he called the "incredulity construction" (p. 236), with examples like: *My mother ride a motorcycle!* He wrote that this construction "is very odd from the point of view of the majority of English sentence-level constructions because the subject is in the accusative case . . . and the verb is non-finite" (p. XX). He somehow wants to remove this construction from the "core" of the language. He seems unaware of the fact that the construction has been discussed (sometimes at length) in many OI papers, and that the ACC case *follows* from the nonfiniteness of the main verb. For example, in languages with NOM default case, the subjects of this construction are NOM, despite the nonfinite verb. For Tomasello, the construction is just some strange thing that does not obey grammatical rules—he thinks it is special to English. But its ubiquity and lawlike behavior make it understandable within UG analyses.

[12]In a way, the intention learning model's lack of specification of a learning theory is in line with the historical foundations of such theories in psychology. The most famous (radical) behaviorist of all, B. F. Skinner, wrote a famous article in which he argued that theories of learning are not necessary.

(15) *Unique Checking Constraint (UCC)*: Children can only check once against the D-feature (the Determiner feature, i.e., the feature that characterizes noun phrases, NPs) of their subjects, whereas adults can do this more than once.

UCC is a developmental constraint on the computational system of language; it holds of young children and fades out over time (it is not a constraint on the adult grammar, UG). Moreover, UCC is not subject to parametric variation, and it is not that some adult languages have UCC and others do not and the child has to learn whether UCC holds. UCC is simply a constraint on children at a particular immature time. Think of it as parallel to constraints that do not allow children to walk at a particular time. See Wexler (1998) for a full discussion of UCC.

But, how does UCC work to predict NS/OI? First, as mentioned earlier, Schütze and Wexler (1996) argued that the OI stage is best described by the AGR/TNS Omission Model (ATOM). There are two inflectional functional categories, AGR (Agreement) and TNS (Tense). ATOM says that in the OI stage, either AGR or TNS is omitted by the child. This yields OIs, because many inflectional morphemes on verbs cannot be inserted without both AGR and TNS being present, the result being the infinitival morpheme, and thus the OI. For example, *s* in English specifies both agreement (third person singular) and tense (present). If AGR or TNS is omitted, *s* cannot be inserted, and the nonfinite morpheme (the phonetically empty morpheme in the case of English, *en* in Dutch, etc.) is inserted on the verb. Schütze and Wexler argued for ATOM on the basis of the particular constellation of effects of subject case errors.

Why does ATOM hold? Wexler (1998) argued that ATOM follows from UCC. Syntactic theory (Chomsky, 1995) argues that functional categories like AGR and TNS have D-features, and these D-features (unlike the D-features of NPs) are uninterpretable. Therefore, to obtain a coherent meaning, the uninterpretable features must be eliminated. This is done by checking the uninterpretable D-features of AGR and TNS against the D-feature of a NP (the subject NP). The idea is that a subject NP has to check the D-features of both AGR and TNS. For the child, UCC prevents this from happening. Therefore, children omit AGR or TNS. Thus, the UCC implies that the OI stage exists and is described by ATOM. In other words, the OI stage results from the difficulty in the child's computational system of checking some syntactic features.

Informally, UCC prevents subjects from moving to both AGR and TNS, and if subjects have not moved to these functional categories, they are ill-formed: All verbal functional categories demand to see a nearby subject. Thus, the child has to eliminate either AGR or TNS, so as to make a well-formed sentence. The child's grammar, like adult grammars, will not tolerate AGR or TNS without a local subject.

An Italian-speaking child should, and generally does, have the same difficulties due to UCC. However, in Italian, AGR does not have to be checked
against, because it itself is interpretable as the subject of the sentence (the
traditional idea about null subject languages). That is, in Italian the D-
feature of AGRS is interpretable. Thus, the subject NP in Italian only has to
check against TNS, not AGR, and this amount of checking is not too much
and does not violate UCC. So the Italian-speaking child (or a child learning
any null subject language) does not have to omit AGR or TNS in order to
satisfy the UCC. Thus, all features are specified in productions of the Italian-
speaking child. There is no OI stage, which is why NS/OI holds.

Using the same informal analogy, the subject only has to move to TNS in
Italian, not to AGR at all (there is grammatical evidence that this is correct).
This is because AGR itself operates like a subject in null subject languages.
Only one movement is necessary, so UCC is not violated; the child has no
reason to omit either AGR or TNS, and keeps both. Thus, the finite morpheme, which depends on both AGR and TNS, can be inserted, and the
child does not produce an OI.

UCC will still have an effect on children speaking languages like Italian,
but they will not produce main clause infinitives, for reasons just given.
However, they are predicted to omit auxiliaries (for reasons given in
Wexler, 1998), and they do, during the OI age range.

CROSSLINGUISTIC VARIATION IN DEVELOPMENT

Although the description in the last section of the underlying theory of the
OI stage (the UCC) was very brief, its introduction serves to demonstrate
the character of the explanation. But why does UCC hold and how does it
go away as children age? Given UCC as a constraint on young children, it is
obvious why the OI stage exists, and also why many languages do not go
through the OI stage.

In other words, there is an interaction between developing principles of
the computational system of language (e.g., the UCC) and the actual language the child is learning. Children are such excellent learners of parameters (VEPS; also see Wexler, 1998, for arguments that the child learns correctly from very early whether or not the language is a null subject
language), they know whether or not their language is a null subject language, that is, whether or not AGR has to be checked. Therefore, UCC does
not come into play in a language where children are not checking AGR. It is
the interaction of universal developing principles and what is learned in a
particular language that determines the linguistic behavior observed.

Note that the model does not say that children learn the parameters of
Italian better than they learn the parameters of English or Dutch. The rele-

vant parameters are all learned quickly and well (VEPS). It just turns out that once the child has learned the parameter values in different languages, these values interact differently with the universal developing principles to which both English- and Dutch-speaking children are subject (e.g., UCC).

This is quite a different picture than the traditional one in generative grammar-oriented studies of linguistic development, and also of more traditional studies. It is a picture that assumes (and shows) that children are excellent learners of language-particular properties of language. But there are some universal constraints on the developing child that might not exist on the adult, and these interact with the principles to form what looks like very different behavior. But, in no way is it a *learning* deficit. After all, the detailed learning (of parameter values, of default case, of agreement and other inflectional forms) is exquisitely precise. Children are excellent learners of language-particular facts and they know universal grammar principles. However, they have some particular computational limitations as a result of their immaturity.

In fact, there are a wide variety of developmental differences across languages explained by the OI model. Some effects are quite interestingly subtle—for example, effects on rates of OIs, as opposed to the presence or absence of OIs. In particular, there are large differences in OI rates across languages that do have OIs in the appropriate age range. These effects are understood by the interaction of the particular morphology of the language with the ATOM, which describes the OI stage. For example, English children in a particular age range show a larger rate of OIs than do Dutch children at the same age. These results are understood by an analysis of the verbal morphology of the two languages, and the application of ATOM to this morphology. The differential rate is predicted. See Wexler, Schaeffer, and Bol (in press) for the analysis and data. There are quite a few other cases like this, which are too lengthy to discuss here.

The UCC has been applied to explain an even more diverse range of phenomena in the OI age range. Hagstrom (2000) and Baek and Wexler (2000) explained a particular well-known word order error in the development of Korean using the UCC. Namely, in the so-called short form negation structures, *an/not* normally appears after the object, yielding the word order in (16a) in this SOV language:

(16) a. Subject Object an V
      b. *Subject an Object V (child form)

Children, however, often produce the form in (16b). Although well-documented as an existing error, there has been no satisfactory explanation of why children go strongly against the input and create the wrong form. Hagstrom and Baek and Wexler proposed that in adult Korean, the object raises, checking twice. Thus, the UCC prevents this second checking, forcing the object to remain in a lower position, and thereby creating the word order error in (16b).

Baek and Wexler showed that a predicted correlation holds, namely, that when the child fails to raise the object (16b), he never inserts ACC case, although he often inserts ACC case when he does raise the object (16a). There are a number of other phenomena that are predicted and tested, and a detailed syntactic theory is given. The point is that a constraint on child grammar that explains the OI stage (and the failure of the OI stage to hold in some languages) also explains a completely different type of error in an unrelated language. Developing constraints have effects throughout the grammar. What looks to be unrelated phenomenologically is in fact the result of the same cause. There is no (phenomenologically) comparable kind of error in English because English does not have the same double checking process of object raising.

The implications of the method and results are striking. It is a truism of research in developmental psycholinguistics that children's behavior looks quite different in different languages. Of course, it is expected that different developing languages will exhibit properties that are different simply because the languages themselves differ. But the errors look different too. The general problem in the field is very old and it had been hard to figure out its solution. Why should children subject to universal principles make a different kind of error, even when the error is not simply the missetting of a parameter?

Furthermore, we have a picture in which strikingly different effects in child language are seen to be due to the same cause (e.g., the subsumption of the Korean word order error to the UCC). There is no need to search for a different cause for every different kind of child error, a particularly unhappy situation for a field that aspires to be a science. The field of child language begins to take on the hope that it might aspire to the theoretical, empirical, and methodological standards of the more traditional "hard" sciences.

IS THE OI STAGE DUE TO LEARNING?

The big question is, why the OI stage? Take the OI stage to be accounted for by the UCC from the last section. Why does it hold of children? What causes the OI stage to end? The answer is that the UCC goes away. But what causes the UCC to go away?

According to traditional approaches to language acquisition, including traditional generative grammar approaches, the children learn to leave the OI stage, or that the UCC does not hold. This traditional answer cannot be right. Learning is, by definition, a change in the cognitive system due to the informational content of experience; for example, children learn to spell *the* in English; they do not learn to have teeth (even if it turns out that teeth are strengthed by use; there is no informational content in using teeth). Learning is the picking up of information from the environment, which is influenced by many variables. Learning implies that the behavior under discussion follows the laws of learning, for example, that learning changes to match the input and lots of clear input will result in learning that matches the input well. Emergence from the OI stage cannot be the result of learning. There are at least four excellent reasons; more are discussed as we find further sources of evidence in studies of the causes of learning, in behavioral genetics, and in studies of impaired development.

Problems for the Hypothesis That Learning Is the Cause of the Fading Away of the OI Stage

First, the evidence available to the child for finiteness being required in main clauses is enormous, existing in all input sentences. Children hear thousands of finite sentences, and very few sentences with main clause nonfinite verbs. There is a tendency to speak shortly to children (Newport, H. Gleitman, & L. Gleitman, 1977), so that children hear fewer subordinate, potentially infinitival clauses than adults. At any rate, all sentences have a finite verb in the main clause. It is difficult to see what kind of a learning mechanism could be so faulty that it takes several years to learn that finiteness is required. This is especially so because there is excellent evidence that children know the inflectional morphemes, with their grammatical and semantic properties, in the OI stage. For example, they know that *s* in English can be used only with third person singular present tense verbs. So they have easily learned the properties of *s*—except for the one stating it is obligatory rather than optional.

Second, if it is a question of learning, why should children start out mostly with forms that are not the most common forms in the input? Consider for example, the 83% OI rate in Dutch children from age 1;6 to 2;0 in Table 1.1. Children hear many finite verbs, so if a learning mechanism is responsible for emergence from the OI stage, then how did children ever get into the stage? Why don't they overuse the finite morphemes, which are used so often? Children essentially never substitute a finite morpheme where an infinitival morpheme is required. (See, e.g., Guasti, 1994, for Italian.) Yet, this is what would be expected if it were a question of learning which morpheme goes where. Remember that in most languages studied, the equivalent of infinitival *to* in English is not used; rather the infinitival verb is used, for example, *kopen/buy (nonfinite)* in Dutch (6). So the infinitival verb follows the direct object in (6). But finite verbs also follow the direct objects in embedded clauses—they too occur at the end of sentences.

So why don't children make the "learning" error of deciding that finite verbs can substitute for nonfinite verbs? They do not. There just does not seem to be a learning mechanism with the properties that will capture the empirical facts.

The problem is even more acute in languages like Danish, Norwegian, or Swedish. These are languages without surface agreement. There is only one form for present tense, and it occurs in every present tense sentence, and it does not vary with the features of the subject. So this one present tense form is extremely frequent. Yet, in these languages, there is a very high rate of OIs in young children. Because the same present tense form is so frequent, why isn't it substituted for the infinitival form rather than the other way around? Again, what learning mechanism could possibly have the required empirical properties?

Third, basic sentence and inflectional parameters are learned extremely early and extremely well, with almost no observable error (VEPS). That is, parameter learning for these parameters is completed successfully by the time the child enters the two word stage, around age 18 months. There is evidence in some children that learning of basic sentence parameters (such as V2) is successfully completed at a somewhat younger age than 18 months. Given that children's learning abilities are so outstanding that they have learned basic parameter values perfectly at such a young age, what is it about their learning mechanisms that is so poor and leaky that the obligatoriness of finiteness is only mastered a couple of years later? It is simply difficult to put together the exquisite early learning of parameter values with the late learning of obligatory finiteness, if only one learning mechanism is to account for both properties.

Putting these (and many other arguments) together sheds light on the great value in studying parameter setting empirically in children. Namely, parameters are language specific, and their values vary depending on the language. Thus, there is unanimous agreement among nativists and empiricists (even behaviorists) that the parameter values (or whatever accounts for this variation) have to be learned from experience; there is no question of that. I believe that there is excellent evidence (both theoretical—e.g., learnability arguments, see Wexler & Culicover, 1980—and empirical) that many principles are genetically programed. But empiricists deny this claim; they think that principles (to the extent they believe that principles exist) are learned (for more discussion on learning, see Conti-Ramsden, sect. II in this volume). So at the very least the evidence is arguable, if for no other reason than that it takes an argument to claim that a principle is genetically programed. But the claim that parameters are learned is incontrovertible.

So parameters are a perfect testing ground in which to study learning because they must be learned. If someone wants to study learning, parameters (or other aspects of language where it is known that there is variation, e.g., varying properties of the lexicon) are the place to study them.

This study in OI analyses showed that children are brilliant, precocious learners. It was no surprise to anybody who studies the OI stage to see the results of Saffran, Aslin, and Newport (1996), which showed that 8-month-old children could learn some distributional properties of stimuli. What other than the ability to learn from such kind of evidence could underlie the ability of children before age 18 months (as measured by production data) to set their parameters correctly? It would be surprising if the ability emerged suddenly at, say, 15 months, resulting in correct parameter settings in production at 18 months. (There are studies in some languages showing some word order patterns are produced correctly at 15 months.) Children have to be able to attend to varying order of words and morphemes and perform calculations, including learning calculations, on these. It is good to have confirming experimental evidence at a somewhat younger age, because it makes the world consistent. But if somebody carried out an experiment showing that children could not learn distributional information at an age somewhat before 18 months, then the conclusion would be that either the experiment did not appropriately tap their learning ability, or the materials presented were too far from a languagelike situation. The evidence from the production data that children are excellent learners of this kind of information, at least in a languagelike setting, is vast and overwhelming, so there is no way that this evidence could be consistent with a lack of learning ability.

Fourth, if the OI stage is the result of a general human learning mechanism, then the OI stage would be expected to show up in second language learning by adults. It would simply be the result of applying a learning mechanism to input data. But, in fact, the OI stage does not show up in adults. The growing literature on this topic is relatively recent, but the evidence is already quite good. See, for example, Haznedar and Schwartz (1997), Prevost and White (1997), and Ionin and Wexler (2000, 2002). Adult L-2 learners do use root infinitives sometimes, but they have very different properties from OIs. For example, they often appear in second position in V2 languages, which is something that never happens to OIs (Prevost, 1997). Five- to 10-year-old L-1 Russian speakers often consider finite forms of *be* to be a kind of tense marking, using *be* together with a stem form, *he is go* (Ionin & Wexler, in press), something that children in the OI stage almost never do (Rice & Wexler, 1996). Haznedar and Schwartz (1997) showed that even a young child (L-1 Turkish) learning English continues giving lots of what appear to be OIs, but does not use null subjects along with them, contrary to the behavior of children in the OI stage. Ionin and Wexler replicated this result with their 5- to 10-year-old L-1 Russian learners of English. There is not enough space to discuss this literature in any detail here, but the best hypothesis is that adult L-2 learners have much more difficulty than young child L-1 learners in learning the exact properties of inflections (Prevost and White's hypothesis that adult L-2 learning has trouble with learning surface forms). Ionin and Wexler concluded that there is no OI stage in adult L-2 learning. Adults do show some error-filled, slow acquisition of morphemes and their properties that learning theories would expect. So, at many points, child L-1 learning and adult L-2 learning diverge— the OI stage is not replicated in adults.

IS IT GENETICALLY GUIDED MATURATION?

Fortunately, there are two answers available in science for what causes immature forms to grow into mature forms. Although learning plays a role in some instances, genetically guided maturation is even more basic, and presumably more common. So the obvious hypothesis to make about the withering away of the OI stage, of the UCC, is that it matures away, under genetic guidance. In other words, the genetic system determines that at birth (or whenever the language system comes online) the UCC is in place and the genetic system also insures that the UCC dies out over time. The maturing away of the UCC is a matter of genetically timed development, as are so many other aspects of development in both human and nonhuman biology.

Borer and Wexler (1987, 1992) made the classic arguments for maturation of the linguistic capacity in the generative tradition, and since then there has been a lively debate on the topic. Here, consider what evidence exists for the proposition that it is genetics that guides the withering away of the UCC and thus of the OI stage.

First, all the problems raised for the learning hypothesis in the previous section are easily dealt with by the hypothesis that the development is genetically guided. Yes, children are excellent learners, as seen in their excellent abilities at learning the properties of inflectional morphemes like *s*. Children use their learning abilities to learn the features of *s* perfectly and early. But the UCC affects the child's ability to mark every root verb as finite. Genetic inheritance causes the UCC to be part of the young child's computational system of language (or to constrain it in some way), until it withers away, again under genetic guidance. So OIs can persist even though learning of features of morphemes (not constrained by the UCC) is finely tuned. This solves the first problem.

The second problem asks why the child starts out with such a large proportion of OIs. Assume that the genetic system specifies that the UCC constrains the very young child's computational system of language and that it dies away over time, under genetic guidance. At the youngest age, the child is most susceptible to the UCC, and the result is large OI rates—

the input did not cause the OI rates, which are orthogonal to the input. This is exactly what is expected from genetically guided systems. Forcing hard food into a child's mouth will not cause it to grow teeth, just as saying lots of finite forms to the child at a very young age will not force the child to leave the OI stage. In general, maturational systems play out over time, in a graded, not usually discontinuous manner. Teeth grow; they get bigger. Similarly, the effects of the UCC die away over time, so that OI rates will gradually diminish. See Lenneberg (1967) for examples of maturational curves in biology.

The third problem is likewise not a problem under the current view. Children set parameters correctly because their learning systems are so good, but this learning system will not solve the problem for them that the UCC in their brains (via genetically based heredity) calculates that a sentence in need of double checking is ungrammatical, and they therefore have to omit AGR or TNS, producing an OI. Infants are capable of learning much; they cannot "learn" to grow teeth before their biology requires or allows it.

The final problem also vanishes under the view that the UCC is a developmental constraint. Because adults (or older children) are not subject to the UCC, second language acquisition by these older children or adults will not result in the properties of the OI stage. Whatever errors exist in learning a second language at an age past the OI age range will be due to other factors, for example, the difficulty in learning language-particular material that adults show, which is a difficulty not shared by very young children.

FURTHER EVIDENCE THAT THE OI STAGE DIES AWAY UNDER MATURATIONAL GUIDANCE

So far the discussion has covered a number of empirical arguments from phenomena concerning facts of normal language development that show that the OI stage (the existence of the UCC) dies away under genetically guided maturation. There is evidence from a wide variety of additional sources that shows that development must essentially be genetically guided maturation, and not a process of learning from experience. Again, it is important to point out carefully that the child does do a good deal of learning from experience; some of the most striking evidence showing how good the child is at this process has already been discussed. But development out of the OI stage is too slow, too delayed, and too at odds with the input to be an event of learning. The phenomenology of the OI stage is so striking when set alongside the background of the phenomenology of parameter setting (learning) that it calls out for a different explanation. The "empirical footprints" of learning and maturation are fundamentally different (Babyonyshev et al., 2001).

Some additional arguments for maturation bring in a wide array of alternate methodologies and fields, and help to integrate broadly across different empirical approaches to a major problem. At the same time, the last piece of evidence concerns specific language impairment (SLI), so that we can even integrate impaired development into the picture, in an important way, and show how its properties flow from and contribute to knowledge of normal development.

Additional Empirical Arguments That the UCC Is Genetically (Maturationally, Developmentally), Guided

Variables That Affect Learning. The usual variables that affect learning of learned material, including learned material in language, do not affect the development of the UCC. Learning is influenced by many variables, as psychologists have shown for more than 100 years. Many of these variables are related to input and its properties. For example, richness of input leads to faster learning. If growth out of the OI–UCC stage is due to learning, this growth would be expected to be influenced by the same variables that affect learning in general.

It has already been argued earlier that it does not make sense to think that growth of finiteness is affected by richness of input. Nevertheless, the question can be asked anyway. Perhaps the relevant property that makes input "rich" has been missed. Perhaps there is some mysterious property of the input that does not always exist, and the child is waiting for this mysterious property to appear.

By adopting the strategy of finding out what variables affect learning in other domains of language, it will be possible to see if those variables affect the learning of obligatory finiteness. If they do not, then growth out of the OI–UCC stage is not caused by learning, by any psychologist's definition of learning. Learning must obey the laws of learning; if it does not, then it is not learning. For example, the growth of teeth is not a case of learning; this growth is not affected by experience the way learning theory expects. So if the approach to the question of learning is conducted in an objective, scientific fashion, then a question arises: Do the variables that affect learning also affect the learning of obligatory finiteness?

Rice, Wexler, and Hershberger (1998) carried out this study in English. They had Rice and Wexler's sample of approximately 60 children (40 normal, 20 SLI) who had been studied longitudinally for several years—the normal children from age 3;0 to 6:0, the children with SLI from age 5;0 to 8;0. They asked the question: What variables affected the growth of the obligatory nature of finiteness? It was straightforward to quantify this variable; it is the percentage of finite forms used in obligatory contexts over a range of contexts, all of which are predicted to be sometimes nonfinite in the OI stage—for example, omission of third person singular *s*, omission of *be* forms. Their results held for both normal children and children with SLI, so those are not separated out here. The focus returns to the children with SLI when discussing the nature of SLI.

Rice, Wexler, and Hershberger, considering what variables to study as potential causes of the growth of finiteness, decided to test the variables that had been shown to strongly affect and to be predictive of the growth of vocabulary size. These variables had been taken to be important variables in causing learning to take place.

One variable was the amount of the mother's formal education. This *mother's education* variable had been shown to be quite predictive of growth of vocabulary in previous research (Huttenlocher, Haight, Bryk, Seltzer, & Lyons, 1991). And it makes a lot of sense. After all, vocabulary growth takes place in an item-by-item manner; it is normally thought to be influenced by number of presentations of the item, by the contexts in which it is presented, by the drawing of attention to objects and events, and by richness of input in various ways. And the amount to which a parent does all these things is thought to be influenced by degree of education, not categorically of course, but statistically, over the population. Vocabulary growth needs input, and each item needs input. Individuals cannot learn a word they have not heard or seen. So there is no question that growth of vocabulary is influenced by learning, at least a significant part of it is learning, and this is constant, because each item must be learned.[13] Mother's education was chosen because it was the most significant environmental variable found in vocabulary studies.

A second variable, *child's IQ*, that has been shown to have an effect on rate of vocabulary group in studies of growth of vocabulary the IQ of the child. This makes sense because IQ is considered to be related to general ability to learn. Vocabulary growth has a large component that has to be learned and each item has to be learned, so child's IQ would be expected to be predictive of rate of vocabulary growth, and it is.

Rice, Wexler, and Hershberger did hierarchical linear modeling—as was done in the studies of vocabulary growth—to see the effect of these variables. The results showed that (in strong contrast to the results on vocabulary growth done using the same methodology) neither mother's education nor child's IQ were significantly predictive of the growth of the rate of finiteness. In fact, these two variables together with three other variables, includ-

---

[13]There is very good reason to believe that much about the lexicon is part of UG and is genetically programmed (Jerry Fodor makes the extreme argument that everything about the lexicon is innate except phonetic spell-out). But no matter how much of the structure of the lexicon is innate, the phonetic spell-out plus the choice of which items are spelled out in the lexicon has to be learned item by item (short of productive rules, in the lexicon, what are sometimes called *lexical redundancy* rules).

ing whether the child was in the normal or SLI group, together accounted for only .3% of a reduction in variance in the growth of finiteness, less than a third of one per cent!

This is a remarkably strong result, using just the kind of data and method needed to test the idea of whether the growth of finiteness follows the laws of learning, that is, is influenced by variables that influence learning. What the results tell us is that if you look at two children, with the same level of finiteness (in obligatory contexts), but one of whom has a higher IQ and a mother with more education than the other, you will know nothing at all about how to predict which of the two children has a faster rate of growth in finiteness! Finiteness grows independently of the mother's education or the child's IQ. The two children will likely grow at different rates because growth is not identical across children. But you won't know anything given the other variables about how to predict which will grow faster. The growth of finiteness simply contradicts the laws of learning; the growth is not learning.

The situation is comparable to the following. Suppose there are two children of the same age. Would knowing the IQ of the child and mother's education level put a researcher in a better position to predict which child's hair will turn gray earlier? Maybe there is an effect, but it would not be expected intuitively; it would be no surprise if mother's education and child's IQ did not influence when hair turned gray. The reason no one would be surprised is that people do not believe that the hair's turning gray is a process of learning; it does not follow the laws of learning, so variables that affect learning should not necessarily affect the hair's turning gray.

What variables do affect growth of finiteness? Simply, the answer is time. A linear function of the time that has passed reduces the variance in finiteness rate by 72% and adding in a quadratic function reduces the variance more than 87%. That is, it is possible to know almost everything there is to know about a child's finiteness rate if it is known at what level the child was when the child was measured for the first time and how much time has passed since then. If there are two children with the same finiteness rate, and then their finiteness is measured a year later, they will be very close in finiteness at the later measure; there is very little random fluctuation in growth, given the 87% reduction due to time. (If this number were 100%, then any two children who have the same rate at time t_1 would have to have the same rate at a later time, t_2—there would be no statistical flux at all. So the 87% figure is huge.)

Of course, the fact that the passage of time is the major factor (almost a complete factor) in growth of finiteness, and other variables are not factors at all, is exactly what is expected on a maturational model. As the passage of time occurs, and the child ages, the genetic system carries out its functions. The UCC dies away as time goes by, uninfluenced by the variables that affect learning, simply influenced by the passage of time, the effects of which arise from the genetic system.[14]

What is particularly beautiful, almost surprising even to a theorist who believes that the principles of language grow rather than are learned (as Chomsky has often written) is the extent to which the empirical data, gathered via traditional quantitative psychological studies of longitudinal data, confirm the essential growth character of the demise of the OI–UCC stage. This looks like science; it looks like biology. It looks the way Eric Lenneberg's classic *Biological Foundations of Language* (1967) expected language development to look, although the developmental evidence did not exist at the time. Perhaps we should think of it as Lenneberg's dream.

Behavioral Genetics. The UCC develops more similarly in identical (monozygotic) twins than in fraternal (dizygotic) twins. Turning to the behavioral genetic data, we can ask the same question just discussed, but turned on its head. In studying the question of which variables affect growth of finiteness, what is being asked is (this is simplified) if two children start out with the same rate of finiteness, then what predicts differential rates of growth? Behavioral genetics asks, if two children are identical in genetic system to such and such an extent, then how much does this genetic identity predict a growth similarity compared to the growth similarity of two children who are less identical?

Ganger, Wexler, and Soderstrom (1997) used the standard behavioral genetic method of studying a group of identical (monozygotic) and fraternal (dizygotic) twins. MZ twins share 100% of their genes and DZ twins share 50% of their genes over a population. Ganger et al. studied the growth of finiteness in sets of these twins. To the extent that genetic factors affect the growth of finiteness, it would be expected that the MZ twins will be more similar in their development than the DZ twins.

The reason that the twin methodology is used in behavioral genetics is that it is assumed that both members of a pair of twins will grow up in a fairly similar environment, so that effects of the environment may be controlled. More essentially, it is assumed that whatever environmental differences there are between identical twins will not be exaggerated for frater-

---

[14]In principle, it is possible that orthogonal factors are responsible for the demise of the OI stage. For example, perhaps the OI stage is due in some way to an immature pragmatic system. As this system develops, the OI stage goes away. Although this is conceptually possible, there are severe empirical hurdles for such a proposal. For example, why don't children developing null subject languages like Italian show the same pragmatic deficit, thereby producing OIs in their language? Even if the empirical challenge can be met by some refined theory, it will still be necessary to ask the learning/development question of the pragmatic system. Can it be learned? Or is itself subject to maturation and to developmental constraints? At the moment there are no proposals that solve these problems, or a sufficient body of empirical analysis (e.g., what variables influence the development of pragmatics?), but the question is ultimately an empirical one.

nal twins. The methodology rests on that assumption. After all, siblings share the same proportion of genes (50% over a population). But the crucial assumption/hope is that fraternal twins, being twins of the same age, living in the same family environment at the same time, are treated as similarly as identical twins, who also are twins of the same age, living in the same family environment at the same time.

There are certainly cases where it is reasonable to question that assumption. To take an extreme case, suppose it is discovered that identical twins tend to dress more identically than fraternal twins. We wouldn't conclude that how one dresses has a genetic component, because it seems reasonable to guess that parents of identical twins might try to exaggerate their identicalness by dressing them alike, so that choice of dress is influenced by an environmental variable, parental training.

The argument of behavioral genetics rests on the assumption that it is a different kind of case, one in which the dependent variables being tested are such that the parents of identical twins are not any more likely to treat them similarly than are the parents of fraternal twins. Thus, for vocabulary growth, say, the assumption would be that parents of identical twins are not more likely to give their twins a similar environment that is related to training on vocabulary than are the parents of fraternal twins. One can question this assumption and critics of behavioral genetics have often questioned the assumption, reasonably in many cases.

Vocabulary growth is a good example of how it might be possible for parents to affect the similarity of twins. It is conceivable, at least, that parents try to introduce words to each of two identical twins in a similar manner, and they have a much smaller tendency to do this for fraternal twins.

So all behavioral genetic data and analysis should be approached with a reasonable degree of skepticism. However, if there is any cognitive or linguistic area where the crucial assumption is warranted, it might be the growth of finiteness. Conceptual arguments explaining that training differences should not be relevant to growth of finiteness have already been presented—there are so many exemplars given to any child in a reasonably normal environment. What would the child do with more examples? The OIs do not come from what parents do, so it is not as if parents choose a rate of OIs they are going to use and parents of identical twins would use a similar rate of OIs in talking to their two twins, whereas parents of fraternal twins would not do so. Moreover, there is good data that shows that the intuitively plausible environmental variables do not affect growth of finiteness. These variables include mother's education, which is presumably a surrogate for the things that a mother actually does to affect the child's environment. So it looks as if environment, in the standard sense, does not have any effect on rate of growth of finiteness. Thus, to the extent that one accepts the behavioral genetic methodology at all, the growth of finiteness is exactly the kind of variable that can be studied relatively worry free that a fundamental assumption of the method is being violated.

Ganger et al. studied a set of MZ twins and a set of DZ twins and measured how closely the twins in a pair attained a criterion in the use of obligatory finiteness. The measure was the difference of age of the twins when they reached the criterion. Zero weeks would mean that the twins reached the criterion at exactly the same time, and as the number grows, the more different the twins are in reaching criterion. The result turned out to be 13 weeks for the DZ twins and 3 weeks for the MZ twins. In other words, the identical twins attained a criterion for a rate of finiteness on the average (over the set of identical twins) only 3 weeks apart; this number shot up to 13 weeks for the DZ twins.

Although preliminary, because it is the first behavioral genetic study of the growth of a property tightly bound up with early grammar, the result is quite promising. Ganger (1998) provided more evidence on this issue, using the same twin method. Much remains to be done, but to the extent that there is any evidence from behavioral genetics, it is evidence for the proposition that genetic variation affects rate of growth of finiteness. It can be concluded that rate of growth of finiteness is affected by the genetic system. This is what would be expected on a maturational (growth) view of the development of grammar. Some children develop faster because their genetic systems develop somewhat faster.

It should go without saying that there is no reason to think that children whose genetic systems cause their rates of finiteness to grow faster than other children's are superior in any way, or that their linguistic systems are superior. The situation is just like with rate of growth of bodily organs. All normal children develop; the rate of growth varies a bit. There is no question of superiority. Moreover, unlike continuous variables (e.g., height), the use of obligatory finiteness rises to the same rate—100%—for the approximately 95% (see a later section on SLI) of normal children. Unlike height, use of finiteness at maturity does not show a normal distribution. The phenomenology is more like that for having a heart, with all its parts. Short of pathology, people develop hearts. Some grow faster than others, but people get there.

Specific Language Impairment. The UCC's withering away is greatly delayed in SLI, perhaps it never goes away. Moreover, children with SLI are excellent learners of material in language that needs to be learned. SLI, by definition, is an impairment that is specific to language; children are not considered to be children with SLI if they have any kind of cognitive, auditory, or speech deficit. There seems to be a group of such children, encompassing approximately 5% of the developing population according to a large epidemiological study (Tomblin, 1996).

Many chapters in this volume review the literature on SLI. This one describes its central features, and relates these features to the fact that the UCC remains active far longer in children with SLI than in normal children despite the fact that children with SLI are excellent learners of linguistic material. It turns out that SLI is an impairment that strongly supports the genetically guided maturational basis of the growth out of the OI–UCC stage, so the concentration is on those features relevant to these questions.

One of the focus points of this volume is the study of SLI and the connection of this study to linguistics. As was pointed out at the beginning of this chapter, to study impairment in some domain of language, there must be a good idea of normal development, its technical features, its structures and how they are attained, and what mechanisms drive this development. The study of the OI–UCC stage has all these features; it is understood better in technical detail, with the integration of a range of empirical material, than any other domain of early linguistic development. Moreover, there is more clear empirical information (much already discussed) about the mechanisms that drive the growth of language in this domain than in other domains.[15] As both linguistic theory and researches in language acquisition itself conclude, much of linguistic growth, outside of the domain of experienced-based language variation, like parameters, is driven by genetically based growth.

Thus when I decided with Mabel Rice to undertake a study of SLI, it seemed only natural to ask whether the children with SLI were in the OI stage for too long a period, and how much of their behavior could be accounted for by this very simple hypothesis. This is the *Extended Optional Infinitive Hypothesis* (also see Rice, chap. 2 in this volume), which says that children with SLI are just like normal children except they go through the OI period for a much longer time than normal children, perhaps never really emerging from it. Given that the OI period is more accurately (on the current theory discussed here) a period in which the UCC holds, it could be called the Extended Unique Checking Constraint (EUCC) period. The name does not matter, but the assumption does. According to this hypothesis, whatever causes the OI stage is present in children with SLI for a much longer time, perhaps indefinitely.

---

[15]In general, there is a better understanding of developmental properties of language that have been described within the principles and parameters approach than those which have not. The idea of genetically driven maturation of parts of the computational system of language was actually introduced into language acquisition studies with the results on passives and related structures (Babyonyshev et al., 2001; Borer & Wexler, 1987, 1992; Lee and Wexler, 2001; Miyamoto, Wexler, Aikawa, & Miagawa, 1999). But in the case of the OI stage, there is a great deal of added quantitative evidence about variables that cause learning, behavioral genetics, impairment studies, detailed relations to second language acquisition, and so on. Part of the reason for this is the simplicity of the phenomena; I fully expect that the same kind of evidence will be available for more complex cases as research proceeds.

This was a natural choice because I had already decided that the best hypothesis about normal development was that the OI stage was the result of a genetically driven maturational stage. Thus, it was natural to believe that the genetically driven event that caused the demise of the OI–UCC stage did not take place or took place late in children with SLI. The mistiming of genetic events is well-known enough to have a name in the genetics literature: heterochronology. So it was a natural enough biological possibility.

Of course, the naturalness of the idea did not mean it was true. It was almost too much to hope that such a simple idea could turn out to be true. Wouldn't it be more likely that SLI grammar was far more different from normal grammar than just in the processes that underlie the OI stage? This was a brute empirical question, and it received a very simple and clear answer in the work that I've done with Mabel Rice in English. The EOI does characterize SLI.

In order to demonstrate that the EOI characterizes SLI, researchers must show much more than that children with SLI produce too many OIs for their age. That result is necessary but not sufficient. Recall that the OI–UCC stage is characterized by a number of features. One of the central properties of the OI–UCC stage is that parameters have been correctly set. Another of the properties is that major inflectional morphemes in the verbal system have been learned correctly together with their syntactic and semantic features. In other words, in the OI stage children show a particular deficit (e.g., the production of nonfinite verbs in many languages) together with a range of excellent competence in other aspects of the computational system of language. (Of course, NS–OI predicts that SLI in null subject languages will not show OIs). It is crucial to determine that children have this knowledge/competence alongside the specific deficit if it is to be argued that children are in the OI stage.

Following this reasoning, Rice and Wexler decided to study the EOI stage by both studying the phenomena that were predicted to show a deficit (finiteness marking on verbs) and the phenomena that were not predicted to show a deficit. In the latter we chose as the first piece of competence to look at the question of subject-verb agreement. Children in the OI–UCC stage get subject-verb agreement right, in the sense that if a child uses a finiteness morpheme, then the subject almost always agrees with this morpheme.

This was first shown for German by Poeppel and Wexler (1993). For example, Poeppel and Wexler's data and other data in the literature (Clahsen, 1986) showed that when a German-speaking child used third person singular *t* the probability was greater than .97 that the subject was third person singular. When the child used the morpheme on the verb for first person singular, the probability was similarly great that the subject was first person singular. The child knew the agreement morphemes and their features, so that the subject always agreed with the verb. This was an essential part of the OI stage.[16] The essential property is that the child has stored the verbal morpheme together with its correct (adult) features.

Similarly, Harris and Wexler (1996) showed that English-speaking children in the OI stage never used *s* with anything other than a third person singular subject. Very young children learn correctly the features that go with verbal suffixes.

Rice, Wexler, and Cleave (1995), in the first empirical study of SLI in terms that took account of the OI stage, showed that two central properties of the OI stage held in children with SLI who were much older than the normal OI range.

(17) English-speaking children with SLI at an older age than normal children
    a. produce OIs, and I
    b. when the verb is finite, they produce a subject that agrees with it, almost all the time.

These phenomena were unknown. In a rough manner, the production of OIs (17) might have been thought to be known; after all, SLI was supposed to be having trouble with morphology, and leaving out verbal morphemes was one way that this happened. It was not thought of as lacking finiteness, nevertheless the phenomenon itself was not surprising.

But, (17b) was not only not known in the SLI literature, but it went against the received opinion that said children with SLI had trouble with morphology, and they had a learning deficit concerning morphology. For if children with SLI really did have a learning deficit in morphology, they would be expected to produce agreement errors. Because they sometimes used finiteness/agreement morphemes (like *s*), to have a learning deficit would mean on any kind of computational model that they had stored *s* with potentially incorrect features, that it were used at least sometime in a random manner so that the subject might not agree with it; the children might say **I goes* or **they goes*. But, as Rice, Wexler, and Cleave showed, this is exactly what does not happen in SLI. Children with SLI were like normal children in this regard.

The EOI is quite different from the suggestion that children with SLI drop morphemes to get shorter forms. That might work for some phenomena in

---

[16]Given the ATOM, there can be more subtle predictions about a language. See Wexler, Schaeffer, and Bol for a discussion of how ATOM might predict agreement errors in Dutch OI children, for example. But even on this latter analysis, the child has inserted into her lexicon the verbal agreement morpheme together with its correct features (person, number). But agreement or tense features may be omitted from the structure, producing the errors.

English, but it does not work in other languages. Remember that young normal Dutch produce large numbers of OIs (see Table 1.1)? These OIs are not shorter forms than the correct agreement forms, they just substitute a different suffix morpheme (*en*) for the finite morpheme. (8) repeated as (18) is an example, with *en* added to the stem *wass*:

(18) pappa schoenen wassen
      daddy shoes wash-INF
      'Daddy wash (non-finite) shoes'

In fact, for the first person singular, the agreement morpheme is Ø, the inaudible, phonetically zero morpheme. So when children use OIs instead of first person singular verbs (there are large numbers of these; see data in Wexler, Schaeffer, and Bol, in press), they are complicating the verb, and adding material to it in a surface sense. So there is no empirically reasonable notion of "surface shortening" in SLI or in normal children in general (thus no empirically adequate defense of the "surface hypothesis" of Leonard, 1989, or of the ideas on "morpheme omission" in Bishop, 1997). The notion of "shortening," or "omission," of surface material was a pure accident of overconcentration on the study of English, where the infinitival morpheme is phonetically zero. As soon as the range of study is expanded out to even the closest related languages (e.g., the Germanic languages, the Romance languages), it may be seen that shortening is not empirically correct.

So the general idea of the EOI (and ultimately of the EUCC) is that the UCC has not been eliminated via genetically driven maturation in children with SLI, despite the fact that they are at the age where it is eliminated in normal children. But other grammatical development is intact.[17] Thus, it may be predicted that children with SLI (a) Use OIs in languages where

---

[17]Actually, there is one other strongly natural possibility. It is quite possible that children with SLI are delayed not only in the OI–UCC, but also in other areas where normal children are themselves maturationally delayed. That is, it is possible that SLI shows delay from normal children on grammatical property P if and only if P is itself a property that matures in normal children. Call this the "Hypothesis of Delay in All Maturational Properties." For examples, there is good evidence that A-chains mature over time (until around age 5) (the *A-chain Deficit Hypothesis* of Babyonyshev et al., 2001; Borer & Wexler, 1987, 1992; Lee & Wexler, in press; Miyamoto et al., 1999); this is a very well-known area of maturational delay in the computational system of language. If the hypothesis of delay in all maturational properties is correct, then children with SLI would be expected to be seriously delayed from normal children in the representations of A-chains, for example, verbal passives, being able to give verbs a correct unaccusative analysis, and so on. There is preliminary evidence in unpublished research that Mabel Rice and I are doing that there is not much serious delay in verbal passive of children with SLI (certainly they are not delayed compared to language[MLU]-matched controls, whereas the central results of Rice, Wexler, and Cleave (1995), Rice and Wexler (1996), and many others is that children with SLI are delayed on finiteness rates relative to language[MLU]-matched controls). To the extent that English-speaking children with SLI are not delayed on verbal passive and similar structures, the strict EOI/EUCC is correct—it is only UCC-implicated structures on which children with SLI are

TABLE 1.4
Finiteness/Position Contingency Children with SLI

All children with SLI	V2	V_{final}
Finite	1,071 (99.8%)	16 (5%)
Nonfinite	2 (0.2%)	335 (95%)

Note:

younger normal children do, and (b) show the same patterns of grammatical knowledge as normal children.

But it is probably easier to describe the logic of establishing the EOI–EUCC by considering a language with the kinds of properties that the original OI languages had—with surface infinitival morphemes and with processes of parameter-set verb movement that allowed for strong predictions of morphology/word order correlations.

Consider Dutch. Table 1.1 shows that normal children in Dutch go through an OI stage that is largely over in the 3;0–3;6 age range; in that interval, there are only 7% OIs. Wexler, Schaeffer, and Bol also studied 20 children with SLI. In the 6;0–8;2 year range, the children with SLI still had 15% OIs (50 of 334). The OI stage persisted much longer in the children with SLI.

But especially striking is the correlation between verb second position and morphology. This was shown for normal children in Table 1.2. Table 1.4 from Wexler, Schaeffer, and Bol is for children with SLI.

The data is remarkable because the children with SLI are so obviously excellent at the essential correlation. Observe that 99.8% of all V2 verbs are finite. But only 5% of final verbs are finite. This is beautifully precise, with very little having to be accounted for by performance or measurement error—at most 18 items out of 1,424 items (again, only nonambiguous data cases were counted). Children with SLI are essentially perfect at the correlation, they are essentially just like normal children. This is exactly what was predicted—it is an essential part of the OI stage.

This has to come as a surprise to any model of children with SLI that says they are lacking grammar, or lacking the ability to learn surface morphemes. (How could they get this correlation so perfectly right if there was something they had not "learned" about a surface morpheme?) Note that there is no question even of "omitting" morphemes. The nonfinite forms have an *en* ending. The finite forms have a *t* ending in second and third per-

---

delayed. To the extent that children with SLI are delayed on verbal passive and similar structures, there will need to be a loosening of the EOI hypothesis to allow for delay on A-chains and similar. The logic of the two hypotheses is quite clear; they are both natural. Future research will decide which is more correct. At any rate, the fact that children with SLI are OI–UCC delayed is quite well-established.

son singular, of which there are plenty (see detailed tables in Wexler, Schaeffer, and Bol). Only the first person singular finite forms have a zero ending, and these are in second position because they are finite. So the OIs actually make some verbs longer. And, moreover, they get put in final, unmarked position, where nonfinite verbs go.

So the Dutch children with SLI are clearly in the EOI–UCC stage. They get agreement perfectly right; there is excellent evidence that they have stored the agreement morphemes with the correct features.

Considering only the English and Dutch cases, we now know much in technical detail about the nature of knowledge and nonknowledge in children with SLI. Moreover, much is known about the effect of a *learning deficit* on SLI. With respect to the computational system of language, there is no learning deficit, because Dutch children with SLI have set their parameters completely correctly. They get the V2/finiteness correlation perfectly; they behave completely correctly with respect to the *yes* setting of the V2 parameter, which Dutch exhibits. No SLI child has failed to learn that value of this parameter, and they hardly even show any noise on behaving with respect to the correct parameter value.

So children with SLI are *brilliant learners*, just as normal children. They learn the language-particular properties that have to be mastered. They do not have a learning deficit.

Dutch- and English-speaking children with SLI *are* delayed. There is a maturational delay in a property that is not learned, the property of obligatoriness of tense. That is, there is a delay in the demise of the UCC. Children with SLI at a much older stage are still governed by the UCC.

This Dutch and English data on SLI thus provide a strong argument that the development out of the OI stage is genetically driven maturation. The children do not have a learning delay (parameters, agreement morphemes). When they have to learn, they learn, early, quickly, and well. They pay attention; there is no attention deficit with respect to grammar. After all, they have to pay attention to learn parameter values.

How is it possible to draw such strong conclusions about the ability of children with SLI to learn linguistic properties in a field that has traditionally characterized children with SLI as having a learning deficit with respect to language? The whole idea started with a clear idea of what was particular (parameters) and universal (principles) in language, and then the question was asked: How do children perform on aspects of language that uncontroversially are learned—parameters? Children with SLI learn parameters essentially perfectly; if there is a piece of language-particular information that normal children learn well, then so do children with SLI. As has happened so often, in every science, drawing fundamental distinctions (in this case between the definitely learned and the possibly/probably not learned) gave a clear answer to a fundamental question. It is now known that children with SLI do not have a learning deficit.

CLINICAL MARKERS FOR SLI: CROSSLINGUISTIC VARIATION

It is crucial to have clinical markers for SLI in order to determine which children have SLI, both for scientific and practical reasons. Rice and Wexler did extensive research arguing that rate of fineness is by far the most correct and sensitive clinical marker for SLI that has been proposed. There is virtually no overlap at a given relevant age between normal children and children with SLI on rate of overall tensing. See Fig. 1.1 from the data in Rice and Wexler (1996).

The sensitivity and specificity of this grammatical marker for SLI argues for its usefulness. It is extremely rare in studies of cognitive abilities to have such a powerful cognitive marker. Of course, these results argue even more for the EOI nature of SLI.

It is intriguing, however, that it follows from the underlying theory of the OI stage that the EOI stage will show extremely different surface properties in different languages. For example, suppose Italian children with SLI undergo the EOI stage in Italian. It has already been shown that Italian children in the OI age range do not produce root infinitives, and this follows from the interaction of the UCC with the parameter settings of Italian (the null subject parameter setting, in particular). It has been argued that children with SLI learn their parameters very well, and without a deficit, so it would be expected that Italian-speaking children with SLI will have correctly set the null subject parameter to *yes*. Suppose Italian-speaking children with SLI are subject to UCC at a much older age than normal children. Given their null subject parameter setting, however, the UCC predicts that

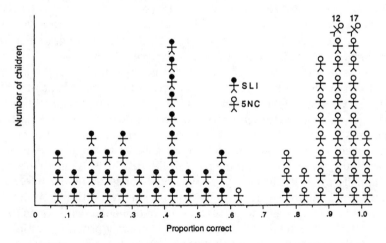

FIG. 1.1. The rate of overall tensing for normally developing and children with SLI.

these children will not produce a significant number of OIs. This is a startling prediction: English-speaking children with SLI produce huge numbers of OIs; tense appears to be a problem. But the prediction is that Italian-speaking children with SLI, because they have learned the null subject nature of Italian, will not produce such. It is a real test of theory.

What would be predicted to mark SLI in Italian? Should SLI exist at all in Italian? The answer is that any nonadult utterance caused by the UCC should mark SLI at a fairly late age in Italian (or any other language). Wexler (in press) argued that one such error is the omission of object clitics. An object clitic is a pronoun whose thematic role is related to object position (after the verb), but that appears in preverbal position, a clitic phrase (ClP). Some element (the clitic itself, or in current theories more often an invisible noun phrase, *pro*) starts out in object position and winds up in ClP. But because the clitic must be checked for case (ACC case or DATIVE case), the invisible noun phrase also has to pass through an intermediate position (known as AGR-Object on some accounts), which assigns ACC case. So on standard accounts, *pro* moves and checks twice, to AGR-Object, and then to ClP. These movements can be thought of as checking the D-feature of the empty element, checking it twice, with AGR-Object and with INFL. Wexler argued that UCC prevents this from happening, often resulting in the omission of ClP and thus of the clitic. Informally, the double movement is not allowed by the UCC. But, if both movements do not occur, then there is something wrong with ClP; it does not have a NP with the right object features in local relation to it (*pro*). So ClP (and thus the clitic) must be omitted to obtain a good structure. Thus, omission of Romance object clitics is predicted to be a consequence of UCC and omission of object clitics for an extended period of time is predicted to be a marker of SLI.

Here are the predictions about Italian SLI:

1. NO OIs for main verbs
2. Nevertheless, omission of auxiliaries (see Wexler, 1998, for the argument for normal children, which carries over to SLI).
3. Good agreement (because children with SLI learn well)
4. Major omission rates of object clitics

The fact that SLI seems to present so differently in different languages has made the whole problem seem intractable. But there are fundamental reasons why there should be differences in SLI behavior in different languages, based on a clear understanding of particular properties of grammar, variation among grammars, children's learning abilities, and children's maturational states. Taking all of these properties into account, with independent evidence for each one, gives a clear picture. All that remains is to decide whether it is true. So, how about Italian SLI?

Bottari, Cipriani, and Chilosi (1996) presented a study of OIs in Italian children with SLI with some normal controls. Of 27 children with SLI with expressive-receptive deficits (thus matching the standard definition of SLI, e.g., those used in the Rice and Wexler studies), 20 of the children produce no OIs at all![18] This is already major information, as children with SLI in English and Dutch produce many OIs. Of the 7 children who do produce OIs, quantitative estimates are only available for 3 of them, and the percentage of OIs (with age of child in parenthesis) is 7.5% (6;2–6;11), 8.8% (8;7), and 11.6% ((8;0). Although they are larger than the numbers for the 3 control children who were studied, they are extremely small by standards of the OI languages. Moreover, it is crucial to remember that 20 of the 27 produced no OIs at all. If we calculate 0% for the 20 participants with no OIs, and these numbers for the 3 participants who OIs whose rate is measured, we find a mean of 27.9/23 = 1.2% OI use per child! The authors wrote:

> If RIs [= Root Infinitives, another name for OI's], produced by Italian children with SLI were to be accounted for in terms of [a hypothesis that the Italian OI's are accounted for by the same mechanism as non-null-subject language OI's] their frequency would have to parallel the frequency of RIs produced by children with SLI speaking English, French or German. This prediction is completely falsified by the English and German data. (p. 81)

They went on to argue that the few OIs that do exist in Italian children with SLI are something else, not the product of the OI stage. At any rate, there is a huge disparity in rate of OIs between Italian, on the one hand, and English or Dutch, on the other. In Italian children with SLI, there are almost no OIs; they have to be sought out. In non-null subject languages, they are an obvious strong phenomenon.

The prediction of the UCC plus the hypothesis that children with SLI (like normal children) set their parameters correctly is strongly confirmed. Children with SLI behave strikingly different in Italian than in English, and this difference is expected.

Bottari, Cipriani, and Chilosi went on to show that Italian children with SLI essentially get verbal agreement close to perfect, as the hypotheses predicted.

An earlier part discussed why Wexler (in press) argued that UCC predicts that object clitics should be omitted during the OI (UCC) stage and that extensive clitic omission should be a marker of Italian SLI during this stage. Bottari, Cipriani, Chilosi, and Pfanner (1998) showed that there is extensive clitic omission by Italian children with SLI. The 11 children with SLI (M = 6;3, range: 4;2–10.7) omit clitics at a mean rate of 41.1%, whereas the 2

---

[18]Unfortunately, the authors do not tell the ages of these children, but the ages of the seven children who do produce some OIs are from 6;5 to 9;1.

much younger normal controls omit many fewer clitics (10.1% at age 32–34 months for Raffaello and 20.8% at ages 27–29 months for Martina). Basically (see Wexler, in press, for a review of the empirical evidence across a number of languages), the clitic omission stage is pretty much over in the third year for normal children, but it is still huge for children with SLI of mean age 6;3.

As expected, the phenomenon of extensive object clitic omission in SLI is also characteristic of French SLI (see Jakubowicz, Nash Rigaut, & Gerard, 1998).

As has been discussed, the UCC does predict that auxiliaries will be omitted in the OI stage, even though infinitival main verbs will not be produced. Thus, Italian SLI would be expected to show a large amount of auxiliary omission. This is confirmed for children with SLI in Bottari et al. (1998). The children (M = 6;3) omit auxiliaries at a 67% mean rate, strongly confirming the prediction. (Compare this with the 1.2% OI rate discussed earlier.) The two (much younger) normal younger in Bottari et al. (1998) also omitted auxiliaries, but fewer than the children with SLI, as expected. The predictions of the EOI/EUCC model are strongly confirmed. Italian children have their own pattern of deficit, which follows from the UCC restrictions, principles of grammar, and the parameter values for Italian that they have learned so well.

In general, different SLI behavior would be expected in different languages, and researchers must be on the lookout for the phenomena that might be predicted by the theory.[19] Thus, the clinical marker of SLI in Italian would be expected to look quite different from the one for English, or for Dutch. The clinical marker should follow from the theory and the nature of each language. It is no surprise to the theory that children with SLI present so differently (on the surface) in different languages. Underneath, they suffer from a common impairment, the extra restrictions on their computational systems caused by the UCC. On the surface, they look different.

This is no more surprising than that different molecules have different properties, although they all obey chemical law. The structure of a molecule will lead to different behavior, consistent with universal physical prin-

---

[19]For example, in Danish (and French) the UCC predicts other interesting patterns (e.g., the use of null subjects with finite verbs in these nonnull subject languages; Wexler, 2000), which are well-confirmed (Hamann & Plunkett, 1997). So this might play a role in the clinical marker for Danish SLI. In Korean, as discussed, Baek and Wexler (2000) argued that the word order error between *an/not* and the direct object was the result of the UCC. So although Korean does not even have an infinitive (and we would not necessarily expect OIs, because Korean might be a null subject language), we might expect to see *an* misplacement errors as a strong feature of Korean SLI. I don't know whether these predictions are true. If they are not, it would argue that the UCC analysis given of these phenomena is wrong; this shows how impairment data can affect analysis of normal language development.

ciple. It is fair to say that the structure of the theory discussed and its precise empirical verification make the science look more and more like chemistry, rather than like traditional psychology or the other social sciences. It is good to know that it is possible to understand with such predictive precision what appeared to be possibly intractable problems. And, best of all, the answers are not just some kind of statistical agglomeration coming out of a simulation that allows no insight. Rather, the empirical answers, combined with the theoretical analysis, allows us to hope to be able to understand—perhaps for the first time—the exact role of learning and the exact role of genetics and heredity in development, including SLI development.

GENETICS AND SLI

There is evidence that SLI has a strong heretibility component (Rice, Haney, & Wexler, 1998). We are currently engaged in a search for the genetic locus of SLI. If it is found, it might help with the extremely difficult question—on which no discernable progress has been made—about the neuroscience of SLI: What happens in the brains of children with SLI? Perhaps if researchers can learn what genes are involved with SLI, then they might be able to figure out what proteins these genes code for and then to understand what happens structurally. At the moment, this sounds almost like science fiction, but who knows when the right breakthrough will be made. If it does happen, the kind of detailed work, clarifying every aspect of what SLI and normal children are capable of, distinguishing development from learning, comparing languages, and so on, will be of the utmost importance. The biological basis of SLI cannot be uncovered until its computational basis is understood. The fact that SLI is a genetic event (or lack of one, the withering away of the UCC) is quite consistent with the observed genetic influence on the likelihood of having SLI. The world is consistent so far, but no doubt there are all sorts of scholars working away to make it (temporarily) inconsistent, and thus to push the field in new directions.

REFERENCES

Babyonyshev, M., Ganger, J., Pesetsky, D., & Wexler, K. (2001). The maturation of grammatical principles: Evidence from Russian Unaccusatives. *Linguistic Inquiry, 32*, 1.

Baek & Wexler (2000). The Role of the Unique Checking Constraint in the Syntax and Acquisition of Korean Negation. 2000. *Natural Language and Linguistic Theory.*

Bertolo, S., Broihier, K., Gibson, E., & Wexler, K. (1997). *Cue-based learners in parametric language systems: Application of general results to a recently proposed learning algorithm based on unambiguous "superparsing."* Unpublished manuscript, Department of Brain and Cognitive Sciences, MIT.

Bishop, D.V.M. (1997). *Uncommon understanding: Development and disorders of language in comprehension in children.* East Sussex, England: Psychology Press.

Borer, H., & Wexler, K. (1987). The maturation of syntax. In T. Roeper & E. Williams (Eds.), *Parameter setting* (pp. 123–172). Dordrecht: Reidel.

Borer, H., & Wexler, K. (1992). Bi-unique relations and the maturation of grammatical principles. *NLLT, 10,* 147–189.

Bottari, P., Cipriani, P., & Chilosi, A. M. (1996). Root Infinitives in Italian SLI children. In A. Stringfellow, D. Cahana-Amitay, E. Hughes, & A. Zukowski (Eds.), *BUCLD 20* (pp. 75–86). Somerville, MA: Cascadilla Press.

Bottari, P., Cipriani, P., Chilosi, A. M., & Pfanner, L. (1998). The determiner system in a group of Italian children with SLI. *Language Acquisition, 7*(2–4), 285–315.

Bromberg, H., & Wexler, K. (1995). Null subjects in child Wh-questions. In C. Shutze, J. Ganger, & K. Broihier (Eds.), *Papers on language processing and acquisition* (MIT Working Papers in Linguistics, 26). Cambridge, MA: MIT Press.

Brown, R. (1973). *A first language.* Cambridge, MA: Harvard University Press.

Chomsky, N. (1995). *The minimalist program.* Cambridge, MA: MIT Press.

Clahsen, H. (1986). Verb inflections in German child language: Acquisition of agreement markings and the functions they encode. *Linguistics, 26,* 79–121.

Clark, R., & Roberts, I. (1993). A computational model of language learnability and language change. *Linguistic Inquiry, 24,* 299–345.

Dresher, B. E. (1999). Charting the learning path: Cues to parameter setting. *Linguistic Inquiry, 30,* 127–167.

Fodor, J. D. (1998). Unambiguous triggers. *Linguistic Inquiry, 29,* 1–36.

Fox, D, & Grodzinsky, Y. (1998). Children's passive: A view from the by-phrase. *Linguistic Inquiry, 29,* 311–332.

Ganger, J. (1998). *Genes and environment in language acquisition: A study of vocabulary and syntactic development in twins.* Unpublished doctoral dissertation, MIT.

Ganger, J., Wexler, K., & Soderstrom, M. (1997). The genetic basis for the development of tense: A preliminary report on a twin study. In E. Hughes, M. Hughes, & A. Greenhill (Eds.), *BUCLID 21* (pp. 224–234). Somerville, MA: Cascadilla Press.

Gibson, E., & Wexler, K. (1994). Triggers. *Linguistic Inquiry, 25*(3), 407–454.

Guasti, M. (1994). Verb syntax in Italian child grammar: Finite and nonfinite verbs. *Language Acquisition, 3,* 1–40.

Hamann, C., & Plunkett, K. (1997). Subject omission in child Danish. In E. Hughes, M. Hughes, & A. Greenhill (Eds.), *BUCLID 21* (pp. 220–231). Somerville, MA: Cascadilla Press.

Hamburger, H., & Wexler, K. (1973). Identifiability of a class of transformational grammars. In K. H. H. Hintikka, E. Moravcsik, & P. Suppers (Eds.), *Approaches to natural language* (pp. XX). Dordrecht: Reidel.

Harris, T., & Wexler, K. (1996). The optional-infinitive stage in child English: Evidence from negation. In H. Clahsen (Ed.), *Generative perspective on language acquisition* (pp. XX). Philadelphia: John Benjamins.

Haznedar, B., & Schwartz, B. (1997). Are there optional infinitives in child L2 acquisition? In E. Hughes, M. Hughes, & A. Greenhill (Eds.), *BUCLID 21* (pp. 257–268). Sommerville, MA: Cascadilla Press.

Huttenlocher, J., Haight, W., Bryk, A., Seltzer, M., & Lyons, T. (1991). Early vocabulary growth: Relation to language input and gender. *Developmental Psychology, 27,* 236–248.

Ionin, T., & Wexler, K. (in press). L1-Russian children learning English: Tense and overgeneration of "Be." In the *Proceedings of the Second Language Research Forum,* Madison, WI.

Jakubowicz, C., Nash, L., Rigaut, C., & Gerard, C. L. (1998). Determiners and clitic pronouns in French-speaking children with SLI. *Language Acquisition, 7*(2–4), 113–160.

Lee, & Wexler (in press). Nominative case omission and unaccusatives in Korean acquisition. (have e-mailed HyoJinn)

Lenneberg, E. (1967). *Biological foundations of language*. New York: Wiley.

Leonard, L. B. (1989). Language learnability and specific language impairment in children. *Applied Psycholinguistics, 10*, 179–202.

Loeb, D. F., & Leonard, L. B. (1991). Subject case marking and verb morphology in normally developing and specifically language-impared children. *Journal of Speech and Hearing Research, 34*, 340–346.

MacWhinney, B., & Snow, C. (1985). The child language data exchange system. *Journal of Child Language, 12*, 271–296.

Manzini and Wexler (87). Parameters, Binding theory and Learnability. *Linguistic Inquiry, 18*(3), pp. 413–444. Mahwah, NJ: Erlbaum.

Maratsos, M., Fox, D., Becker, J. A., & Chalkley, M. A. (1983). Semantic restrictions on children's early passive. *Cognition, 19*, 167–191.

Miyamoto, E. T., Wexler, K., Aikawa, T., & Miagawa, S. (1999). Case dropping and unaccusatives in Japanese acquisition. In A. Greenhill, H. Littlefield, & C. Tano (Eds.), *BUCLD 23*, (pp. 443–452). Sommerville, MA: Cascadilla Press.

Newport, E., Gleitman, H., & Gleitman, L. (1979). Mother, I'd rather do it myself. Some effects and non-effects of maternal speech style. In C. E. Snow & C. A. Ferguson (Eds.), *Talking to children* (pp. 109–149). New York: Cambridge University Press.

Prevost, P. (1997). *Truncation in second language acquistion*. Unpublished doctoral dissertation, McGill University.

Poeppel, D., & Wexler, K. (1993). The full competence hypothesis of clause structure in early German. *Language, 69*(1), 1–33.

Rice, M., Haney, K. R., & Wexler, K. (1998) Family histories of children with SLI who show extended optional infinitives. *Journal of Speech, Language and Hearing Research, 41*, 419–432.

Rice, M., & Wexler, K. (1996). Toward tense as a clinical marker of specific language impairment in English-speaking children. *Journal of Speech and Hearing Research, 39*, 1239–1257.

Rice, M., Wexler, K., & Cleave, P. (1995). Specific language impairment as a period of extended optional infinitive. *Journal of Speech and Hearing Research, 38*, 850–863.

Rice, M., Wexler, K., & Hershberger, S. (1998). Tense over time: The longitudinal course of tense acquisition in children with specific language impairment. *Journal of Speech, Language and Hearing Research, 41*, 1412–1431.

Saffran, R., Aslin, R. N., & Newport, E. L. (1996). Statistical learning by 8-month-old infants. *Science, 274*, 1926–1928.

Sano, T., & Hyams, N. (1994). Agreement, finiteness and the development of null arguments. In M. Gonzalez (Eds.), *Proceedings of NELS 24* (pp. 543–558). Amherst, MA: GLSA.

Schütze, C. T., & Wexler, K. (1996). Subject case licensing and English root infinitives. In A. Stringfellow, D. Cahana-Amitay, E. Hughes, & A. Zukowski (Eds.), *BUCLD 20* (pp. 670–681). Somerville, MA: Cascadilla Press.

Schütze, C. T., & Wexler, K. (2000). An elicitation study of young English children's knowledge of tense: Semantic and syntactic properties of optional infinitives. In S. C. Howell, S. Fish, & T. Keith-Lucas (Eds.), *BUCLD 24* (Vol. 2, pp. 669–683). Somerville, MA: Cascadilla Press.

Soderstrom Wexler & Jusczyk 19 month-olds Sensitivity to Negation/Tense Dependencies. Poster presented at the annual meeting of the Soc. For Cognitive Science. U Penn Aug. 2000.

Tomasello, M. (2000). Do young children have adult syntactic competence? *Cognition, 74*, 209–253.

Tomblin, J. B. (1996). Genetic and environmental contributions to the risk for specific language impairment. In M. Rice (Ed.), *Toward a genetics of language* (pp. 191–210). Hillsdale, NJ: Lawrence Erlbaum Associates.

Wexler, K. (1982). A principle theory for language acquisition. In E. Wanner & L. Gleitman (Eds.) *Language acquisition: The state of the art* (pp. 288–315). Cambridge, England: Cambridge University Press.

Wexler, K. (1990, August). *Optional infinitives, head movement and the economy of derivations in child grammar.* Paper presented at the annual meeting of the Society of Cognitive Science, MIT, Cambridge, MA.

Wexler, K. (1992). *Optional infinitives, head movement and the economy of derivation in child grammar* (Occasional paper No. 45). Center for Cognitive Science, MIT, Cambridge, MA.

Wexler, K. (1994). Optional infinitives, head movement and the economy of derivations. In D. Lightfoot & N. Hornstein (Eds.), *Verb movement* (pp. 305–350). Cambridge, England: Cambridge University Press.

Wexler, K. (1998). Very early parameter setting and the unique checking constraint: A new explanation of the optional infinitive stage. *Lingua, 106,* 23–79.

Wexler, K. (2000). Three problems in the theory of the optional infinitive stage: Stage/individual predicates, eventive verbs and finite null-subjects. In R. Billery & B. D. Lillehaugen. *WCCFL 19 Proceedings* (pp. 560–573). Somerville, MA: Cascadilla Press.

Wexler, K., & Culicover, P. (1980). *Formal principles of language acquisition.* Cambridge, MA: MIT Press.

Wexler, K., & Hamburger, H. (1973). On the insufficiency of surface data for the learning of transformational languages. In K.H.H. Hintikka, E. Moravcsik, & P. Suppes (Eds.), *Approaches to natural language* (pp. 16–179). Dordrecht: Reidel.

Wijnen, F. (1998). The temporal interpretation of Dutch children's root infinitivals: The effect of eventivity. *First Language, 18,* 379–402.

2

A Unified Model of Specific and General Language Delay: Grammatical Tense as a Clinical Marker of Unexpected Variation

Mabel L. Rice
University of Kansas

The central topic of this volume is language competence across populations. The population of interest here is children with specific language impairment (SLI), a condition conventionally defined as one in which children seem to have the necessary developmental precursors to support language acquisition but nevertheless show language delays. This condition is sometimes described as "unexpected and unexplained variation" in language acquisition. This chapter focuses on the nature of variation within the language system, the ways in which affected children do and do not vary from unaffected children, the ways in which children with SLI are similar to and different from children with Williams syndrome (WMS), and the interpretation of a possible grammatical marker as indicative of either a general language delay or a selective delay in addition to the general delay. At the most general levels, the chapter takes up the issues of variation within elements of language, developmental variation as children move toward the adult linguistic system, variation in onset mechanisms versus asynchronous elements within the linguistic system, and variation across different clinical populations of children with language impairments.

The adult grammar, comprised of the underlying architecture and principles of clausal structure, is relatively intolerant of variations across individuals. It is the common knowledge of the structural principles of clauses that allows language users to convey messages of intended meanings from one person to another. Certain properties are obligatory, and if the clause does not follow the obligatory properties, then the structure will be ungrammatical.

Decades of studies have documented that children's utterances do not begin as fully formed, adultlike sentences. This is a form of developmental variation in which children's language does not seem to be fully adultlike for some time. The reference for "unexpected" variation for affected children, then, must be placed in the developmental trajectory of variation between children's and adult's grammars, and the expected convergence of child grammar with the adult grammar.

This chapter examines variations in the language development of English-speaking children with SLI and control groups of unaffected children, and comparisons to children with WMS, in the period from age 3 to 8. The focus is on obligatory properties of grammatical tense marking,[1] knowledge that is emerging during this period for unaffected children, and is a fundamental element of the adult knowledge of clausal structures. In addition, grammatical acquisition is compared to children's lexical acquisition, two linguistic domains that show different patterns of variation over time. The comparison of SLI and WMS groups of children helps clarify possible lines of dissociation across elements of grammar.

The chapter draws heavily on empirical evidence gathered as part of a longitudinal program of investigation carried out in collaboration with Ken Wexler, with funding from the National Institute of Deafness and Communicative Disorders. The intent is to place the empirical evidence associated with a grammatical tense marker of language impairment in the broader context of variations across language elements, and across affected and un-

---

[1]The theoretical context for grammatical tense marking is the optional infinitive (OI) model of Wexler (1994; see chap. 1 in this volume), which is framed in the minimalist model of Chomsky (1996). Technically, the focus of the OI model is on the features of TNS and AGR, and the feature-checking properties of morphosyntax. More recently, the OI model has been revised to the agreement tense omission model (ATOM) in analyses of the relation of pronoun case and TNS–AGR (cf. Wexler, Schutze, & M. Rice, 1998). For the purpose of this discussion, it is sufficient to note the following assumptions of the theoretical framework: (a) TNS and AGR are assumed to be functional heads that serve as landing sites for movement operations in clause structure; (b) TNS has interpretable elements (past vs. present meanings) and uninterpretable elements (thought to require an overt subject in nonnull subject languages, and to license case on its specifier, which is typically the subject); (c) TNS is independent of the selection of the allomorph to mark, for example, past tense; (d) TNS includes forms such as auxiliary Do, which is a semantically empty morpheme inserted in English to carry out the TNS-marking functions; (e) the morphosyntactic properties of TNS are distinct from the semantic elements of a clause (i.e., logical form), which includes elements such as nouns, verbs, adjectives, and adverbs. In this context, grammatical tense marking can be generally glossed as uninterpretable elements of the TNS/AGR feature cluster that are obligatory elements of morphosyntax that occupy a site in the architecture of the phrase structure, control movement rules, are distinct from the phonological elements of the morphemes, and are distinct from meaning elements found in nouns, verbs, adjectives, and adverbs.

affected children, within a developmental perspective. This is not a full research review of the available literature, or an attempt to evaluate the outcomes vis-à-vis alternative theoretical accounts of language impairment. It is an initial sketch of an overarching model of language delays in the context of individual and group differences, and in the context of natural partition lines within the linguistic system, drawing on an extensive empirical data base collected over time from the same children. Such an attempt has value for investigators interested in how the condition of SLI may be related to other conditions of language impairment, which is a topic largely overlooked in the available studies of children with language impairment. According to the premise of this chapter, comparisons of language impairments across clinical populations can be revealing of the ways in which the underlying linguistic system can be selectively robust or weak. The attempt is also relevant for investigators interested in the way in which elements of the linguistic system come "online" in children, whether in the relatively rapid acquisition of a well-synchronized system in typically developing children or in the more protracted and less synchronized system of children with language impairments.

The sequence of topics is as follows: The chapter begins with an examination of the notions of variation that are evident in the previous literature, and two kinds of variation across children that are identifiable and relevant here (i.e., *normative* variation in the form of a bell-shaped distribution of individual differences, and variation that shows a *bimodal* distribution of individual differences, in which children can be clearly distinguished as low or high in performance levels). An integrative model of language delay is described via a train analogy, which differentiates a *general delay* of language acquisition, versus a *selective delay*, where an element of the grammar lags behind the other elements of language acquisition. This model is referred to as a *delay-within-delay model* to capture the fact that there are two possible senses of delay, one general and a second more specific. This is followed by a summary of evidence of variation in the timing mechanisms for the acquisition of grammatical tense marking in young affected English-speaking children as compared to control groups. Concurrent with the manifestations of individual variation in grammatical tense marking, other morphology shows invariance in performance levels, suggesting that protracted acquisition is not a general property of morphology per se. Evidence from various lexical indices is then reported, which shows that children's lexical acquisition displays individual and group variations during this same time period that are unlike those of grammatical tense marking. Growth trajectories of morphosyntactic and morphophonological components of tense marking differ, supporting the assumption that these two elements of the grammar have different properties. This conclusion is supported further by a series of analyses to examine predictors of growth, which show similarity for tense marking indices, but differences from the morphophonological index. Cross-clinical comparisons between children with SLI and children with WMS provide another way to examine the relation of grammatical tense marking, general language delay, and lexical acquisition, revealing further the ways in which these factors vary and covary across children. Two methodological notes highlight measurement issues, showing, on the one hand, the relative stability of mean length of utterance (MLU) as a developmental measure during the age range of 3–8 years, and on the other hand, the need to focus on percentage correct in obligatory contexts as a morphological index that can reveal variations in knowledge of the obligatory properties of tense marking.

The final section lays out some implications for models of language acquisition, specific and nonspecific delay, and the distinction between a general delay outcome of language acquisition versus a delay-within-delay outcome. The delay-within-delay model places the grammatical tense marker in the more general context of two possible relations: as a marker of a general delay or as a marker of a delay-within-delay (and not necessarily the only possible such marker). The grammatical tense marker as a marker of a delay-within-delay outcomes, it is concluded, reflects relatively specific elements of morphosyntax that can be dissociated from lexical acquisition in children's language acquisition, although the technical details across languages remain to be worked out.

SOME BACKGROUND REMARKS

The Assumption of Uniform Robustness

Much of the normative literature on children's acquisition has focused on the ways in which children are invariant, in the observation that all normal children acquire language effortlessly, and seem to follow the same timing mechanisms and the same general sequence of acquisition. An important advantage of this assumption is that it emphasizes the relatively invariant properties of language acquisition across a wide range of environmental circumstances, and thereby brings some helpful constraints to the empirical generalizations that must be captured by a given theory.

This assumption is most cogently expressed by Pinker (1984, p. 29): "In general, language acquisition is a stubbornly robust process; from what we can tell there is virtually no way to prevent it from happening short of raising a child in a barrel." Although there were advantages to this perspective, it did not meet the test of empirical validity. There were, in fact, children who did not acquire language effortlessly, even though they were reared according to conventional childrearing practices.

The Updated Assumption of Variable Robustness

By the early 1990s, there was widespread recognition that otherwise apparently normal children (reared in normal circumstances) can have language impairments. The existence of the condition of SLI was, of course, known before then to students of language impairments and in the field of speech pathology. The advent of modern genetics helped shift attention from the ways in which individuals are uniformly robust to the ways in which individuals are variably robust in language acquisition, and broadened the scientific interest in affected children beyond the scope of practitioners who provided clinical services. Investigations of possible sources of genetic etiology are intrinsically focused on individual differences (i.e., ways in which affected individuals can be identified as different from unaffected individuals). As is apparent from the evidence summarized later, one of the most interesting aspects of the emerging evidence of variable robustness is that the loci of individual differences across children can be seen in relatively invariant properties of morphosyntax, the very elements of clausal structure that are essential to the formulation of grammatical sentences. As it turns out, then, the updated assumption of variable robustness applies to elements of language as well as individual differences.

KINDS OF VARIATION ACROSS CHILDREN

Normative Variation

Understanding of children's development is greatly influenced by the concept of *normative variation*. This is typically referenced to age expectations. Imagine, for example, a group of 5-year-old children. If they are administered a conventional test of language acquisition, such as the lexical comprehension test, the Peabody Picture Vocabulary Test–Revised (Dunn & Dunn, 1981), the collection of obtained scores will be distributed as the well-known bell-shaped curve, as is shown in Fig. 2.1. This curve has some remarkably robust psychometric properties that allow for the prediction of the distribution of individual scores as a function of the group mean and variances from the mean. The conventional definition of language impairments has been cast in terms of the distance of an individual's score from the expected group mean, given the observed variance within the group. This is usually in the neighborhood of one to two standard deviations below the mean, roughly in the bottom 5th–15th percentile, indicated by a line at the lower tail of the distribution in Fig. 2.1. Conventionally, the condition of SLI involves the further exclusionary criteria of documented performance within or above normal range on assessments of nonverbal intelli-

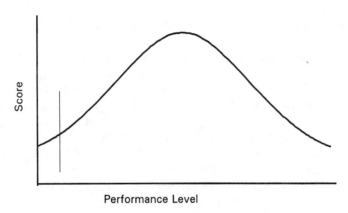

FIG. 2.1. Bell-shaped curve.

gence, with the caveat that the precise criteria for exclusionary criteria are subject to current discussions and debate (Tager-Flusberg & Cooper, 1999).

A Grammatical Marker

The bell-shaped curve, however, is not applicable to all elements of language acquisition. Compare, for example, the same 5-year-old children in their knowledge of morphosyntax, such as their use of copular and auxiliary forms of BE. The expected distribution of percentage correct in obligatory contexts would show a different pattern, one of a markedly skewed distribution with most of the children at adultlike levels of performance and only a few children showing lower levels of accuracy, as shown in Fig. 2.2.

Thus, there are two different ways in which children with SLI could show unexpected variation when compared to other children of the same age. One variation would be evident as a lower relative level of performance on a measure of language acquisition that shows variation across children of a given age, where variation is continuously distributed in the form of a bell-shaped curve. The second possible variation would be a low level of performance on a property of the grammar where variation across individuals is not expected.

The notion of a clinical marker has been useful in the medical literature, when referring to a symptom that is diagnostic of a particular medical condition. The idea of a marker for language impairment has appeared in the recent literature in investigations of the etiology of language impairments, and the need to be able to identify affected individuals for the purpose of studying possible inherited contributions to the condition. Note that a distribution such as that in Fig. 2.2, where low performance is clearly differenti-

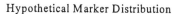

Hypothetical Marker Distribution

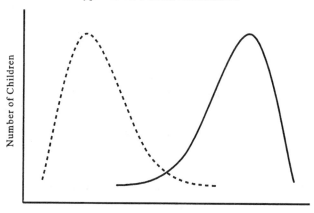

Performance Level

FIG. 2.2. Bimodal curve.

ated from high performance, would be felicitous for the identification of a clinical marker of language impairment, in effect a grammatical marker of language impairment.[2]

Variation in Onset Timing

A long-standing differentiation in the literature on language impairments is the distinction between a *language delay* and a *language deviance* (Lee, 1966; Leonard, 1972; Menyuk, 1964; Morehead & Ingram, 1973). A language delay means that children could be delayed in the onset of their language system, which sometimes (but not always) takes on the related meaning that they remain similar to younger children for a protracted period of time, and may or may not ever reach mastery levels. Such children are sometimes referred to as "late talkers," when the language delay is the only apparent developmental delay. The likelihood that they would "outgrow" such a delay, and when such a jump would be expected, remains a matter of ongoing investigation and some controversy in the literature (cf. Thal & Katich, 1996).

In contrast, children with language impairments could show a delayed onset, and a linguistic system that is "deviant" or unlike that of younger children. This possibility (originally proposed by Menyuk, 1964) was, follow-

---

[2]Note the subtle difference in meaning between a grammatical marker, which refers to a grammatical symptom of language impairment, and marking a grammatical feature, as in tense marking, which refers to the computational processes involved in morphosyntax.

ing the available linguistic models, first thought of in rather general terms of rather pervasive differences in possible grammars for affected children.[3]

Investigations of language impaired children often employ a three-group design in order to evaluate delay versus deviance interpretations, involving two crucial group comparisons: one in which the affected group of children is compared to a control group based on chronological age, where differences between affected and control children would reveal areas of language delay; and a second in which the affected group of children is compared to a control group based on linguistic equivalencies (often on the basis of mean length of utterance), where differences between affected and control children would reveal areas of linguistic differences not accounted for by a younger level of mean length of utterance, for example.

In light of the evidence summarized later, an elaborated version of the delay notion is proposed, in a model that recognizes possible late activation mechanisms of two sorts: one more global and another more localized within certain elements of the grammar, referred to as a delay-within-delay model. This model recognizes different rates of development within the elements of the linguistic system.

A train metaphor illustrates the general notions, shown in Fig. 2.3. The expected emergence of language early in a child's development can be thought of as a train, where the "language train" early on shows clear organizational composition of lexical, syntactic, morphological, and computational elements, perhaps roughly analogous to the alignment of cars, wheels, connections between cars, engine, drive shafts, and so on, of the train example. These elements are constrained to follow a developmental trajectory, perhaps roughly analogous to the tracks of the train that constrain the route of forward motion.

For most children, the train begins to move (i.e., departs the station) at an expected time, roughly when the child is between age 12 and 24 months, and then moves forward in an expected rate and trajectory of acquisition, as indicated in Panel A of Fig. 2.3. In contrast, for other children, the start-up of language acquisition may be delayed, as in Panel B. That is to say that the train may not leave the station at the expected time, although the train is configured in the same way as the train in Panel A. Such a delayed start could fol-

---

[3]Recently Leonard (1998) proposed a five-way set of distinctions: (a) *delay*, consisting of a late start; (b) *plateau*, showing leveling off before mastery levels are achieved; (c) *profile difference*, in which the difference in performance between two morphemes, such as *-s* for plurals and third person singular present tense, may be greater for children with impairments than for unaffected children; (d) *abnormal frequency of error*, in which a greater number of errors of a given type, such as that of pronoun case, are seen for affected children; and (e) *qualitative difference*, such as phonological processes evident in affected children unlike those of unaffected children (a category that Leonard noted is highly unlikely). The delay-within-delay model presented here places the delay distinctions within a framework of linguistic domains, and a delay-within-delay that plays out differently across different linguistic elements and different measurements.

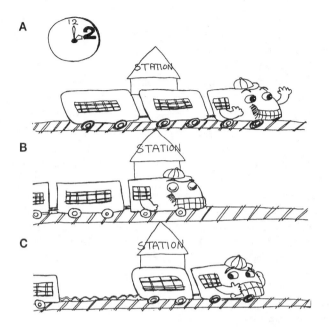

FIG. 2.3. Train.

low the same trajectory and speed (rate of acquisition) as that of typically developing children, and could possibly remain behind the train of Panel A by a steady distance throughout the language acquisition period, or, for unknown reasons, may eventually speed up to catch Train A at a later time, thereby reducing the gap generated by a different start-up time. This scenario corresponds to the conventional sense of a language delay. A third possibility is that a late-starting language system also has a localized difference in linguistic elements, as shown in the train of Panel C, where perhaps coupling or computational relations between elements are not the same as the expected alignments. Such a language system could start late, and perhaps some elements might eventually catch up to those of unaffected children, or perhaps some elements remain delayed relative to that of the rest of the language system. Whether or not they are ever fully integrated into the language system would be an important matter to determine.

The point of the train metaphor is to distinguish between individual differences between children in general onset timing for language acquisition and individual differences attributable to a selective delay within the linguistic system, a delay-within-delay, even though there are inherent constraints and configurational properties of the language system that are intact for both kinds of individual difference. Within this view, a grammatical marker could be part of a general delay (Panel B), or part of a selective delay in addition to the general delay (Panel C). Refer to Panel C as a delay-within-delay model, for a second delay in excess of the initial delay in onset of the general language system. Another possibility is that, in principle, a grammatical marker could be the only area of delayed onset (i.e., that most of the components of the language system emerge at the expected time and proceed in the expected acquisition trajectory but there is a selective and single area of delay in certain areas of the grammatical system). Such youngsters under current clinical practices would not necessarily be regarded as having a language impairment.

Under the delay-within-delay model, individual differences in language acquisition would entail possible differences in timing of acquisition mechanisms, and possible differences in the relative robustness of elements of the linguistic system. Conversely, to the extent that in some children's growth elements of the linguistic system are selectively delayed relative to other elements, evidence of individual differences would be relevant to models of the structure and principles of language.

GRAMMATICAL TENSE MARKING IN CHILDREN AGES 3 TO 8 YEARS

In this section, generalizations will be laid out drawn from the available evidence. The generalizations are indicated in italicized font.

Children with SLI start using grammatical tense markers at a later age, and show slower acquisition, although the change in acquisition over time follows an upward path toward the adult grammar that is not different from normal controls. This conclusion is based on data reported in Fig. 2.4 (from M. L. Rice, Wexler, & Hershberger, 1998). This figure represents the outcomes of a longitudinal study comprised of three groups of children: A group identified as SLI who were age 5 years, on average, at the outset, and who met criteria as having receptive as well as expressive language delays, and no apparent other developmental impairments. They also passed a phonological screening. There were two control groups, one of equivalent chronological age (labeled as "5N," for "5-year-old normal group"), and the second, younger group of equivalent language development (indexed by their mean length of utterances). The language control group was, on average, 2 years younger than the SLI group of children at the outset (hence labeled "3N"). The children were followed for 7 times of measurement, at 6-month intervals, encompassing the full age range of 3 to 8 years. Figure 2.4 plots the children's performance on a "composite tense" measure, which is an arithmetic mean of their percentage use in obligatory contexts of a target set of morphemes thought to require grammatical tense marking (i.e., third person singular -*s*, regular past tense -*ed*, Be copula and auxiliary in statements and

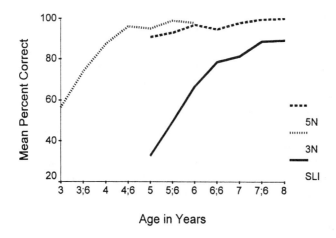

FIG. 2.4. Composite tense. Data from "Tense Over Time: The Longitudinal Course of Tense Acquisition in Children with Specific Language Impairment," by M. L. Rice, K. Wexler, and S. Hershberger, 1998, *Journal of Speech, Language, and Hearing Research, 41*, pp. 1412–1431. © American Speech-Language Hearing Association. Reprinted by permission.

questions, and Do auxiliary in questions). The data are from spontaneous utterances and elicitation probes. Detailed analyses found no difference in methods of measurement (spontaneous vs. probes) and the same general outcomes held for each individual measure, so the summary index is representative of the individual data components.

It is clear from the figure that at the first time of measurement the affected children at age 5 years, as indexed by their group mean, were performing below the language control group who were 2 years younger at the outset. Furthermore, this group difference held throughout the entire longitudinal period of study (see M. L. Rice et al., 1998, for detailed analyses). Thus, even though the younger children were still acquiring this area of grammar in the period from 3;0 to 4;6, their performance exceeded that of the older affected group. In terms of the train metaphor, the affected group follows the train in Panel C, the delay-within-delay model (i.e., in this part of the grammar, the affected group of children is slow getting started, and seems to show a delay beyond what would be expected for their general language level). At the same time, children of the same age level are functioning at adultlike levels. Growth curve analyses found that for both the SLI and 3N groups, the path of upward improvement was described by linear and quadratic components in the equation, and further examined the following possible predictors of the children's growth on the composite tense variable: mother's education, nonverbal intelligence, receptive vocabulary, and mean length of utterance. Growth in this area is not predicted by mother's education, nonverbal intelligence, or receptive vocabulary, and is weakly predicted by the children's mean length of utterance at the outset, suggesting that the grammatical marker is relatively independent of the sorts of differences in a child's home environment associated with differences in mothers' education levels, and of the child's levels of nonverbal intelligence (within the broad range of "normal" or above) and the child's understanding of vocabulary. That is to say that the part of the "train" devoted to tense marking is to some interesting extent separable from other parts (i.e., receptive vocabulary, nonverbal intelligence, and even mean length of utterance). Detailed analyses of the children's utterances found that overt errors of sentence formulation, or morphological forms, were rare, and almost all the errors consisted of omissions of the target forms, thereby suggesting that even the affected children knew about basic rules of sentence formulation, even as they were likely to omit obligatory elements of the grammar. This observation, in combination with the fact that the growth curve is the same for the affected children as the younger control children (although offset at lower levels of performance, and a probable later time of emergence), suggests that the two groups' language acquisition does not differ in fundamental ways (i.e., that the "train" is probably configured in a similar way, and follows the same tracks forward).

One possibility is that the production data shown in Fig. 2.4 indicate a problem that the affected children might have in formulating the production of utterances, perhaps in a memory buffer that is crucial for morphemes such as those involved in grammatical tense, instead of an underlying grammatical weakness (cf. Bishop, 1994). In order to evaluate this possibility, a grammaticality judgment task was developed that paralleled the production tasks. In this task, children were asked to judge sentences that included tense markers, such as *He drinks milk* and *He is hiding* and sentences in which tense markers were omitted, such as *He eat toast* and *He running away*. These contrasts were labeled as an optional infinitive (OI) grammar, following Wexler's terminology for the phenomenon of grammatical tense markers being absent in children's utterances (cf. Wexler, chap. 1 in this volume), under the interpretation that a child who judged sentences with omitted tense markers as acceptable was operating according to the representations of an OI grammar. The responses were summarized as A' (referred to as "A prime"), an index that controls for children's greater likelihood of saying "yes" than "no." This index can be interpreted as mathematically similar to the percentage correct in a two-alternative forced choice task (i.e., as if a child was asked "which is grammatically acceptable?" and given both choices simultaneously). Figure 2.5 reports the A' means for the groups' performance on the grammaticality judgment task, which was first administered when the affected children were age 6 years (and the younger controls were age 4 years; cf. M. L. Rice, Wexler, &

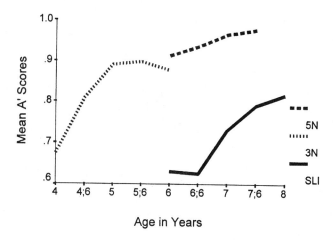

FIG. 2.5. A′ adult versus OI grammar.

Redmond, 1999). The general pattern of outcomes is the same for the judgment data, which did not require children to produce forms, as for the production data. This is to say that the affected children performed below that
of the younger language control group (as well as below that of the age control group) at each of the five times of measurement; growth change over
time was very similar for the affected and younger language control group
(growth curve analyses yielded linear and quadratic components of the
equation for both groups); and the same outcomes as for the production
data were found in the analyses of predictor relations (i.e., neither mother's
education, the children's receptive vocabulary nor the children's nonverbal
intelligence levels predicted growth on the judgment tasks), but there was a
small effect for MLU. The findings for judgment, therefore, also are consistent with the delay-within-delay train of Panel C, and support the interpretation that the source of the grammatical marker is to be found in underlying
grammatical representations.

*Young children show individual variation in grammatical tense marking that
disappears by age 5, as they arrive at the levels of the adult grammar.* The previous section considered variation evident in groups of children of different
ages, and in a comparison of children with SLI with age or language equivalent groups of children. The reported group means indicate the central tendency (i.e., the average score calculated across the members of the group).
Here the variation in performance of children within the groups is examined. This is reported in Fig. 2.6 for the composite tense scores for the SLI
group and the younger language-equivalent control group (note that for the
unaffected age control group the children show little variation; i.e., all are at
high levels, across the ages sampled, so that group is not included in the
figure). The box plot depicts the full range of scores of the children in the

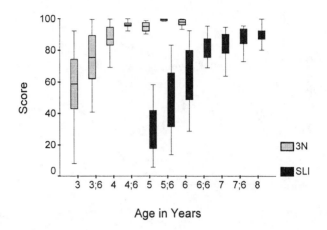

FIG. 2.6. Within-group variation in composite tense over time.

group, shown by the end of the "whiskers" at each end of the colored boxes; the scores that fall in the 25th to 75th percentile of the group, shown by the filled in boxes; and the median values for the group, shown by the lines in the middle of the boxes. The age-related trends are obvious. The same group of children (i.e., the 3N group) shows more variation in performance levels across the children when they are young, and as they age the variation across children disappears as they uniformly adopt the obligatory properties of the adult grammar. This same generalization holds for the children with SLI as well, although the variability is greater within this group throughout. In other words, among the children who at the outset met the criteria for diagnosis as "receptive/expressive SLI," there was a wider range of performance levels. This seems to be attributable to two slightly different outcomes: One is differential rates of growth, such that some children follow steeper slopes to high levels of performance than do other children in the group, and, second, some children show a less consistent upward trajectory of change as they waffle around a midlevel plateau of optional use (between ages 5 and 6 years) before moving upward to the final level of performance. At the same time, even though there are individual differences, the overall trajectory is clearly upward for all the affected children. Figure 2.7 shows that a very similar pattern of individual differences within groups is apparent for performance on the OI grammaticality judgment tasks.

At age 5 years, variation in levels of grammatical tense marking within a group of SLI children is likely to be in a range below the variation expected in unaffected children. Given the fact that, during the early childhood period, children who are typically developing show variation in their progress toward the obligatory properties of tense marking, even at the same age levels, it is very important not to confuse the ordinary variation across chil-

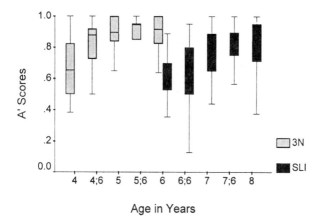

FIG. 2.7. Within-group variation in OI A′ over time.

dren with the variation that may be indicative of a language impairment (i.e., the likelihood of a protracted period of language acquisition of either a general delay in language acquisition or a delay-within-delay outcome). It is very important to show that the performance levels of affected children are in fact likely to be below those of their age group (i.e., to show that, at the same age level, the affected children cluster at the bottom end of performance, whereas the unaffected children cluster at the top end of performance, as depicted in Fig. 2.2).

The distribution of performance levels of two groups of 5-year-old children, one group of 37 children identified as expressive/receptive SLI and a control group of the same age (cf. M. L. Rice & Wexler, 1996), is depicted in Fig. 2.8, which reports their performance on a composite tense marking score (collapsed across regular third person singular -s, past tense, Be and Do). It is obvious that the affected children, with the exception of one child, cluster at the bottom end of the performance levels, and the control children, with the exception of one child, cluster at the top end. One way to describe the outcomes is to note that 97% of the affected children score below 80% (sometimes referred to as the *sensitivity index* of the level of detection of the true cases of affectedness) and 98% of the control children score above that level (the *specificity index* of the level of identification of the true cases of nonaffectedness).

More extensive data collection was recently carried out for the development of a standardized test version of the experimental grammatical marker tasks, involving 393 children between ages 3;0 and 6;11 whose language skills were considered normally developing (with a broad definition of normal including children diagnosed with attention deficit disorders) and 444 children between the ages of 3;0 and 8;11 who had a diagnosed language disorder (which included a mixture of children with expressive-only

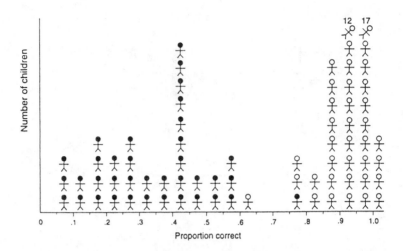

FIG. 2.8. Distribution of individual children's performance on a composite tense marking score: 5-year-old SLI and age controls.

language impairments as well as the expressive/receptive criteria used in the experimental studies reported earlier). In this broad sampling, for children ages 4;6 to 4;11, the sensitivity of the composite tense marking index at a level of 80% was .94 and specificity was .82; at 5;0 to 5;5, sensitivity was .90 and specificity was .80; and at 5;6 to 5;11, sensitivity was .90 and specificity was .90 (cf. M. L. Rice & Wexler, 2001).

NONVARIATION IN THE ACQUISITION OF MORPHOLOGY

Under some models of specific language impairment, such as the low phonetic salience account (Leonard, Eyer, Bedore, & Grela, 1997), it is predicted that morphemes that share phonological properties, such as -s affixes, would be likely to be jointly affected by a grammatical delay. A test case for this prediction is the level of performance of the regular plural -s, which shares phonological properties with third person singular -s. Figure 2.9 reports the levels of performance on the percentage correct use of regular plural -s in spontaneous speech samples for the 5N, 3N, and SLI children of the longitudinal study, which shows that throughout this period of time all three groups of children, including the affected children, perform at high levels of percentage correct in obligatory contexts. This constitutes further evidence of the ways in which the language acquisition system of children with SLI is robust and similar to that of unaffected children, and works against a model that posits that -s omissions for the third person singular af-

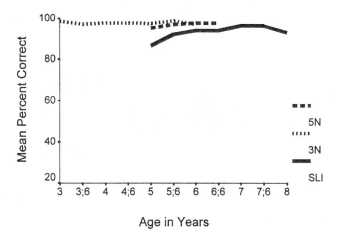

FIG. 2.9. Regular -s plurals.

fix are attributable to the phonological properties shared with regular plural -s. It is still possible that there may have been a delay in the onset of plural marking for the affected children at an age period earlier than that of the
study, which has been resolved by the time the children are, on average, 60
months old. It would be interesting to know, in the event that such an early
delay exists, if the extent of the delay was part of a general language delay,
consistent with expectations indexed to MLU, or if it showed a selective delay as well. It remains for studies of young children with SLI to investigate
this possibility.

LEXICAL ACQUISITION AS AN AREA OF GENERAL, NOT SPECIFIC, DELAY

A number of analyses have been carried out on the lexical acquisition of
the participants in the longitudinal study to determine if there were differences between the SLI group and the younger control group. If such differences were observed, then it would suggest that a grammatical marker
would be joined by a lexical marker in the selective delay of language. If no
such differences appear, then it would be consistent with a model of general delay of lexical elements of language acquisition (i.e., that the levels of
acquisition of the children with .SLI were quite similar to that of younger
children, of equivalent levels of MLU).

A number of different lexical variables show the same general outcomes:
the SLI group performs at levels very similar to that of the unaffected younger control children. The number of different word roots (collapsed across
all form classes) in children's spontaneous language samples are reported

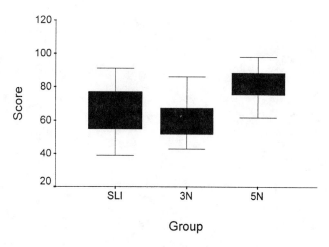

FIG. 2.10. Number of different word roots.

in Fig. 2.10, from samples at the first time of measurement, when the affected children were age 5 years, for the three participating groups; the number of different lexical verb types in Fig. 2.11 is reported for the first time of measurement and again at the second time of measurement, 6 months later, for the SLI and 3N groups; the number of verb tokens (total lexical verb use) is reported in Fig. 2.12 for the first and second time of measurement for the SLI and 3N groups; Fig. 2.13 reports on the percentage of general all-purpose (GAP) verbs in the children's spontaneous samples at the first and second times of measurement, where GAP verbs are defined as the small set of lexical verbs used more than the average number of times (the previous four variables are reported in M. L. Rice, Tweed, &

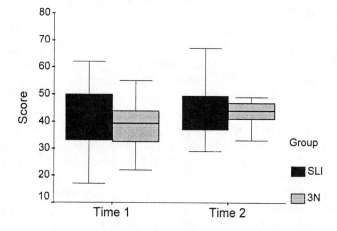

FIG. 2.11. Verb types.

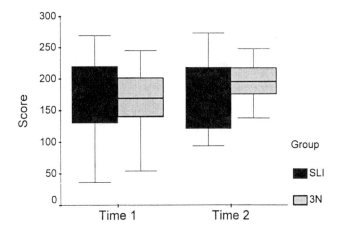

FIG. 2.12. Verb tokens.

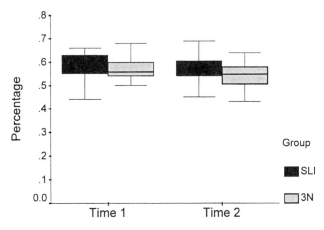

FIG. 2.13. Percentage GAP verb use.

Higheagle, 2000); and Fig. 2.14 reports the raw scores on the Peabody Picture Vocabulary Test–Revised (Dunn & Dunn, 1981) at each age level for the four times of annual testing for the 3N and SLI groups (K. J. Rice, M. L. Rice, & Redmond, 2000).

Statistical analyses reveal that for each of these variables the children with SLI do not differ in level of performance from the younger control group. The conclusion is that the affected children's acquisition of lexical items shows a general delay, which remains parallel to the language acquisition of a group of children about 2 years younger than the affected group of children. This generalization is complicated somewhat by the fact that on tasks of word learning in naturalistic circumstances, children with SLI per-

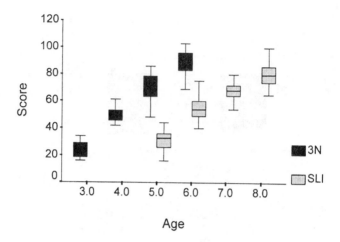

FIG. 2.14. PPVT raw scores.

form less accurately than younger language control children (cf. M. L. Rice, Buhr, & Nemeth, 1990). A reduced capacity to learn new words quickly, relative to the younger control children, may be a major factor in the SLI group's general language delay, although the details of the process, and associated limitations, are not yet worked out, and there are mixed outcomes in the literature. What is highly relevant here is that, in the lexicon, the level of understood vocabulary items and the diversity of use of vocabulary items in spontaneous utterances follows a general delay pattern for the children with SLI.

MEAN LENGTH OF UTTERANCE AS A PART OF A GENERAL DELAY

Since the work of Brown (1973), the mean length of spontaneous utterances of children has served as a conventional general descriptor of young children's language acquisition. In his investigation of three children at the beginning stages of language acquisition, Brown suggested that around the level of 4.0, MLU may become less stable, and therefore less reliable for interpretation. In the intervening years since Brown (1973), other studies document that MLU is highly associated with age below and above the 4.0 level (cf. Conant, 1987; Scarborough, Rescorla, Tager-Flusberg, & Fowler, 1991).

Because MLU is used as a matching variable in studies of children with SLI, and as a diagnostic criterion for identification of affected children, measurement stability and validity are important attributes. Gavin and Giles (1996) reported high levels of test–retest reliability for MLU derived from spontaneous speech samples of unaffected children between 31 and

46 months, for sample sizes of 175 or more complete and intelligible utterances. On the other hand, based on their literature review, Plante, Swisher, Kiernan, and Restrepo (1993) challenged the use of MLU as a matching variable for English-speaking children. Elsewhere, Bol (chap. 10 in this volume) challenges the validity of the MLU index. It is therefore of interest to examine the developmental trajectory of MLU values in the children studied in the longitudinal study described here. In seven times of assessment, the levels of MLU were calculated from the spontaneous utterances of the children in the SLI and the 3N groups. They are reported in Fig. 2.15, where it can be seen that the MLU levels show a strong association with age in the form of steady upward progression (although the within-group variation stays fairly constant, unlike the restricted variation at upper ages that is evident for the obligatory morphemes). Furthermore, as is evident from the figure, the levels of MLU of the SLI and 3N groups stay very similar throughout the period of investigation. Statistical tests show that the two groups are equivalent in their levels of performance, at each age level. Such outcomes are strong indicators of stable and valid measurement properties of the MLU index, which in the case of the data reported here are based on sample sizes of more than 175 complete and intelligible utterances, with careful attention to consistency of scoring criteria.

Once again, the MLU outcomes are consistent with a general delay of language acquisition for the affected group, one in which it must be assumed that the affected children continue to follow the same underlying acquisition mechanisms of children 2 years younger, over a period of 3 years' observation, in the kinds of language growth indexed by the MLU. Detailed

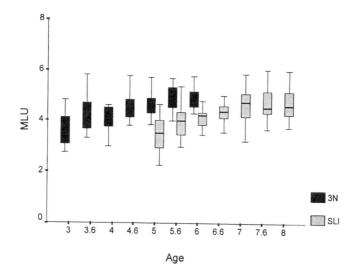

FIG. 2.15. MLU in morphemes.

analyses of the children's utterances reveal relatively rare and apparently unsystematic occasional errors of word order or other sentential errors. The children are not "off the track," but instead seem to lag behind their normal peers in their ability to increase the length of their utterances.

LINGUISTIC DIFFERENCES IN SELECTIVE VERSUS GENERAL DELAYS

The way in which affected children fall behind their younger controls is in the *consistency* with which they mark grammatical tense in obligatory contexts. They occasionally use the target morphemes in contexts where use is required, and in doing so they demonstrate that they know a great deal about the phonological representations of given morphemes, and the contexts in which use is required. This distinction is apparent when alternative methods of evaluating grammatical acquisition are examined (see K. J. Rice, M. L. Rice, & Redmond, 2000, for a more complete report of the outcomes described later).

The index of productive syntax (IPSYN; Scarborough, 1990) is a morphology measurement system for children's spontaneous utterances, in which a child's use of target morphemes, such as those included in the grammatical tense marker, are scored as "0" if there is no use of the morpheme, "1" if the morpheme appears once, and "2" if the morpheme appears more than once. The total score is highly associated with age, and has proven to be a helpful summative measure for general morphological development. Figure 2.16 reports the outcomes of an IPSYN analysis for the three groups of the longitudinal study at the first time of measurement. The dependent measure is the verb phrase subscale, which includes prepositions, verbal particles (such as "put the hat *on*"), and modals, as well as the tense marking morphemes included in the grammatical marker assessed in Figs. 2.4–2.8. As is clear from the box plots in the figure, the affected group does not differ from the younger control group in their level of performance on verbal morphology indexed by the IPSYN, an impression supported by statistical analyses that found no significant difference between the two groups. This is taken to mean that the affected youngsters do not differ from the younger control group in their occasional use of morphology, and/or that the broadly defined cluster of morphemes included in the verb phrase subscale includes morphemes that are not part of the selective grammatical delay as well as morphemes that are part of the selective delay, a mixture that could obscure the underlying grammatical marker.

Another index is sometimes used to describe children's grammatical development, the Developmental Sentence Scoring (DSS) scale (Lee, 1974). Under this system, each utterance is given a total score based on accumulated

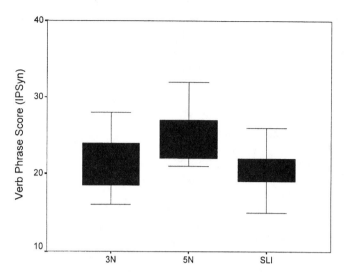

FIG. 2.16. Distribution of verb phrase scores.

well as morphemes that are part of the selective delay, a mixture that could obscure the underlying grammatical marker.

Another index is sometimes used to describe children's grammatical development, the Developmental Sentence Scoring (DSS) scale (Lee, 1974). Under this system, each utterance is given a total score based on accumulated points within eight scoring categories (indefinite pronouns, personal pronouns, main verbs, secondary verbs, negatives, conjunctions, yes/no questions, and wh questions). The DSS was calculated for the same children in

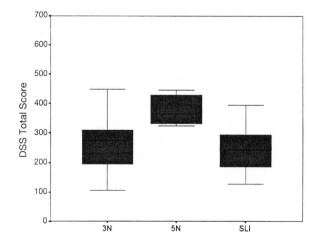

FIG. 2.17. Distribution of DSS scores.

from younger children. Two elements are essential in the measurement system: items that tap into tense marking in the morphosyntax, and an estimate of the likelihood of use in obligatory contexts (i.e., occasional use of a few instances will not capture the optionality dimension of the selective delay of the grammatical marker).

TIMING OF ACQUISITION FOR MORPHOSYNTACTIC AND MORPHOPHONOLOGICAL COMPONENTS OF TENSE MARKING

The studies of the grammatical marker summarized thus far have focused on the morphosyntactic properties (i.e., the children's use of the target forms in obligatory clausal contexts) and follow-up detailed analyses of errors to determine if there were overt errors of usage. Another important element of morphology is the morphophonological learning that allows a youngster to acquire the phonological forms of a given morpheme. The contrast between regular and irregular English past tense forms allows for consideration of the two dimensions. For a given irregular past tense form, such as "ran," a youngster could produce a bare stem form of the lexical verb in an obligatory context (i.e., "run"), suggesting that the morphosyntactic requirement of past tense was not honored; or a youngster could produce the expected past tense form, "ran," showing that the child had two items in his lexicon (i.e., "run" and "ran"), and the past tense context required "ran;" or a youngster could produce the regular morphology instead of the irregular form (i.e, "runned"), showing that the child understood that past tense must be indicated but by the erroneous choice of the *-ed* affix, indicating that the child had not yet completed the morphophological learning of the irregular stem exceptional phonological patterns.

The outcomes of the longitudinal study are illustrated by performance of the SLI group of children, reported in Fig. 2.18, from M. L. Rice, Wexler, Marquis, and Hershberger (2000). This figure shows three indices of past tense acquisition over time: The top line is the percentage correct on the regular past tense probe items, such as "walked"; the bottom line is the percentage correct on the irregular past tense probe items, such as "caught"; and the middle line is a measure of finiteness, which credited an overregularization of the regular *-ed* morpheme as an attempt at marking past tense. In these data, children's responses almost always fell into one of three categories: an unmarked bare stem form of the target verb (which appeared for both regular and irregular past tense forms), the correct adult form, or an overregularized irregular verb. The bare stem responses were interpreted as lacking tense marking, and the overregularized verbs were interpreted

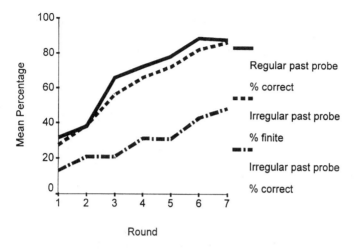

FIG. 2.18. Past TNS probe: SLI group.

as having tense marking that did not follow the adult morphophonological patterns.

Inspection of Fig. 2.18 reveals that responses sharing the property of tense marking, regardless of morphophonological accuracy, align over time, whereas the dimension of morphophonological accuracy trails at a lower level of performance, for the elicitation task, during this period of acquisition. In other words, the likelihood of "walked" and "catched" is similar, whereas "walked" and "caught" are less well associated. The performance of the 3N and 5N groups also follow this pattern.

Growth curve analyses helped further clarify the similarities and differences across measures. Recall that growth curve analyses for composite tense marking, reported earlier, found linear and quadratic components of the predictor equation and, among the predictors, mother's education, the child's nonverbal intelligence, and the child's receptive vocabulary were all nonsignificant, with MLU as the only predictor (and a relatively weak one at that). Growth curve analyses revealed the same set of outcomes for the finite past tense measure (i.e., the index that credits overregularized forms of irregular past tense). In contrast, the outcomes for the percentage correct irregular past tense, which required morphophonological accuracy, yielded linear growth only for both the SLI and 3N groups, and found that the children's initial levels of nonverbal intelligence and receptive vocabulary predicted subsequent growth, in addition to MLU.

The outcomes add further evidence to the generalization that not all elements of the linguistic system are in synchrony in children's acquisition trajectories. In this case, elements of morphophonology for past tense marking are learned at a rate different from that of the obligatory properties of past tense marking. This example of dissociation of surface phonology from morphosyntax is complementary to the earlier example of the same phonology yielding different patterns of acquisition for different morphological functions (i.e., regular plural -s vs. third person singular -s).

Interestingly, the SLI group performs below the younger language control group on the percentage finite (i.e., morphosyntactic) measure throughout the period of study, but on the percentage correct irregular past, the morphophonological measure, the affected group performs at a level equivalent to the younger control group. In other words, the general delay holds for the morphophonological elements, whereas the additional selective delay holds for the tense-marking elements.

A COMPARISON OF SLI CHILDREN AND WMS CHILDREN RELATIVE TO MLU EXPECTATIONS

Children with Williams syndrome (WMS) offer an informative contrast to children with SLI, for the purpose of examining the possible lines of dissociation across elements of grammar. Roughly speaking, the two clinical groups can be thought of as mirror conditions relative to language abilities (i.e., children with SLI seem to have the general developmental prerequisites available for language acquisition and nevertheless show language impairments, whereas children with WMS seem to have cognitive limitations that would preclude grammatical strengths; see the descriptions of WMS provided by Levy, chap. 14; Mervis & Robinson, chap. 9; Clahsen & Temple, chap. 13 in this volume, for more detail). M. L. Rice, Mervis, Klein, and K. J. Rice (1999) carried out an investigation of the spontaneous utterances of a sample of 29 children with WMS (M = 7;7 years) who were at equivalent levels of MLU to the sample of 37 5-year-old children with SLI and 40 3-year-old MLU-equivalent children studied by M. L. Rice, Wexler, and Cleave (1995). There were an additional 45 children in the 5-year-old age-control group. See Fig. 2.19 for the box plots of MLU levels within groups, which show that the MLU levels were equivalent for the SLI, 3N and WMS groups, and somewhat higher for the 5N group. The children's spontaneous utterances were coded for percentage correct of the following morphemes: regular past tense -ed, third person singular -s, Be copula and auxiliaries, plural -s, and the prepositions in and on. The past tense, third person singular -s and Be forms were considered to share the function of grammatical tense marking, whereas the plural -s and prepositions were considered to serve nontense marking functions.

The children's performance is illustrated in Fig. 2.20 for the percentage correct use of Be copula and auxiliary forms in obligatory contexts in spontaneous utterances. Although the MLU levels are equivalent for the SLI, 3N,

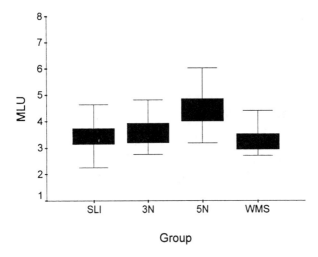

FIG. 2.19. Mean length of utterance.

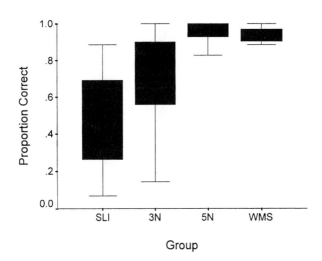

FIG. 2.20. BE, spontaneous.

and WMS groups, there are striking differences in levels of performance: a mean of 91% for the WMS group, 70% for the 3N group, and 47% for the SLI group (and 96% for the 5N group). Statistical analyses found that the WMS group level exceeded that of the other two MLU matched groups and was equivalent to the 5N group; the SLI group was lower than each of the comparison groups. Similar findings held for the other morphemes in the tense marking set, whereas the groups did not differ in their performance on plural -s or the prepositions.

These outcomes suggest that in the domain of grammatical tense marking, it is possible for children to be selectively advanced, relative to general language acquisition indices such as MLU, as well as for children to be selectively delayed in this domain. In some important ways, the tense marking element of children's emerging linguistic systems can be relatively discrete, allowing tense marking to be either relatively poorly developed or relatively strongly developed.

IMPLICATIONS FOR MODELS OF LANGUAGE ACQUISITION AND SPECIFIC AND NONSPECIFIC DELAY

The delay-within-delay model sketched here, and longitudinal evidence of variation across children and across elements of language and change over time during the 3- to 8-year-old age period, places the grammatical tense marker of SLI in the broader picture of general delays of language acquisition. This context may prove to be helpful in evaluating the diversity of characterizations that appear in the literature with regard to children with SLI (e.g., whether or not they have impairments in lexical acquisition, or lexical components of the grammar, or general principles of clause construction). If affected children are compared to their age mates, or to the adult grammar on any given dimension of language, then the conclusion could be that they have an impairment in a particular dimension of language acquisition. Although this is an important observation, it is valuable to sort out whether or not an observed difference is part of a general language delay, in which the linguistic system of a given youngster is globally like that of a younger child, in effect, a general immaturity of language growth, which probably included a late onset as well as a generally off-set (i.e., lower, as in the growth curves of the figures reported here) level of performance relative to age expectations. Note that differentiation of a delay versus delay-within-delay requires recognition of the expected variation within normal children as they move from a child to an adult language system (i.e., a delay should not be confused with variation in acquisition evident in unaffected children).

Low performance on a grammatical tense marker could be diagnostic of a general language delay, or of a selective language delay-within-delay. In order to differentiate these two possibilities, it is necessary to collect further information about the child's general language status, on measures of lexical development, mean length of utterance, and other elements of the emerging grammar. It is possible that children with other conditions, such as autism or Down syndrome, will show a selective delay in grammatical tense marking relative to their general levels of language acquisition, even if those general levels of acquisition are quite depressed relative to age expectations for emergence and mastery over time. Roberts, M. L. Rice, and Tager-Flusberg (2000) reported that in a sample of 51 children with autism, omission of tense marking was evident in their responses to an elicitation probe, in the form of bare stem responses for third person singular present tense -s and past tense forms. The children were subgrouped according to their levels of performance on the Peabody Picture Vocabulary Test–Revised (PPVT–R). The children's performance was closely associated to their performance on the PPVT–R (which was generally parallel to their performance on nonverbal intelligence testing), although even the highest group had performance below age expectations (see Tager-Flusberg, chap. 12 in this volume, for further discussion of autism).

Miller (1996) argued that children with Down syndrome show selective difficulty with grammatical acquisition, relative to their cognitive levels. It could well be the case, although it is as yet untested, that children with Down syndrome would show selective difficulty with tense marking as part of a grammatical deficit. The point of these observations is to note several possibilities. One possibility is that there is overlap in the clinical groupings of SLI and autism, a generalization that may have some clinical validity but would have the interpretive limitation that it would not capture the observations from children with Down syndrome, if they prove to have difficulties in tense marking relative to their MLU levels, or the observations of relative sparing of tense marking in children with WMS. The second possibility is that tense marking can be a marker of a general language delay, such that, relative to age expectations, limitations in tense marking can be consistent with a general level of language delay and concomitant with other elements of language acquisition (e.g., vocabulary development and nonverbal intelligence), which could be the case for children with autism. The third possibility is that a grammatical tense marker can be part of a selective language delay-within-delay, either without general cognitive deficits (as in SLI) or in addition to general cognitive deficits (as in Down syndrome). If there is a possible disconnect in the synchronicity of cognitive and language development (as indicated in the WMS and SLI children), then the disconnect could also be evident in relative levels of cognitive and language development in the case of Down syndrome.

With regard to the synchronization of elements of the linguistic system as children grow, it is obvious from the evidence reported here that there are some important natural partition lines between the lexical system, grossly defined in terms of how many words children know (what can be regarded as semantic/conceptual knowledge under some models) and the morphosyntactic system, comprised of nonsemantic elements of clause structure with associated computational principles and processes. Performance in the lexical system does not predict performance in the grammatical tense marking elements of the morphosyntactic system (i.e., early lexical growth does not predict individual growth curve outcomes for tense marking for either affected or unaffected children). Furthermore, children at equivalent levels of lexical development and equivalent levels of MLU can differ in levels of morphosyntactic development.

The empirical outcomes reported here that indicate a partition between growth in the lexical and morphosyntactic systems are consistent with adult linguistic theoretical distinctions between the lexicon, on the one hand, and the grammar (including morphosyntax), on the other hand. These distinctions are described in more detail in Wexler's chapter (chap. 1 in this volume). The outcomes reported here support the generalization that a relatively discrete morphosyntactic system emerges in children, and some children show selective delays in the system that exceed the delays that can be evident in lexical development. In the theoretical model guiding the investigation reported here, that of the extended optional infinitive (EOI) model (cf. Wexler, chap. 1 in this volume, for more explication), the tense marking system is regarded as central to the morphosyntactic delay, in the form of an underspecified tense marker, a locus of impairment that captures the systematic relation that exists across the multiple morphemes that mark tense in English, and the fact that the selective delay is not evident in affixation processes in general or in surface similarities in phonological structure, or in general principles of clausal structure, and the fact that patterns of overt errors of sentence structure unrelated to tense/agreement are rare. At the same time, other elements of morphophonological learning such as mastery of the irregular past tense morphology, seems to be part of a general language delay (i.e., the morphophonological learning mechanisms of the SLI group of children reported here is equivalent to that of younger language controls). Although the EOI model captures a wide range of empirical observations (one of the criteria of a scientifically useful model), it does not entail the assumption that grammatical tense marking is the only possible symptom of a delay-within-delay acquisition outcome. Other such clinical markers may exist, and may ultimately yield to further investigation.

At the level of etiology, the delay-within-delay model suggests that there may be different etiological factors at work in the global language delay than in an area of specific delay, such as grammatical tense marking. Certain critical cognitive/neuro/genetic/social factors are operative at the time of language emergence. Returning to the train metaphor, there is a need to get the train to leave the station on time. Although the expected time of emergence is one of the strongest assumptions of what is known about language acquisition, the underlying trigger for onset is unknown. A complete account of language delays in children ultimately must specify what is in volved in activating the language system. For many, if not most, children with language delays, the onset is delayed and, as the condition of SLI makes clear, factors outside the linguistic system per se are not likely to be sole causal agents.

There may well be maturational mechanisms specific to the linguistic system. Elsewhere, a maturational component of the selective delay evident in the grammatical tense marker has been advocated by M. L. Rice and Wexler (1996). The delay-within-delay model suggests that a two-phase maturational process may be implicated, one for onset and a second for grammatical tense marking (or any other marker found to lag behind the global language acquisition trajectory). Investigations to date strongly suggest that it is the obligatory property of tense marking in English that is implicated in the selective delay, an empirical observation that remains to be more fully explicated theoretically.

The studies reported here are carried out with English-speaking children. Much work remains to be done to determine whether a delay-within-delay is evident, or detectable, across multiple languages. The empirical challenges are many, given the need to have relatively robust measures of global language acquisition in order to be able to estimate the variation evident in given linguistic domains across unaffected children of given ages, developmental indices that are not available for all languages. At the same time, the variations across languages are essential for clarification of the ways in which language delays can be manifested, whether the delays seem to be restricted to delays in language (as in the condition of SLI) or are associated with other conditions, such as autism, WMS, or Down syndrome. Central to the crosslinguistic comparison are the ways in which the lexical and morphosyntactic requirements of a given language interact with a child's language acquisition propensities. The contributors to this volume add significantly to the knowledge base in these matters. Ultimately, this is all a part of a collective movement toward a better understanding of the ways in which children have inherent differences in aptitude for language acquisition, and the ways in which the linguistic system is designed to unfold as children mature.

ACKNOWLEDGMENTS

The work reported in this chapter was funded by awards from the National Institute of Deafness and Other Communicative Disorders (R01 DC01803; T32 DC00052). Special appreciation is expressed to Patsy Woods for her assistance with manuscript preparation, and to Karla Barnhill for her assistance with data analysis.

REFERENCES

Bishop, D.V.M. (1994). Grammatical errors in specific language impairment: Competence or performance limitations? *Applied Psycholinguistics, 15*, 507–550.

Brown, R. (1973). *A first language: The early stages*. Cambridge, MA: Harvard University Press.

Chomsky, N. (1996). *The minimalist program*. Cambridge, MA: MIT Press.

Conant, S. (1987). The relationship between age and MLU in young children: A second look at Klee and Fitzgerald's data. *Journal of Child Language, 14*, 169–173.

Dunn, A., & Dunn, A. (1981). *Peabody Picture Vocabulary Test–Revised*. Circle Pines, MN: American Guidance Service.

Gavin, W. J., & Giles, L. (1996). Sample size effects on temporal reliability of language sample measures of preschool children. *Journal of Speech and Hearing Research, 39*, 1258–1262.

Lee, L. (1966). Developmental sentence types: A method for comparing normal and deviant syntactic development. *Journal of Speech and Hearing Disorders, 31*, 311–330.

Lee, L. (1974). *Developmental sentence analysis*. Evanston, IL: Northwestern University Press.

Leonard, L. B. (1972). What is deviant language? *Journal of Speech and Hearing Disorders, 37*, 427–446.

Leonard, L. B. (1998). *Children with specific language impairments*. Cambridge, MA: MIT Press.

Leonard, L., Eyer, J., Bedore, L., & Grela, B. (1997). Three accounts of the grammatical morpheme difficulties of English-speaking children with specific language impairment. *Journal of Speech and Hearing Research, 40*, 741–753.

Menyuk, P. (1964). Comparison of grammar of children with functionally deviant and normal speech. *Journal of Speech and Hearing Research, 7*, 109–121.

Miller, J. F. (1996). The search for the phenotype of disordered language performance. In M. L. Rice (Ed.), *Toward a genetics of language* (pp. 297–314). Hillsdale, NJ: Lawrence Erlbaum Associates.

Morehead, D. M., & Ingram, D. (1973). The development of base syntax in normal and linguistically deviant children. *Journal of Speech, Language, and Hearing Research, 16*, 330–352.

Pinker, S. (1984). *Language learnability and language development*. Cambridge, MA: Harvard University Press.

Plante, E., Swisher, L., Kiernan, B., & Restrepo, M. A. (1993). Language matches: Illuminating or confounding? *Journal of Speech and Hearing Research, 36*, 772–776.

Rice, M. L., Buhr, J., & Nemeth, M. (1990). Fast mapping word learning abilities of language delayed preschoolers. *Journal of Speech and Hearing Disorders, 55*, 33–42.

Rice, M. L., Mervis, C., Klein, B. P., & Rice, K. J. (1999, November). *Children with Williams syndrome do not show an EOI stage*. Paper presented at the Boston University Conference on Language Development, Boston.

Rice, K. J., Rice, M. L., & Redmond, S. M. (2000, June). *MLU outcomes for children with and without SLI: Support for MLU as a matching criterion*. Paper presented at the Symposium on Research in Child Language Disorders, Madison, WI.

Rice, M. L., Tweed, S., & Higheagle, B. (2000, June). *GAP verbs of children with SLI: Longitudinal observations*. Paper presented at the Symposium on Research in Child Language Disorders, Madison, WI.

Rice, M. L., & Wexler, K. (1996). Toward tense as a clinical marker of specific language impairment in English-speaking children. *Journal of Speech and Hearing Research, 39*, 850–863.

Rice, M. L., & Wexler, K. (2001). *Rice/Wexler Test of Early Grammatical Impairment*. San Antonio: Psychological Corporation.

Rice, M. L., Wexler, K., & Cleave, P. L. (1995). Specific language impairment as a period of extended optional infinitive. *Journal of Speech, Language, and Hearing Research, 38*, 850–863.

Rice, M. L., Wexler, K., & Hershberger, S. (1998). Tense over time: The longitudinal course of tense acquisition in children with specific language impairment. *Journal of Speech, Language, and Hearing Research, 41*, 1412–1431.

Rice, M. L., Wexler, K., Marquis, J., & Hershberger, S. (2000). Acquisition of irregular past tense by children with SLI. *Journal of Speech, Language, and Hearing Research, 43*, 1126–1145.

Rice, M. L., Wexler, K., & Redmond, S. M. (1999). Grammaticality judgments of an extended optional infinitive grammar: Evidence from English-speaking children with specific language impairment. *Journal of Speech, Language, and Hearing Research, 42*, 943–961.

Roberts, J. A., Rice, M. L., & Tager-Flusberg, H. (2000, June). *Tense marking in children with autism: Further evidence for overlap between autism and SLI.* Paper presented at the Symposium on Research in Child Language Disorders, Madison, WI.

Scarborough, H. S. (1990). Index of productive syntax. *Applied Psycholinguistics, 11*, 1–22.

Scarborough, H. S., Rescorla, L., Tager-Flusberg, H., & Fowler, A. E. (1991). The relation of utterance length to grammatical complexity in normal and language-disordered groups. *Applied Psycholinguistics, 12*, 23–45.

Tager-Flusberg, H., & Cooper, J. (1999). Present and future possibilities for defining a phenotype for specific language impairment. *Journal of Speech, Language, and Hearing Research, 42*, 1275–1278.

Thal, D. J., & Katich, J. (1996). Predicaments in early identification of specific language impairment. In K. N. Cole, P. S. Dale, & D. J. Thal (Eds.), *Assessment of communication and language* (pp. 1–28). Baltimore: Brookes.

Wexler, K. (1994). Optimal infinitives, head movement and the economy of derivations. In D. Lightfoot & N. Hornstein (Eds.), *Verb movement* (pp. 305–350). Cambridge, MA: Cambridge University Press.

Wexler, K., Schutze, C. T., & Rice, M. (1998). Subject case in children with SLI and unaffected controls: Evidence for the Agr/Tns omission model. *Language Acquisition, 7*(2–4), 317–344.

3

Two of a Kind?
The Importance of Commonalities
and Variation Across
Languages and Learners

Martha Crago
McGill University

Johanne Paradis
University of Alberta

This chapter addresses the meaning of the term *specific* in specific language impairment (SLI) in a broader way than is customary. Usually this term denotes the specificity of the impairment within the individual child. SLI has been defined as the atypical development of language that cannot be attributed to other disabling factors such as hearing impairment, emotional, neurological, or intellectual deficits (Leonard, 1998). In the case of specific language impairment, specific has been used to signify the definition of this impairment by exclusionary criteria (see also de Villiers, chap. 17 in this volume).

Yet, there may be other ways in which specific language impairment is not so specific. For instance, are the morphosyntactic deficits caused by SLI specific to particular languages or are they common across all languages even if the languages have different structural properties? Are these morphosyntactic deficits specific only to children with specific language impairment or do they exist in other language learners, that is, younger children with typical development and second language learners? In other words, just how universal and just how specific is this form of childhood impairment? This chapter addresses these aspects of its specificity by describing commonalities and variation in the manifestation of SLI in three languages that are structurally quite different (English, French, and Inuktitut) and across three learner groups (children with typical development, children with SLI, and children who are acquiring a second language).

COMMONALITIES AND VARIATION IN SLI ACROSS
THREE LANGUAGES

In establishing commonalities and variation in SLI across languages, the description will be limited to the deficits that children with SLI have in their verbal morphology. In particular, the existence of an extended optional infinitive stage (EOI) is examined (Rice & Wexler, 1996; see also Rice, chap. 2 in this volume; Wexler, chap. 1 in this volume). The concept of an extended optional infinitive stage is premised on Poeppel and Wexler's (1993) claims that a maturational stage exists in normally developing children in which finite and nonfinite forms are used optionally because tense (TNS) has not yet been acquired. Rice and Wexler (1996) found that English-speaking children with SLI also used finite and nonfinite forms optionally. Wexler (1998) confirmed that the grammatical structure of a language influences the existence and the nature of an optional infinitive (OI) stage in typically developing children. In languages that permit null subjects, children do not go through an optional infinitive stage. On the contrary, in non-null subject languages, Wexler claimed that a universal checking constraint allows only one determiner feature to be checked, eliminating either TNS or agreement and producing a nonfinite or infinitival form. This chapter focuses on two major forms of variation in how the optional infinitive and the extended optional infinitive stages are manifest in three different languages. One is the relation between the optional use of nonfinite forms as they are produced by children with typical development and as they are produced by children with SLI (i.e. the relation of the OI stage to the EOI stage). The other is the nature of the error form that children use when they do not inflect the verb correctly.

The Relation of OI and EOI in English, Inuktitut,
and Quebec French

English. Rice and Wexler (1996) established that 5-year-old English-speaking children with SLI correctly inflected past tense in less than 40% of the verbs produced in their spontaneous speech. This was considerably less than the typically developing 3-year-old children who were language matched by mean length of utterance (MLU) to the children with SLI. The typically developing 3 year olds inflected their verbs correctly for past tense about 50% of the time. In contrast, Rice and Wexler found that typically developing children who were 5 years old correctly inflected the past tense 90% of the time. The relation between the three groups forms a kind of a staircase pattern with 5-year-old children with SLI on the bottom level, having the most difficulty in correctly inflecting for past tense; 3-year-old language matched, normally developing children are on a middle level, correctly inflecting past tense more often than the children with SLI but less often than the typically developing 5-year-olds. The 5-year-olds are, of course, on the top level, performing virtually at a ceiling level. This pattern of relation between the three groups led Rice and Wexler to coin the term *extended optional infinitive* stage to describe the relative deficit of the children with SLI in comparison with the other two normally developing groups of children. One interpretation of their work is that the English-speaking children with SLI are delayed in their language development. Yet, interestingly enough, their performance is not equal to the control group that was matched on mean length of utterance. Therefore, an alternative hypothesis is that the children with SLI are both delayed and deviant in their production of past tense.

Rice, Wexler, and Hershberger (1998) provided further insights by establishing that English-speaking children with SLI improved in their production of the past tense over time from a mean of 40% correct at 5 years old to between 70% and 80% correct by the time they were 8 years old. However, 8-year-olds could still be considered to have SLI because their percent of correct past tense at age 8 was still significantly less than the 90% correct rate found in typically developing children at age 5. Indeed, Rice and her colleagues demonstrated that children with SLI acquire the inflection for tense over a very slow and extended period of time. At least an additional 3 years is added to the learning curve for these children. However, even more strikingly, Rice and her colleagues showed that the acquisition curves for the correct inflection of past tense for both the typically developing children and those with SLI were very similar. The younger typically developing children improved rapidly from less than 50% correct at age 3 to over 90% correct past tense productions by age 3½. This rapid change over a 6-month time period was mirrored by a similar leap by the children with SLI. Both groups accelerated their performance sharply in less than a year's time. However, in the case of children with SLI, the period of accelerated growth occurred between ages 5 and 6. In contrast, the children who were more typical in their development had their period of acceleration some 2 years earlier than the children with SLI. Moreover, the typically developing children had attained well-developed competency with past tense inflection by age 3 . The children with SLI, on the other hand, did not show the same degree of competency even by age 7. In a sense, it is remarkable that the two groups had this similar a pattern of acceleration, given the lack of similarity in the overall rates of correctness by the group with SLI and the language-matched control group. Yet, just as remarkable was the difference in final level of competency, a level that after 7 years of acquisition remained at the 70% to 80% level in the children with SLI.

Certain questions remain to be answered. When and at what level will the learning of children with SLI arrive at an end state? Hopefully, Rice and her colleagues will be able to continue their studies of children with SLI as they mature to even older ages. The portrait of English-speaking children with SLI is certainly one of an impairment, but yet one with a pattern of learning that is somewhat similar to the pattern demonstrated by normally developing children, at least for certain aspects of the morphosyntax. The difference lies in the timing of the accelerated learning period, in the extent of the learning period, and possibly in the final degree of resolution of the optional use of the infinitive. If the end state achieved by children with SLI is different than that achieved by normally developing children, then it is difficult to describe SLI as simply a delay. In other words, if the extended optional infinitive stage is irresolvable, then this could be taken as indication that something more than delay or extension of a normal period has happened. Indeed, such a difference in end state could signify the deviant nature of language development in children with SLI. In this case, the term *deviant optional infinitive stage* would be a more appropriate description of the nature of the impairment.

Inuktitut. Inuktitut is a null subject, polysynthetic language with extensive inflectional morphology but, interestingly enough, no inflectional form for tense. (See Allen, 1996, and Crago and Allen, 2001, for more extensive detail on Inuktitut grammar.) Crago and Allen (2001) reported their study of language acquisition in five Inuit children with typical development and a single Inuk girl with specific language impairment. The relation between the acquisition of finiteness in Inuktitut by the children with typical development and the child with SLI is strikingly different from the pattern described for English-speaking children. In what ways is it different? Four of the children studied by Crago and Allen were within 1 month of their second birthday. At scarcely 2 years old, they were inflecting verbs in the adult lexicon correctly more than 90% of the time. This rate of production refers to overall verbal inflection because Inuktitut has no inflection for tense. Nevertheless, it indicates a striking difference from the optional inflection of past tense observed in the English-speaking 3-year-olds reported by Rice and Wexler (1996). The pattern of early production of finite forms in Inuktitut adheres to Wexler's (1998) prediction that children speaking null subject languages will show the capacity for early inflection, making an optional infinitive stage either very short or nonexistent. In summary, the normal acquisition of English and Inuktitut involves quite a different starting point for full competency in verbal inflection. The Inuit children are 1 to 1½ years ahead of the English-speaking children in their mastery of finite inflections, demonstrating the impact of different language structures on the nature and timing of the acquisitional process.

Inuktitut does not have a true optional infinitive stage, so what form does SLI take in this language? If, for instance, an Inuktitut-speaking child with SLI optionally produces inflections, then it is not logical to use the term extended optional infinitive stage because there is no normal optional infinitive stage that can be extended. In fact, the single child that Crago and Allen studied did produce inflections optionally. Only approximately 60% of her verbs were correctly inflected at age 5. This could be described as a two-step pattern of acquisition for Inuktitut, in contrast with the three-step pattern for English. There is one level of optional inflection for the child with SLI and a second level of full inflection for the 2-year-olds. Clearly, the problems with inflection that the child with SLI experienced were not similar to a stage of normal development. They represented a deviant or atypical rather then an extended pattern of acquisition for Inuktitut. In this case, it would be more accurate to describe the Inuk child with SLI as being in a stage of deviant optionality. The study indicates that the similarity of the lower rates of past tense inflection observed in younger normally developing children and in English-speaking children with SLI cannot hold for Inuktitut speakers. The variation in this relation across these two languages means that the OI–EOI relation with its implicit concept of extension or delay is specific to certain languages and not universal to all languages. However, the difficulty with inflection experienced by children with SLI seems to be common to both English and Inuktitut, making it a candidate for a universal or nonlanguage specific deficit. In summary, both deviant optionality and extended optionality have similar properties but delay is not one of them. It is the optional nature of inflection that is common to both English- and Inuktitut-speaking children with SLI.

Quebec French. Learners of Quebec French demonstrate both commonalities and differences from learners of English and Inuktitut. Paradis and Genesee (1997) demonstrated that bilingual children learning both French and English simultaneously from birth had different levels of correct verbal inflections in their two different languages. At age 3, over 80% of their French verbs were correctly inflected, whereas only approximately 40% of their English verbs were correctly inflected. It is interesting to note that the 3-year-old bilinguals had a similar rate of correct inflections in their English when compared to Rice and Wexler's 3-year-old monolingual English speakers. The difference lies in the bilinguals' earlier and more complete competency with their French inflections. Yet, the level of mastery of inflection in Quebec French is not as early or as complete as the Inuit children's mastery of inflection in Inuktitut is at a younger age. Children speaking Quebec French are situated somewhere in between the English and the Inuktitut speakers in their degree of mastery of verbal inflection. They normally have a shorter optional infinitive stage with fuller mastery at an earlier age than English speakers, but a longer and later optional infinitive stage than Inuktitut speakers. A possible explanation for the French–English differences lies in the morphological structure of the verb paradigm in French, which is explored in Paradis and Crago (in press). The difference between Quebec French, English, and Inuktitut raises the question of whether speakers of Quebec French with SLI and English-speaking children with SLI will have the same pattern of deficit.

Paradis and Crago (under review) compared three groups of Quebec French language learners: 10 7-year-old children with typical development (7ND), 10 7-year-old children with SLI (7SLI), and 10 typically developing 3-year-old children matched by mean length of utterance to the children with SLI (3ND). All 30 children came from homes and schools where they were exposed exclusively to Quebec French. Once again, as with the Inuit children, the pattern of correct inflection has only two steps for these groups of children. The children with SLI used a significantly lower percentage of finite verbs than the other two groups. The two groups of typically developing children showed no difference from each other, both used over 90% of finite verbs in obligatory context. The children's ages, MLUs, and percent scores for finite verb use are given in Table 3.1. So once again, it is not clear that there is the same relation between OI and EOI for children learning Quebec French as there is for children learning English, at least not by the time the children with SLI are 7 years old. However, one noteworthy aspect of commonality in Paradis and Crago's findings when compared with Rice, Wexler, and Hershberger's study (1998) on tense over time is that the 7-year-old English-speaking children with SLI were producing past tense inflections correctly at about the same rate as the Quebec French speakers of SLI. This rate of production made the English-speaking children with SLI significantly different from the typically developing children who were matched to them by MLU and the MLU matched group was significantly different from the age-matched group of children (Paradis, Crago, Genesee, & Rice, 2001). Furthermore, it is interesting to note that the Quebec 7-year-olds with SLI were matched on MLU to 3-year-olds. This is rather unexpected because English-speaking 5-year-olds with SLI are normally matched by MLU to normally developing children that are 3 years old. This difference presumably reflects the earlier resolution of the optional infinitive

TABLE 3.1
Age, MLU, and % Correct of Finite Verbs for French-Speaking Children

	7SLI	3ND	7ND
Age	7;6	3;3	7;4
MLU (words)	3.977	3.672	5.702
% finite verbs	87.5	94.3	99.5

Note: 7SLI = 7-year-old children with SLI; 3ND = normally developing 3-year-olds; 7ND = normally developing 7-year-olds.

stage in French. Is SLI in Quebec French a pattern of extended optional infinitive or one of deviant optional infinitive? Certainly, there is some form of an optional infinitive stage in Quebec French that has similar properties to the language of children with SLI. However, the verbal inflections of the age and language matched normally developing children resembled each other more than either one of them resembled the performance of children with SLI. This indicates that the pattern of impairment, by age 7, was not one of simple delay and not merely a question of extended learning. It appears as if the learning period was so extended that it could be considered deviant from the normal pattern.

Thus far, in this account of SLI in three languages, the characterization of children with SLI as being in an extended optional infinitive stage suits English-speaking children better than it suits Inuktitut- or French-speaking children. In other words, the difficulty children have with realizing verbal inflection is similar across the three languages, but the relation of the grammatical deficit to a normal stage of development differs because the nature and very existence of an optional infinitive stage in normal learners varies across these three languages. From a simple comparison of SLI in only three languages, it does appear that the term *deviant optional infinitive stage* captures the properties of the grammatical deficit exhibited by children with SLI more aptly over a variety of languages and at older ages of development than the term "extended optional infinitive" does. Needless to say, more well-planned comparative studies of SLI across a larger variety of languages than presented here are needed to elucidate the nature of the relation between OI and EOI and what that relation reveals about language specific and language universal properties of SLI (see Paradis & Crago, in press, for a more complete description of existing research on SLI in a variety of languages).

The Nature of the Error Form in English, Inuktitut, and Quebec French

This section addresses the kinds of errors children with SLI make when they do not correctly inflect a verb. Just how specific is the use of the infinitive as an error form? Rice and Wexler (1996) showed that it is the error form in English, but is it the error form in languages other than English? Crago and Allen (2001) and Paradis and Crago (in press) documented that the error or default form produced by children with SLI differs across languages. A brief overview of the crosslinguistic differences in form is presented in Table 3.2. Inuktitut, for instance, has no infinitive form. Therefore, an infinitival form cannot, by necessity, be the default error form. The Inuk child with SLI studied by Crago and Allen (2001) produced bare root forms, which are virtually nonexistent in the language of typically developing

TABLE 3.2
Form of the Default (Root Infinitive) in SLI Across Languages

Language	Nonfinite Default	Finite Default

ENGLISH
  Rice & Wexler (1996)
	verb stem /infinitive
	present progressive
	  participle [-*ing*]
	perfect participle [-*en*]
		none

SWEDISH
  Hansson (1997)
  Håkansson (1998)
	infinitive [-*a*]
	supine perfect partici-
	  ple [-*t*]
		unknown

NORWEGIAN
  Meyer Bjerkan (1999)
	infinitive (elicitation
	  contexts only)
		present tense
		[verb + *er*]

GERMAN
  Rice et al. (1997),
    Roberts & Leonard (1997)
	infinitive [-*en*]
	(verb stem)?
		(verb stem)?

DUTCH de Jong (1999)	infinitive [-*en*] participle verb stem	present tense (for past) verb stem (in V2)

FRENCH
  Paradis & Crago (2000),
    Jakubowicz et al. (1999)
	infinitive [-*er*, -*ir*, -*re*]
	past participle [-*é*]
		present tense [verb stem + Ø]

ARABIC Abdalla (2000)	none	imperative first singular present (both closest to root form)
INUKTITUT Crago & Allen (2001)	verb root	none

Inuktitut speakers of any age. Quebec French does have an infinitival form. For certain groups of French verbs, the infinitive is homophonous with the past participle (e.g., _marcher/to walk_ and _marché/walked_). However, by inspecting verb groups where the two forms are not homophonous, Paradis and Crago (2000) found that children with SLI used the infinitival form (e.g., _finir/to finish_) less frequently as a replacement for the past tense form than they used the nonfinite past participles (e.g., _fini/finished_). When the past participle was used, the auxiliary was dropped rendering the participle nonfinite. Furthermore, the so-called infinitival form in English is not entirely straightforward because it is the same as the stem form (e.g., _walk_). What all these different forms have in common is that they are nonfinite. However, as indicated in Table 3.2, in some cases a form that patterns like the nonfinite forms in the speech of children with SLI would be considered a finite form in the adult language. These finite root infinitives are typically the most minimally inflected forms in the present tense paradigm. Paradis and Crago (in press) put forth an analysis of finite root infinitives as underspecified for tense features, thus accounting for how they can pattern with untensed forms like infinitives. As such, the substitutes for correctly tensed verbs in the speech of children with SLI might be more appropriately referred to as default forms, rather than infinitives.

In summary, the nature of the nonfinite form that both children with SLI and normally developing children substitute for the finite form of a verb differs across languages. This lack of similarity in the error form is another indication of the lack of universality in the properties of SLI that occur across languages with various structures. In this regard, specific language impairment is more specific than it is universal. In other words, languages with different structures are not necessarily two of a kind when it comes to the particulars of the default error form. Yet, just as importantly, the overall nature of the error in verbal inflection produced by children with SLI is the substitution of a nonfinite form, of one kind or another, for a finite form. In this regard, the overall nature of the error is universal. It is in the specifics of the error form that children with SLI who speak different languages vary. To encompass the full range of error patterns and forms it is worthwhile to consider replacing the term extended optional infinitive with deviant optional default.[1]

COMMONALITIES ACROSS TWO GROUPS OF LEARNERS

This section discusses the specificity of the language learning process in children with SLI. A major preoccupation concerns whether other learners show the same relative lack of proficiency with verbal inflection as children with SLI and whether they make the same types of errors. These issues are explored by inspecting whether second language learners as well as first language learners with SLI pass through an optional or extended optional infinitive stage.

Concurrent with the investigations of the OI stage in normal and impaired acquisition, researchers have investigated the acquisition of functional categories in second language learners. Because of the maturation assumptions in the OI account, an OI stage would not be expected in first language learning in children past the primary acquisition years. However, certain studies have found that that second language learners show many OI stage properties in their intermediate language, such as omission of tense marking coextensive with a paucity of commission errors in agreement (Eubank, 1993–1994, 1996; Gavruseva & Lardiere, 1996; Grondin & White, 1996; Paradis, Le Corre, & Genesee, 1998; Prévost, 1997; Prévost & White, 2000). On the other hand, researchers have found that, unlike normally developing and impaired monolingual speakers, the word order and

---

[1]An idea suggested to Martha Crago 8 years ago by Shari Baum.

finiteness properties along with certain other OI stage properties are not always apparent in second language learners' speech (Haznedar & Schwartz, 1997; Lardiere, 1998; Prévost & White, 2000). Moreover, it appears that there is a difference between child and adult second language learners (Grondin & White, 1996; Prévost & White, 2000) in this regard. Children learning French as a second language, for example, even when producing a nonfinite form for the verb would place it correctly with regard to the negator. This demonstrated that despite having the word order associated with finiteness, the children learning a second language still had trouble producing correctly tensed verbs.

Given this apparent similarity between the grammatical problems of children learning a second language and those with SLI, Paradis and Crago (2000) conducted a study that directly compared the acquisition of verbal inflection in three groups of children: 10 7-year-old children with SLI, 15 similarly aged and language matched second language learners, and 10 7-year-old normally developing children. Later, Paradis and Crago were able to make comparisons with a group of 10 younger monolingual normally developing children who were language matched to both the children with SLI and to the second language learners. The children learning a second language all spoke English as their first language but, at the time of the study, had attended a school for 2 years where they had received instruction exclusively in Quebec French. Moreover, their classmates were monolingual French first language speakers.

The findings of this study show that impaired learners and second language learners have certain commonalities. In fact, they had more in common than either group had with the normally developing children of their age. More surprisingly, they also had more in common with each other than they had with the younger normal learners who were matched to them by mean length of utterance. For example, both the children with SLI and the second language learners had significantly more difficulty inflecting verbs for tense than either the age or language matched normally developing monolingual children had (see Fig. 3.1). The overall accuracy rate was 88% for the children with SLI and 89% for second language learners. This was statistically significantly lower than the normally developing monolingual 7-year-olds whose overall accuracy rate was 99.5%. Furthermore, both groups had more difficulty with inflecting for past tense and future tense than they had with present tense. In fact, of all of the groups, the second language learners had the lowest percent correct for past (48%) and future tense (49%) inflections. This was considerably lower than the children with SLI who inflected past tense correctly at a rate of 74% and future tense at an accuracy rate of 64%. Indeed, at this age and in this stage of their development, the children with SLI and the second language speakers had certain similarities in their use of finiteness. They both had significantly more prob-

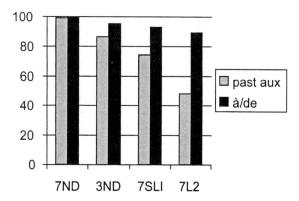

FIG. 3.1. Percent correct in obligatory context for the past tense auxiliary verbs and the prepositions à/de for French-speaking children: 7ND (normally developing 7-year-olds), 3ND (normally developing 3-year-olds), 7SLI (7-year-olds with SLI), 7L2 (7-year-old L2 learners).

lems with producing finite forms than either of the groups of typically developing children, but they varied in the degree of their difficulty with the correct expression of past and future tense forms. The second language learners at this age and stage of language development had a lower overall rate of correct past and future tense than the children with SLI. Yet, the language of both these groups could be characterized as having the properties of the optional infinitive stage. Moreover, in accordance with the predictions of OI theory, the children with SLI and the second language learners had high rates of accuracy with nontense grammatical morphemes, like the French prepositions à and de. Figure 3.1 illustrates the contrast between the monolingual normally developing children, and the children with SLI and the second language learners on the one hand, and between tense bearing and nontense bearing morphemes on the other. The past tense auxiliary in French is a short duration morpheme, as are the prepositions, and the third person singular form of the past auxiliary is homophonous with the preposition à. Both the children with SLI and the second language learners are much less accurate with the past auxiliary than the 7- and 3-year-olds; however, all the children produce prepositions at the rate of 90% or higher.

However, a revealing picture emerged from an analysis of tense errors. Here the two groups of learners part company and no longer appear to be two of a kind. The children with SLI used nonfinite forms in place of correct past and future tenses. In fact, the children with SLI used different nonfinite default forms in different tense contexts. They replaced correct future tense with the infinitival form and almost all of the correct past tense forms with past participles. On the other hand, the second language learners replaced both the correct past tense form and the correct future tense form with an incorrect finite form. It is important to note that there was some overlap in the error patterns between the two groups. In other words, both had finite and nonfinite substitution errors, but the central tendencies of the two groups were interestingly different. Expressed simply, the second language learners appeared to have a greater capacity to use finite forms, although these finite forms are not always correct ones. The children with SLI, on the other hand, gravitated to nonfinite forms to replace the tensed forms they were not capable of producing. In summary, the default forms of these two groups of language learners were, for the most part, different from each other.

This study raises an important theoretical concern. The resolution of the OI stage in normally developing monolingual children has been attributed to neurological maturation. Its existence in children with SLI has inversely been attributed to delayed maturation (Wexler, 1996). How do second language learners fit into a maturational theory of grammatical development? Clearly, at age 7, they are no longer in the primary years for language acquisition. They also do not suffer from any maturational breakdown or delay, having mastered a first language in the typical fashion at the typical age. One possible explanation is that an intermediate stage of language acquisition with properties of optional inflection can occur in various language learners at least through adolescence and possibly well into adulthood. Perhaps it is the intermediacy of the stage and not maturation or biological intactness that is important. The second language learners studied appeared to be moving out of the optional use of tensed forms 1 year after their involvement in our study (i.e., after 3 years of second language learning). However, if SLI does not resolve and if its end state in adulthood still involves the optional production of finite forms, then the grammar of individuals with SLI can no longer be seen as an intermediate stage of development. Instead, the properties of this form of impaired grammar would be more accurately characterized as a deviant and arrested stage of development rather than the extension of a stage through which an individual passes belatedly. If this distinction in the process and timing of resolution is what distinguishes children with SLI from other language learners, then, despite certain commonalities with typically developing children and second language learners, specific language impairment, as its name implies, is indeed a particularly specific form of language learning.

This chapter has raised unsolved but not insolvable questions concerning the universality and specificity of language learning across various types of languages and learners. Old questions of whether SLI is best characterized by deviance or delay remain. To them are added questions about whether SLI is truly an extension of a normal stage or an unresolved stage of acquisition. Comparing SLI across languages and learners has also intro duced the notion of a more inclusive and generic classification of the error form as having default rather than only infinitival properties.

Clearly, there is more to do. Additional studies comparing similar morphological variables for normal developing children and those with SLI across more languages are needed before the universal aspects of morphological development and deficit can be teased apart from those that are language specific. Questions about the resolution of SLI beg for studies on end state learners, in other words, on adults who were considered to be specifically language impaired as children. In addition, other learner populations, such as children with cochlear implants, can help elucidate understanding of the developmental progression of morphological learning at various ages. The nature of the deficit in SLI is still not clear. Attribution of the deficit to a disability in grammatical representation needs to be proven with more certainty. Real-time processing studies comparing individuals with SLI to other learners such as individuals learning a second language will help to confirm the hypothesis that the deficit is one of representation and not one of access or processing. Researchers look forward to the answers to questions, to the building of new theory, the confirmation of old hypotheses, and most of all to strengthening knowledge so that it can be used to improve the communicative opportunities of individuals with SLI.

REFERENCES

Abdalla, F. (2000). *Verbal inflection in Arabic-speaking children with specific language impairment.* Unpublished manuscript, Montreal, McGill University.

Allen, S. (1996). *Aspects of argument structure acquisition in Inuktitut.* Amsterdam, NL: Benjamins.

Crago, M., & Allen, S. (2001). Early finiteness in Inuktitut: The role of language structure and input. *Language Acquisition, 9*(1), 59–111.

de Jong, J. (1999). *Specific language impairment in Dutch: Inflectional morphology and argument structure.* Enschede, The Netherlands: Print Partners Ipskamp.

Eubank, L. (1993–1994). On the transfer of parametric values in L2 development. *Language Acquisition, 3*(3), 183–208.

Eubank, L. (1996). Negation in early German–English interlanguage: More valueless features in the L2 initial state. *Second Language Research, 12*(1), 73–106.

Gavruseva, L., & Lardiere, D. (1996). The emergence of extended phrase structure in child L2 acquisition. *BUCLD 20 Proceedings,* 225–236.

Grondin, N., & White, L. (1996). Functional categories in child L2 acquisition of French. *Language Acquisition, 5,* 1–34.

Håkansson, G. (1998). Language impairment and the realization of finiteness. In A. Greenhill, M. Hughes, H. Littlefield, & H. Walsh (Eds.), *BUCLD 22* (pp. 314–324). Somerville, MA: Cascadilla Press.

Hansson, K. (1997). Patterns of verb usage in Swedish children with SLI: An application of recent theories. *First Language, 17,* 195–217.

Haznedar, B., & Schwartz, B. (1997). Are there optional infinitives in child L2 acquisition? *BUCLD 21 Proceedings,* 257–268.

Jakubowicz, C., Nash, L., & van der Velde, M. (1999). Inflection and past tense morphology in French SLI. In A. Greenhill, H. Littlefield, & C. Tano (Eds.), *BUCLD 23* (pp. 289–300). Somerville, MA: Cascadilla Press.

Lardiere, D. (1998). Case and tense in the "fossilized" steady state. *Second Language Research, 14*, 1–26.

Leonard, L. (1998). *Children with specific language impairment.* Cambridge, MA: MIT Press.

Meyer Bjerkan, K. (1999, July). *Do SLI children have an optional infinitive stage?* Paper presented at the conference of the International Association for the Study of Child Language, San Sebastian, Spain.

Paradis, J., & Crago, M. (2000). Tense and temporality: A comparison between children learning a second language and children with SLI. *Journal of Speech, Language and Hearing Research, 43*(4), 834–848.

Paradis, J., & Crago, M. (in press). The morphosyntax of specific language impairment in French: Evidence of an extended optional default account. *Language Acquisition.*

Paradis, J., Crago, M., Genesee, F., & Rice, M. (2001, June). *Bilingual children with SLI: How do they compare with their monolingual peers.* Paper presented at the Symposium on Research in Child Language Disorders, Madison, WI.

Paradis, J., & Genesee, F. (1997). On continuity and the emergence of functional categories in bilingual first language acquisition. *Studies in Second Language Acquisition, 6*, 91–124.

Paradis, J., Le Corre, M., & Genesee, F. (1998). The emergence of tense and agreement in child L2 French. *Second Language Research, 14*(3), 227–256.

Poeppel, D., & Wexler, K. (1993). The full competence hypothesis of clause structure in early German. *Language, 69*, 1–33.

Prévost, P. (1997). Truncation and root infinitives in second language acquisition of French. *BUCLD 21 Proceedings*, 453–464.

Prévost, P., & White, L. (2000). Accounting for morphological variation in L2 acquisition: Truncation or missing inflection? In M. A. Friedmann & L. Rizzi (Eds.), *The acquisition of syntax* (pp. 202–234). London, England: Longman.

Rice, M., Ruff Noll, K., & Grimm, H. (1997). An extended optional infinitive stage in German-speaking children with specific language impairment. *Language Acquisition, 6*(4), 255–296.

Rice, M., & Wexler, K. (1996). Toward tense as a clinical marker of specific language impairment in English-speaking children. *Journal of Speech, Language and Hearing Research, 39*, 1236–1257.

Rice, M., Wexler, K., & Hershberger, S. (1998). Tense over time: The longitudinal course of tense acquisition in children with specific language impairment. *Journal of Speech, Language and Hearing Research, 41*, 1412–1431.

Roberts, S., & Leonard, L. (1997). Grammatical deficits in German and English: A crosslinguistic study of children with specific language impairment. *First Language, 17*, 131–150.

Wexler, K. (1996). The development of inflection in a biologically based theory of language acquisition. In M. Rice (Ed.), *Towards a genetics of language* (pp. 114–144). Hillsdale, NJ: Lawrence Erlbaum Associates.

Wexler, K. (1998). Very early parameter setting and the unique checking constraint: A new explanation of the optional infinitive stage. *Lingua, 106*, 23–79.

4

Do Heterogeneous Deficits Require Heterogeneous Theories? SLI Subgroups and the RDDR Hypothesis

Heather K. J. van der Lely

Center for Developmental Language Disorders and Cognitive Neuroscience, Department of Human Communication Science, University College London

The heterogeneity of specific language impairment (SLI) in children is a major issue in current research on the etiology of the disorder. Are these studies looking at one or many disorders? And, what are the relations between co-occurring deficits found in some children with SLI? Determining whether differences between various forms of SLI are qualitative or quantitative would considerably advance understanding of the disorder and could have direct clinical implications. For instance, if there are definable subgroups, with different etiologies, then distinctive theories as well as therapeutic approaches may be called for. Furthermore, such knowledge would provide valuable insight into the development of cognitive function and structure—a focal area of ongoing debate in cognitive science. This chapter first discusses the theoretical and methodological issues raised by the heterogeneity of SLI. Second, it argues for the detailed study of SLI subgroups to complement those of nondifferentiated SLI groups. Third, to illustrate the subgroup approach, consideration is given to the characteristics of the grammatical-SLI (G-SLI) subgroup and the representational deficit for dependent relations (RDDR) hypothesis, which has been advanced to account for the grammatical deficits found in G-SLI.

THE HETEROGENEITY ISSUE

An ongoing controversy surrounds the heterogeneity of the linguistic and cognitive characteristics found in children with SLI and the significance of this for any single account of the cause and nature of the disorder. Although there is a general consensus that a genetic deficit causes SLI (Bishop, 1997b; Bishop, North, & Donlan, 1995; Fisher, Vargha-Khadem, Watkins, Monaco, & Marcus, 1998; Leonard, 1998; van der Lely & Stollwerck, 1996; see also Wexler, chap. 1 in this volume), researchers are far from understanding how genes affect the development of neural pathways to result in an impaired grammatical system or in an impairment in language abilities generally. A further issue in this controversy is whether aspects of language, such as parts of grammar, are under specific genetic control. Some scholars reject the notion that a genetic impairment can lead to specific higher order cognitive deficits (Elman et al., 1996; Karmiloff-Smith, 1998; Tomblin & Pandich, 1999), whereas others contend that this is a viable possibility (Marcus, 1999; Pinker, 1999; van der Lely, Rosen, & McClelland, 1998). This controversy revolves around the domain-general versus domain-specific view of the development of specialized cognitive systems.

The *domain-general*, or *domain-relevant*, perspective puts forward that mechanisms underlying specialized functions are not unique to any one function, but become specialized with the development process and specific environmental interactions (Elman et al., 1996; Karmiloff-Smith, 1998). Moreover, Karmiloff-Smith (1998) contended that any genetic deficit affecting cognitive functioning is likely to result in a cascade of subtle deficits rather than a single higher level one. Furthermore, Karmiloff-Smith (1998) considered that different cognitive disorders lie on a continuum, rather than are truly specific. According to the domain-general perspective, this is because genes cannot target specific mechanisms, because mechanisms are not developmentally specific to any one function (Elman et al., 1996; Karmiloff-Smith, 1998). Thus, the domain-general perspective predicts that developmental domain-specific deficits should not exist. Therefore, the finding of a domain-specific deficit in the absence of any other cognitive impairment would be evidence against this theoretical perspective.

Alternatively, the domain-specific perspective contends that genetically determined cognitive mechanisms could uniquely subserve specialized cognitive functions such as grammar (Coltheart, 1999; Marcus, 1999; Pinker, 1994, 1999; van der Lely et al., 1998). Marcus (1999) argued that by acting as switches, specific "master control genes" could trigger complex hierarchical cascades of genes that elicit widely varying arrangements of cells. Moreover, aspects of language could be under specific genetic control and, for instance, a specific grammatical impairment could reflect the absence of some gene that ordinarily triggers a cascade of events that leads to the construction of machinery that uniquely subserves grammar (Marcus, 1999). Thus, the finding of a consistent co-occurring deficit or deficits alongside a grammatical deficit would provide evidence against this domain-specific perspective.

The issue of the nature of SLI is relevant to basic research as well as to clinical assessment and remediation of children with SLI, because definable subgroups, with different etiologies, may require distinctive therapeutic approaches. Thus, does SLI constitute multiple disorders, which vary subtly in genetic and behavioral characteristics? Does it constitute different and specific deficits, which occur heterogeneously across populations of SLI children? Or, is it a single deficit, which variably manifests itself in cognitive and linguistic deficits?

One approach to address these controversial issues is to study selected, homogeneous subgroups and compare their performance across behavioral measures of grammar, nongrammatical language abilities, and nonverbal abilities. Comparisons within and between subgroups, and between subgroups and groups who are not homogeneous selected SLI subgroups, could yield invaluable insight into whether these are truly qualitatively different forms of SLI, as well as into the developmental relations between aspects of language and cognitive function. Toward this end, the next three sections review data from nonlinguistic cognitive abilities, nongrammatical abilities, and grammatical abilities of an SLI subgroup of children with G-SLI and compare their pattern of performance with those of other groups of SLI children reported in the literature, in order to consider possible interpretations of these data with respect to the nature and cause of SLI.

The G-SLI subgroup is a homogeneous subgroup of children with SLI, who are selected for exhibiting persistent grammatical impairment. These children do not display pragmatic language impairments or any consistent nonverbal cognitive deficits (van der Lely et al., 1998). All the children were age 9 or older (up to age 18) when selected. They exhibit grammatical deficits in syntax and morphology, which affect performance on comprehension, expression, grammaticality judgments, and sentence-picture judgment tasks. G-SLI subjects' speech is clear and intelligible and they do not evince speech (dyspraxic) impairment, although subtle phonological deficits are evident upon detailed testing (Peiris, 2000; van der Lely & Harris, unpublished data, 1999). As with many children with SLI, vocabulary development lags behind normal, but is generally less impaired than their grammatical abilities. In contrast, language abilities that rely on pragmatic skills, such as theory of mind, inferential abilities, or pragmatic-social abilities (understanding what the listener knows and can infer, e.g., in story-telling) are age appropriate (van der Lely, 1997; van der Lely et al., 1998).

SLI IN CHILDREN WITH AND WITHOUT CO-OCCURRING NONVERBAL COGNITIVE DEFICITS

Low IQ scores (less than 85 IQ) alongside language impairment are reported in studies of SLI twins (D. Bishop, Bright, James, S. Bishop, & van der Lely, 2000), in the "KE" family (a large family spanning three generations of which half suffer from SLI; Vargha-Khadem, Watkins, Fletcher, & Passing-ham, 1995), as well as in longitudinal studies of SLI children (Aram, Ekel-man, & Nation, 1984; Leonard, 1998). Some researchers have interpreted this finding as a general measure of cognitive impairment in children with SLI, and as providing support for the domain-general, nonmodular view of cognitive development (Bishop, 1997b; Elman et al., 1996; Karmiloff-Smith, 1998). Thus, it might be expected that those children with co-occurring cog-nitive deficits would have more severe language impairment. However, this does not appear to be the case.

When similar language assessments have been administered to subjects with and without nonverbal cognitive impairments alongside SLI, they show little difference in their language performance. For example, the same test of past tense morphology was administered to the KE family and the G-SLI subgroup (Ullman & Gopnik, 1999; van der Lely & Ullman, 2001). Both sub-jects from the KE family and the G-SLI subgroup were impaired in produc-ing regular and irregular past tense forms, were more impaired relative to control subjects in producing regular forms, and, in contrast to control sub-jects, showed frequency effects for regular past tense production (Ullman & Gopnik, 1999; van der Lely & Ullman, 2001). The affected members of the KE family had a mean performance IQ of 86 (range 71–111), whereas the unaf-fected members had a mean IQ of 104 (range 84–119) (Vargha-Khadem et al., 1995). These data are taken by some scholars to indicate that SLI is a multi-faceted cognitive deficit affecting many cognitive functions (Elman et al., 1996; Karmiloff-Smith, 1998). However, this conclusion seems premature. First, it is noteworthy that there is considerable overlap in IQ in the affected and unaffected members of the KE family, yet no direct relation is found be-tween severity of language deficit and cognitive abilities. Furthermore, de-spite strong similarities between the KE family and the G-SLI children in the test of past tense morphology, the G-SLI subjects' mean performance IQ is 99.09 (range 86–119) (van der Lely & Stollwerck, 1997; van der Lely & Ullman, 2001). Moreover, within the G-SLI subgroup, severity of grammati-cal impairment does not appear to be related in any way to performance IQ; the brightest subjects in the subgroup continue to have severe gram-matical difficulties (van der Lely, 1997; van der Lely et al., 1998). Thus, without a theory of how a particular genetic deficit can cause multiple cognitive impairments—including grammar in some individuals, but se-lected primary grammatical deficits in other individuals—there appears to be little reason to pursue this line of inquiry in its broadest form, as the evidence directly conflicts with the predictions of a broad version of the domain-general perspective.

A narrower version of the domain-general perspective is the long-stand-ing hypothesis that SLI is caused by capacity limitations for processing rap-idly successive auditory verbal and nonverbal stimuli (Tallal, 2000). Indeed,

Tallal et al. (1996), Wright et al. (1996), and colleagues claimed that performance on nonverbal auditory tasks distinguishes normal children from those with language impairment. Moreover, remediation of the nonverbal auditory processing deficit is claimed to improve general language abilities (Tallal, 2000). Evidence showing a consistent deficit in auditory processing in all SLI children would provide convincing evidence for a strong relation between mechanisms involved in nonverbal cognitive abilities and language abilities.

This chapter examines 1 of the 28 studies that Tallal (2000) claimed demonstrates that SLI subjects have deficits with speed of nonverbal auditory processing, and compares their findings with those of auditory investigations of the G-SLI subgroup. Neville, Coffey, Holcomb, and Tallal's (1993) study is particularly interesting to the issues central to this discussion. First, it provides neurophysiological (event-related potentials) evidence alongside behavioral measures. Second, it provides data on nonverbal auditory processing and grammatical sentence processing. And third, it explores individual profiles alongside group data.

Neville et al. (1993) studied 34, 9-year-old children with SLI and reading disabilities who were part of the longitudinal cohort studied by Tallal and colleagues since they were 4 years old and an age matched group of control children. The subjects were administered tests, including the Tallal Auditory Repetition Tests, in which tones of different frequencies were presented at different rates (i.e., by varying the interstimuli intervals, ISI), and the Curtiss and Yamada Comprehensive Language Evaluation–Full, including the syntactic subtests (see Curtiss et al., 1992). ERP recordings of open and closed class words during online sentence processing were also made while the subjects read sentences that ended in a semantically appropriate or anomalous word.

The results revealed that, as a group, the children showed abnormalities in behavioral and neurophysiological measures of these auditory and grammatical abilities—thus, concurring with much previous research (Tallal & Piercy, 1973). However, finer grained analyses revealed that within the group multiple aspects of processing were affected, but the effect was heterogeneous across the group (Neville et al., 1993). ERP components linked to auditory processing were abnormal only in a subset of the children who also displayed abnormal auditory temporal discrimination. Conversely, abnormal ERP components associated with syntactic processing were found for a subset of children who scored poorly on tests of grammar. Neville et al. (1993) pointed out that it is important to note that this second subset of children is not the same as that which displayed auditory sensory processing deficits. Indeed, grammatical impairment was not correlated with the sensory deficits in this study. In sum, Neville et al. (1993) concluded that their data clearly indicate that multiple factors contribute to language processing deficits and these deficits are heterogeneous across populations of SLI children.

Moreover, Bishop and colleagues' studies of monozygotic (MZ) and dizygotic (DZ) twins revealed that environmental factors rather than genetic factors account for auditory impairments in children with SLI, whereas the reverse is the case for phonological abilities and syntactic abilities, which were the same syntactic abilities on which subjects with G-SLI children fail (Bishop, 1997a; Bishop et al., 1999a). These data further indicate that the underlying causes of auditory and grammatical impairments in children are not directly related.

However, it is still necessary to provide detailed analyses of auditory abilities of different subgroups in order to see if auditory abilities are affecting the language disorder in any way. The G-SLI subgroup could be similar to the subgroup in Tallal's cohort who exhibits grammatical deficits. The study tested 15 G-SLI subjects' auditory processing on two tasks, which have been claimed to distinguish normal children from those with impaired language development. First, Tallal and Piercy's (1973) same/different tasks presenting complex tones that vary in fundamental frequency, synthesized *ba–da*, and the second formant (F2) alone from the *ba–da* condition, with varying ISIs (0–400 ms), were used to compare the G-SLI subjects' auditory processing with that of age matched controls and younger children matched on vocabulary abilities or sentence understanding. The *ba–da* sounds are comprised of a number of formants, only one of which (the second formant, or F2) carries the phonemic distinction. Presentation of sounds with the second formant on its own, enabled presentation of sounds that contained the same dynamic spectral information, but were not heard as speech. Both the speech sounds and the nonspeech analogues have the same spectral transitions, but the speech sounds are acoustically more complex (in that they have other noninformative formants present). The nonspeech sounds were also presented on a monotone, to make them even less speechlike—they can be said to sound like quacks. The results revealed that the effect of ISI did not discriminate the groups from each other. Moreover, as a group, the G-SLI subjects' performance did not differ on any condition from that of the language matched controls but was significantly impaired in the tasks in comparison to the age controls. However, calculation of standardized residual (z scores) for each G-SLI subject based on the mean and standard deviation of the age matched controls, revealed that 66% (10/15) G-SLI subjects were normal (within 1.64 *SD*) (range $z = +1.03$ to -1.22) in their auditory processing of the F2 alone condition and 44% (6/15) were normal on the *ba–da* and tone condition (Rosen, van der Lely, & Dry, 1997; van der Lely, Rosen, & Adlard, MS., 2002).

The second set of auditory tests examining absolute thresholds, backward and simultaneous masking in a band-pass noise (Rosen, van der Lely,

& Adlard, 1999) revealed a broadly similar pattern of performance for the groups. The G-SLI subjects performed significantly better than the language matched control groups, but as a group performed worse than the age matched controls. However, once again, individual analysis revealed that a substantial number of the G-SLI subjects (57% 8/14, for backward masking, and 71% 10/14 for simultaneous masking) were within 1.64 *SD* (range: backward masking, $z = -1.59$ to $+1.48$; simultaneous $z = -1.59$ to $+.14$) of the age controls' mean score with 5/14 G-SLI subjects being within 1 *SD* of the age controls' mean score on both tasks. Finally, there was no correlation between performance on auditory tasks and grammatical tasks. The grammatical impairment in G-SLI children did not differ as a function of performance on auditory tasks (van der Lely et al., 1998).

In sum, the findings from investigations of nonverbal cognitive abilities in nondifferentiated populations of SLI children and auditory abilities in the G-SLI subgroup, and those in the Tallal longitudinal cohort of SLI children investigated by Neville and colleagues (Neville et al., 1993) largely concur and, moreover, prove inconsistent with the domain-general predictions.

GRAMMATICAL IMPAIRMENT IN CHILDREN WITH AND WITHOUT NONGRAMMATICAL LANGUAGE DEFICITS

Language impairments in nongrammatical aspects of language, such as pragmatic-social abilities are also variably reported for children with SLI (Bishop, 1997b). Pragmatic-social knowledge, needed for example in storytelling, involves anticipating the knowledge and needs of your listener (intuitive psychology), rather than grammatical rules of a language. Therefore, pragmatic ability is likely to tap memory capacity, inferential abilities (including Theory of Mind), previous world knowledge, as well more general processing and integration of information for online monitoring of the listeners needs (see also Schaeffer, chap. 5 in this volume). Thus, many cognitive capacities are involved in normal pragmatic ability. Therefore, the co-occurrence of grammatical and pragmatic language deficits is unlikely to reflect a domain-specific language deficit of a language system that underlies both abilities, but nothing else.

There appear to be (at least) two subgroups of children with SLI with different linguistic characteristics, who are pragmatically impaired. The first of these is the subgroup, identified by Rapin and Alan (1983) as semantic-pragmatic deficit syndrome. This subgroup is characterized by normal or relatively intact grammar and phonology, but with inadequate conversational skills, selecting inappropriate words, poor maintenance of topic, and so on (Bishop & Rosenbloom, 1987; Conti-Ramsden, Crutchley, & Botting, 1997; Rapin & Allen, 1983). These children exhibit similar pragmatic-language deficits as those of subjects with autism, but without all of the concomitant social-cognitive and behaviors disorders associated with autism. Although it has been suggested that children with semantic-pragmatic disorder have a mild form of autism, the evidence is inconclusive (Bishop, 2000). However, pragmatic-SLI is clearly distinct from G-SLI. G-SLI subjects have normal pragmatic abilities as measured by, for example, their use of pronouns in story-telling and their ability to make conversational inferences (van der Lely, 1997; van der Lely et al., 1998). Conversely, some children with grammatical (syntactic and phonological) impairments also have pragmatic impairments as shown by tests of referential communication skills and story comprehension (Bishop & Adams, 1991, 1992). The dissociation between impairments of pragmatics and grammar, albeit that these disorders can co-occur, indicates the independence of developmental pragmatic and grammatical impairments, and it may be concluded, their underlying cognitive systems (see also Schaeffer, chap. 5 in this volume). This is not to say that when pragmatic and grammatical impairments co-occur in a child, they will not interact and cause a complex, language disorder—clearly they will. However, the manifestation of such a complex language disorder does not necessarily mean that the subcomponents of the disorder are fundamentally related.

Further deficits in nongrammatical language abilities (i.e., in vocabulary development) have also been taken to suggest that more general purpose cognitive systems are important for language but are not restricted to language acquisition (Bates & Goodman, 1997; Tomblin & Pandich, 1999). In particular, Tomblin and Pandich (1999) and other researchers (e.g., Bates & Goodman, 1997) interpret a high correlation between vocabulary and morphology scores as evidence to support the theory that the same mechanism underlies syntactic acquisition and vocabulary development.

Although G-SLI subjects, like many children with language impairment, evince vocabulary impairment (van der Lely & Stollwerck, 1997), an alternative interpretation is that there are (at least) two or three mechanisms involved in word learning (Bloom, 1999, 2000) and G-SLI subject's vocabulary impairment results from their grammatical deficit (van der Lely, 1994). Because many factors contribute to word learning and some of the abilities that contribute to it are specific to language and some are not (Bloom, 2000; Bloom & Markson, 1998), vocabulary impairment can co-occur with many cognitive impairments. Among the abilities needed for word learning Bloom and Markson (1998) argued that children succeed at word learning because they possess certain conceptual biases about the external world, they have the ability to infer the referential intentions of others, and they develop an appreciation of syntactic cues to word meaning. Thus, children with pragmatic-SLI or autism could fail to learn word meaning due to impaired mechanisms underlying inferential abilities, whereas G-SLI children and other children with grammatical impairment fail to learn word meaning because of their grammatical deficit, which affects the use of syntactic cues to word meaning (van der Lely, 1994). Moreover, subjects with G-SLI are normal with respect to logical reasoning and social-pragmatic inference (van der Lely et al., 1998)—the abilities likely to underlie the second mechanisms for word learning listed earlier. Consistent with this alternative, children with G-SLI are impaired in using grammatical cues to learn the meaning of novel verbs (O'Hara & Johnston, 1997; van der Lely 1994), novel collective nouns (Froud & van der Lely, 2002), and are particularly impaired in learning the semantic scope of quantifiers (*every, all*) (van der Lely & Drozd, unpublished data, 1999), and abstract words and relational terms (Leonard, 1998)—exactly those words and aspects of meaning for which grammatical cues are relevant.

In conclusion, the previous data showing language impairments outside the grammatical system do not necessarily provide evidence against a specific and dedicated mechanism underlying grammar. There is evidence from children with SLI and with other cognitive disorders that pragmatic and grammatical impairments dissociate. Further, vocabulary deficits might be predicted in children with grammatical deficit because grammatical cues play an important role in word learning. "Vocabulary" should not be thought of as a core unitary language system per se; and grammatical impairment could cause the vocabulary deficits found in children with SLI.

GRAMMATICAL IMPAIRMENTS IN CHILDREN: VARIATION IN PHONOLOGICAL, MORPHOLOGICAL, AND SYNTACTIC IMPAIRMENT

The distinction between different forms of SLI within the grammatical system is less clear than those between the grammatical system and non-grammatical language systems and nonverbal systems. Caron and Rutter (1991) pointed out that in developmental disorders, the probability of two disorders co-occurring is greater than expected from the population incidence of either disorder alone. Consequently, when impairments within the grammatical system co-occur, as they frequently do, it is less clear whether researchers are looking at comorbidity of two or more different conditions that frequently occur together in the same individual, or variations in the manifestation of the same underlying disorder. Bearing this in mind, first consider phonological impairments and their relation to syntactic impairments.

Primary, specific phonological impairment can be found in children and adults with dyslexia, and it is accepted by many researchers that this reading and writing disorder as well as other related cognitive deficits (e.g., impaired verbal short-term memory) is a consequence of a phonological representational deficit (Snowling, 2000; Snowling & Hulme, 1994). Thus, it seems that developmental phonological impairment can occur without syntactic impairment. However, there is some evidence from longitudinal prospective and cross-sectional studies that expressive or receptive vocabulary may be impaired in children with dyslexia (Gallagher, Frith, & Snowling, 2000; Gathercole & Baddeley, 1989, 1990). Once again, researchers make reasoned arguments that the vocabulary deficits are a consequence later in development of a primary phonological processing impairment (Frith & Happé, 1998; Snowling, 2000).

In contrast to the scant evidence of syntactic or morphological problems in children with primary phonological deficits, many children with SLI, including those classified as G-SLI, have phonological impairment (Bishop, North, & Donlan, 1996; Peiris, 2000; van der Lely & Harris, 1999, unpublished data). One interpretation of this variable co-occurrence of syntactic and phonological impairment is that the phonological deficits are caused by different etiologies in dyslexia and SLI. Consistent with the domain-specific deficit view of G-SLI is that a common grammar-specific proto-mechanism underlies structural relations in syntax and phonology. G-SLI subjects' syntactic abilities reveal particular problems with dependent structural relations (van der Lely, 1998). Further, initial analysis of G-SLI subject's phonological deficits indicates that their expressive phonological abilities break down only with increasing structural phonological complexity (Peiris, 2000). Thus, the evidence so far is consistent with an impairment of domain-specific grammatical mechanism(s) or representation(s) underlying structural relations. However, it is not clear whether a similar deficit could only affect the phonological system in children, as in dyslexia, or whether the origins of phonological impairment in dyslexia is different from that of SLI.

Although the theoretical framework adopted here concurs with specialized mechanisms (e.g., those in syntax, phonology, or morphology) underlying grammar—and as such proto-mechanisms could underlie grammatical structural relations generally—normal phonological (or morphological) development may also rely on mechanisms that are not unique to the grammatical system or to humans. For example, babies appear to be "pre-wired" to attend to and use phonotactic information, prosody, and stress patterns from the speech stream to enable them by 10 months or so to identify "words" in connected speech, although they have no knowledge of word meaning (Jusczyk, 1999). However, these abilities might not be specific to humans but might be shared by other primates (Houser, 1996). Therefore, although these early language detection abilities lay the foundation for later phonological development (Jusczyk, 1999), a deficit with such abilities may not be indicative of a language-specific deficit. In contrast, only humans are capable of forming complex structural syntactic and phonological relations. Thus, as with vocabulary development (phonological deficits may occur for a variety of reasons), only one of them is directly related to a deficit in a specialized dedicated mechanism for grammar in its broader sense, and thus, general mechanisms may also contribute to normal phonological functioning. Further research comparing detailed linguistic analysis of subjects with dyslexia and SLI, if possible, alongside genetic analysis, could lead to a better understanding of the relation between these deficits.

Consider the reported differences in morphological impairments in children with SLI. Although it is widely agreed that morphology is impaired in children with SLI (Bishop, 1994; Clahsen, 1989; Dalalakis, 1994, 1996; Gopnik, 1990; Leonard, 1998; Rice & Wexler, 1996; van der Lely, 1998), the characterization of the deficit varies in different studies of SLI subjects. Some differences may be due to an investigative strategy that focuses on certain aspects of morphology. For instance, most scholars agree that inflectional morphology is impaired—although not uniformly—in SLI, but that derivational morphology is unimpaired (Clahsen, 1989; Leonard, 1998; Rice & Wexler, 1996). However, Dalalakis, (1994, 1996) revealed that when derivational morphology is directly investigated, deficits are evident in English- and Greek-speaking subjects with SLI. It is unclear how extensive deficits in derivational morphology are in the SLI population, because this aspect of language has not received the attention of other aspects of language such as tense or agreement marking (cf. Clahsen, Bartke, & Goellner, 1997; Rice, Wexler, & Cleave, 1995). Thus, until derivational morphology is subjected to more general, detailed investigation, it can only be concluded that the "heterogeneity" in the morphological characteristics of children with SLI is attributable to researchers' investigative strategy, rather than true differences between subjects.

Conversely, using similar investigatory techniques to assess different populations of subjects with SLI, qualitative differences have been revealed in the SLI children's underlying deficits. A clear example of this is two investigations of word formation in noun compounding, both based on Gordon's (1985) study (see also Clahsen & Temple, chap. 13 in this volume, for a similar experiment with children with Williams syndrome). Oetting and Rice's (1993) study of 14, 5-year-old children with SLI found that the majority (11/14) produced irregular plural nouns inside compounds, (e.g., *mice-eater*) but not regular plural nouns (**rats-eater*). Thus, they showed a similar pattern of performance as normally developing children and adults (Gordon, 1985; Oetting & Rice, 1993; van der Lely & Christian, 2000). In contrast, van der Lely and Christian's (2000) study of 16, 10- to 18-year-old G-SLI subjects revealed that the majority of their subjects (14/16) produced regular nouns (*rats-eater*) as well as irregular nouns inside compounds. This indicates that the majority of G-SLI subjects are preferentially storing regular plural forms in their lexicon, rather than computing such forms on the basis of a grammatical rule. It is interesting that, in Oetting and Rice's (1993) study, three subjects with SLI performed in a similar way to the G-SLI subjects, producing regular plural nouns inside compounds. Thus, differences in the subjects' ages cannot account for the differences between the children's performance. These studies suggest qualitative differences between SLI children's morphological representation of words and thus heterogeneity (even) within the grammatical system in the nature of SLI. Replication and substantiation of such findings have implications for the understanding of the disorder and suggest fractionation of impairments within the grammatical system that are revealed in development.

Finally, this section comments on the implications of the finding that syntactic errors made by children with SLI are also found in much younger children who are developing normally. Recent research, particularly that of Wexler and colleagues (Wexler, Schütze, & Rice, 1998), highlights the similarities between SLI grammar and that of much younger children (see also Rice, chap. 2 in this volume; Wexler, chap. 1 in this volume). For example, the use of infinitival verb forms (*jump*) in a matrix clause context when a tensed form would be expected (*jumps, jumped*) is used by both children with SLI and young normally developing children (Rice et al., 1995). More recently, Bishop and colleagues (Bishop et al., 2000; Norbury, Bishop, & Briscoe, 2000), replicating the findings of impaired understanding on passive sentences and assigning reference to pronouns and reflexives previously found for G-SLI subjects (van der Lely, 1996; van der Lely & Stollwerck, 1997), found that young normally developing children (if they make any errors) make errors that show a similar pattern to those of children with SLI. Norbury et al. (2000) interpreted this finding as evidence for general processing limitations and against a modular domain-specific deficit underlying the syntactic errors in SLI grammar.

Although general processing limitations remain a possibility, an alternative is that maturational factors and development within the (domain-specific) grammatical system causes such syntactic errors in young children (cf. Wexler, 1998; chap. 1 in this volume). The difference between children with SLI and those developing normally is that (genetically controlled?) grammatical maturation occurs in children developing normally but not in children with SLI who remain at an early stage in particular areas of syntactic acquisition and thus continue to produce grammatical errors found in young children.[1] Moreover, as a general processing deficit account

---

[1]An alternative explanation within the "Continuity framework" (Radford, 1990) would be that a genetic deficit affects the underlying representations or mechanisms underlying these representations for the parameters within UG, causing later difficulties in determining appropriate parameter setting—hence the deficits in SLI do not show up until later. However, the distinction between the maturational and continuity approaches are not central to the line of reasoning pursued here.

is inconsistent with the selective deficits within syntax found in many children with SLI (see later), a deficit with a genetically determined specialized mechanism, necessary for the normal development of grammar, provides a more parsimonious explanation for the deficits found.

IMPLICATIONS OF HETEROGENEITY IN SLI

The previous sections have provided a snap shot of the available evidence to evaluate whether there is support for consistent co-occurring deficits in nonverbal abilities or nongrammatical language abilities with grammatical deficits. In addition, within the grammatical system in its broader sense (syntax, phonology, morphology), they considered the autonomy versus the association between these grammatical systems in different developmental disorders, as well as illustrated qualitative differences within one grammatical system (morphology) found in different groups of children with SLI.

The data were striking for the fact that despite extensive investigation, no consistent deficit in nonverbal abilities or nongrammatical abilities has been found to occur in all children with grammatical-syntactic deficits. However, many children with SLI show one or more deficits in nonverbal or nongrammatical language abilities that appear unrelated to their syntactic deficits. The occurrence of auditory and cognitive deficits or nongrammatical language deficits in the absence of language impairment, and, conversely, the absence of such deficits in children with G-SLI, strongly indicate the autonomy of these cognitive systems. Thus, these data are inconsistent with the domain-general perspective underlying specialized grammatical abilities. The simplest explanation for the association between disorders is the propensity for comorbidity of disorders in development (Caron & Rutter, 1991).

The autonomy of deficits within the grammatical system is less clear. The evidence for phonological disorder in subjects with dyslexia, in the absence of syntactic disorder, clearly indicates the independence of these grammatical systems. This finding alongside the evidence of underlying phonological deficits in many, if not all, children who evince syntactic deficits attest to qualitatively different causes underlying phonological impairment. The co-occurrence of phonological and syntactic impairments in children with SLI speaks to the extent of the deficit within the grammatical system. Contrary to some scholars' view (e.g., Bishop et al., 2000; Norbury et al., 2000), there appears to be no convincing reason to reject the domain-specific deficit hypothesis on the basis of these data. As already mentioned, phonological structure, like syntactic structure, is hierarchical in nature and involves structural complexity (Chomsky, 1986; Harris, 1994) and is part of the language faculty unique to humans (Pinker, 1994). Thus, it is feasible that a genetically determined specialized mechanism, unique to grammatical systems, is adopted and developed to independently serve both phonology and syntax and thereby can be selectively impaired in children with SLI.

Finally, the apparent fractionation of deficits in SLI, illustrated by differences in the lexical representation of morphologically regular words, further emphasizes the heterogeneous nature of SLI and the need for detailed investigation of a broad range of language abilities in different SLI subgroups, if this disorder is to be fully understood. However, it should be noted that performance on any experimental tests of grammar (syntax, morphology, phonology) measured by behavioral scales (i.e., performance measures rather than neurological measures such as event-related potential) might be subject to postgrammatical, cognitive knowledge and information processes.[2] Thus, a deficit, with a particular syntactic structure could result in different children using different strategies or cognitive abilities to cope with the task. Thus, although the RDDR hypothesis can predict where the problems may or may not occur within the grammar, it does not predict the child's use of nongrammatical cognitive resources.

In sum, the evidence supports the view that genetically determined cognitive mechanisms underlie specialized cognitive functions and can be developmentally selectively impaired. However, the underlying autonomy of deficits within the grammatical system and within each subsystem (e.g., morphology or syntax) requires further research before conclusions can be drawn with any confidence.

The final sections describe, first, the syntactic characteristics of the subgroup of children with G-SLI, and second, the representational deficit for dependent relations (RDDR) hypothesis, which specifies where the breakdown in the syntactic system is occurring, which could lead to G-SLI grammar. These sections aim to illustrate how using a complementary approach to the study of SLI (i.e., studying highly selected homogeneous SLI subgroups) can contribute and advance knowledge of the cause of the disorder.

SYNTACTIC CHARACTERISTICS
OF THE G-SLI SUBGROUP

This section aims to provide a description of the syntactic abilities and disabilities of children with G-SLI. This aim may be contrasted with those who seek to highlight prototypical characteristics or clinical markers of SLI

---

[2]Although measurements of grammar from experimental procedures are potentially subjec to extra grammatical processing, they have the advantage over spontaneous speech analysi where the target utterance is unknown and/or the child simply avoids problematic structures.

such as the incorrect use of optional infinitives (Rice & Wexler, 1996; Rice, chap. 2 in this volume; Wexler, chap. 1 in this volume) or impaired nonword repetition (Bishop et al., 1996).

Subjects with G-SLI evince a broad deficit in aspects of syntax that are normally taken to be core to the human language faculty (Smith, 1999). First, G-SLI subjects show the deficits in tense and agreement marking that are reported in many studies of children with SLI (e.g., Clahsen, 1997; Rice & Wexler, 1996). As with all their grammatical errors, these are found regardless of processing factors. For instance, past tense marking errors, where the infinitival form is used in a past tense context, are found in spontaneous speech, expressive story-telling tasks, elicitation tasks, as well as grammaticality judgments (Gollner, 1995; van der Lely, 1997; van de Lely & Ullman, 1996, 2001). However, G-SLI is not a deficit restricted to inflectional morphology. One of the most reliable findings in G-SLI subjects is problems with assigning theta roles in reversible passive sentences or sentences with complex argument structure, such as dative sentences (van der Lely, 1994, 1996; van der Lely & Dewart, 1986; van der Lely & Harris, 1990). Thus, subjects with G-SLI may interpret *The man is eaten by the fish* or *The man is being eaten*, as either an active sentence (*The man is eating the fish*) or as an adjectival passive (*The eaten man*). Recent research reveals that similar deficits are evinced in other English-speaking and Greek-speaking children with SLI, although some of the children studied do not show such discrete deficits in grammar as the G-SLI subgroup (Bishop et al., 2000; Norbury et al., 2000; Precious & Conti-Ramsden, 1988; Stavrakaki, 2001a, 2001b). G-SLI subject's problems with structural syntactic relations are also revealed when assigning co-reference to pronouns and anaphors in sentences when only syntactic cues are available (e.g., *Mowgli says Baloo is tickling him/himself*), as well as understanding and producing embedded phrases and clauses (*The frog with the blanket . . .*) (van der Lely & Hennesey, 1999; van der Lely & Stollwerck, 1997). Thus, in a story-telling task, subjects with G-SLI produced few, if any, spontaneous embedded or subordinate clauses (van der Lely, 1997). Similar deficits with general structural relations affecting verb structure, noun phrases, as well as clauses and embedded structures are slowly emerging in the literature for other groups of children with SLI (Bishop et al., 2000; Hamann, Penner, & Lindner, 1998; Ingham, Fletcher, Schelletter, & Sinka, 1998; Jakubowicz, Nash, Rigaut, & Gérard, 1998; Norbury et al., 2001; Stavrakaki, 2001a, 2001b). Thus, although deficits in syntactic structural relations are not typically reported, this may well be due to an artifact of an investigative focus on inflectional morphology. As recent research indicates, the SLI deficit is much broader in the general SLI population as well as in subjects with G-SLI.

Finally, G-SLI subjects, like many children with SLI, show both correct and incorrect performance for the same syntactic structure. Thus, it is rare for any structure to be "missing" per se from G-SLI grammar, although many structures are certainly problematic. In sum, the G-SLI subgroup inconsistently manipulates core aspects of syntax. The RDDR hypothesis provides a precise account of the deficit within the syntactic system.

THE REPRESENTATIONAL DEFICIT
FOR DEPENDENT RELATIONS HYPOTHESIS

The representational deficit for dependent relations hypothesis (RDDR) hypothesis, developed over a number of years, aims to account for the broad range of deficits found in G-SLI subjects that are at the core of the syntactic system. The RDDR account identifies the underlying deficit in the computational syntactic system—that is, in the syntax proper (van der Lely, 1994, 1998; van der Lely & Stollwerck, 1997). As a working hypothesis, the RDDR hypothesis assumes that although much of language might arise from general cognitive capacities, certain aspects of grammar have an autonomous psychological and neural basis. Investigations into G-SLI children aim to provide a further step toward identifying which aspects of the grammatical system are autonomous. The RDDR account is not tied to the linguistic minimalist program (Chomsky, 1995, 1998, 1999), but uses it to provide a precise definition of G-SLI grammar. The RDDR account contends that the core deficit responsible for G-SLI grammar involves "movement" (Chomsky, 1995). And, more specifically, whereas the basic grammatical operation/rule "move" in normal grammar is (by definition) obligatory, in G-SLI grammar it is optional. Thus, G-SLI children's grammar may be characterized by "optional movement" (van der Lely, 1998). Within the minimalist perspective (Chomsky, 1998, 1999), long distance dependencies necessitate movement, where movement is construed as attraction by a noninterpretable feature (e.g., tense, case) for the purposes of feature checking.

In other words, a dependent structural (syntactic) relation is formed in a sentence for the purpose of linking and checking (matching, copying, or moving) grammatical features associated with lexical items (or constituents). For instance, the inflectional (Infl) functional category with tense features "attracts" the verb in order that the verb's tense features can be checked (i.e., V to I movement). Thus, in more theory neutral terms, this syntactic dependency occurs when one sentence constituent "looks for" a "sister constituent" for feature checking/matching/copying. Although Chomsky (1995, 1998, 1999) defined this syntactic dependency operation as "movement," the terminology to describe this operation may change with developing linguistic theories. However, it is this basic operation of syntactic dependency and the resulting grammatical operations/processes (feature checking/matching/copying) that is central to the RDDR account of G-SLI and, indeed, central to syntax.

The optionality, rather than the absence, of movement characterizing G-SLI subjects' grammar indicates that the operation or rule "Move F" (a feature) is available to them. Thus, the underlying deficit is not in the operation move itself, but the implementation of the operation (van der Lely, 1998). R. Manzini (personal communication, 10th February, 1998) suggested that the locus of the deficit is with the economy principles (Chomsky, 1998). Van der Lely (1998) explored this suggestion and concluded that of the various principles or properties of economy (e.g., minimal link condition, last resort) that a deficit within last resort provided a parsimonious explanation of the data. Formally, Chomsky (1995) defined last resort as "Move F raises F (a feature) to target K only if F enters into a checking relation with a sublabel of K." Last resort may be thought of as comprising two principles (R. Manzini, personal communication, 10th February, 1998). The first principle, economy 1, ensures that the operation move is permitted only if it satisfies a feature-checking relation. Thus, move F occurs only if there are features to be checked. The second principle, economy 2, forces movement (and thus checking) if the target has not had its features checked. Thus, economy 2 principle of last resort insures that movement operations are obligatory (van der Lely, 1998). Van der Lely (1998) contended that the economy 2 ("Must-Move") principle of last resort is missing in G-SLI grammar and this accounts for the optionality of movement. From a computational, mechanistic viewpoint, this could be interpreted as an impaired (specialized) algorithm, underlying movement representations or operations in G-SLI, such that movement can occur, but, in contrast to normal grammar, is not "automatic" (whereby a 'steady state' has occurred) and thus, compulsory. Conversely, features that can be checked via "merge" (Chomsky, 1999) may be realized correctly—merge being the basic operation whereby a category is inserted into the derivation and unlike move does not form further structural relations with other categories that are in nonlocal relations.

Problems with head-to-head movement (e.g., V to I) can account for G-SLI subjects' deficit with tense and agreement marking. Further, problems with A(argument)-movement can account for G-SLI subjects' difficulties in assigning thematic roles to noun phrases, particularly in passive sentences (van der Lely, 1994, 1996; van der Lely & Dewart, 1986; van der Lely & Harris, 1990). Thus, the RDDR can account for the range of deficits found in G-SLI subject, whereas other accounts of the linguistic deficits in children with SLI, such as the extended optional infinitive account (Rice & Wexler, 1996; Wexler et al., 1998), or the agreement deficit account (Clahsen et al., 1997) can only account for their tense and agreement errors (see van der Lely, 1998). Note that it falls outside of the scope of the focus of here to further discuss alternative accounts of these data (see van der Lely, 1998, for discussion of this issue).

The RDDR hypothesis makes clear predictions with respect to weaknesses and strengths in G-SLI grammar. For example, it predicts that G-SLI subjects would have problems with Wh-operator movement, and Q-feature (do-support) movement in question formation. Conversely, based on the RDDR hypothesis, Davies (2001) predicted that insertion of negative particles (***not*** do***n't***) would not be problematic, because no movement occurs in the syntax, although I-C movement problems may cause auxiliary and copular forms to be omitted (e.g., *They ___ not running*). Van der Lely and Battell (1998, 2001) investigated 16, 11- to 18-year-old G-SLI subjects' production of 36 subject and object questions balanced for *who, what*, and *which* words and compared their performance with that of 5- to 9-year-old, language matched control children. The G-SLI subjects were significantly impaired in producing subject and object questions, and in contrast to the language controls, produced fewer correct object questions. An error analysis revealed that all the G-SLI children produced both wh-operator, such as gap filling or no movement of the wh-phrase (e.g., **What something in Mrs Brown's desk? *Which Mrs Peacock liked jewellery?*) and Q-feature movement errors (e.g., **What cat Mrs White stroked? *What did they drank?*).

In contrast, Davies' investigations of the same subgroup of G-SLI subjects, using an elicitation task revealed that the noncontracted or contracted negative particle was never omitted in 288 sentences (e.g., *They are not running, He's not on the skateboard, He isn't skipping, They aren't on the skateboards*), although the predicted omissions of auxiliary and copular verbs were found (**They not wearing hats. *He not on the skateboard*) (Davies, 2001; Davies & van der Lely, 2000).

CONCLUSIONS

The extensive and detailed exploration of G-SLI subjects' grammatical abilities, in the context of knowledge of their nongrammatical and nonverbal cognitive abilities, has revealed a domain specific but broad deficit with structural relations within the grammatical system. Preliminary research indicates that the structural deficit in G-SLI grammar extends to phonology and morphology. However, further investigations are required to fully explore and define the phonological and morphological characteristics of G-SLI. The RDDR hypothesis provides a characterization of the syntactic deficit in G-SLI, and in so doing enables strengths and weaknesses of G-SLI grammar to be predicted. Moreover, it lays the foundation for further research to evaluate whether core deficits within the grammatical system are directly related or whether they reflect comorbidity of disorders. Such research will elucidate whether there truly are qualitative differences in the nature of SLI in different children, who may or may not manifest deficits in other cognitive abilities. Thus, the significance of the heterogeneity of SLI may be revealed, and thereby, further understanding of SLI in all its manifestations.

ACKNOWLEDGMENTS

Acknowledgments for their help and cooperation are due to all the children, speech and language therapists, teachers, and parents at Moorhouse and Dawnhouse schools, Thornhill primary school, Glebe Infant school, Newent, and the London Oratory school who participated in the studies reported herein. The preparation of this chapter and the studies reported in this chapter were supported by a Wellcome Trust Career Development Fellowship (044179/Z/95) and a Wellcome Trust Project grant (059876) awarded to Heather van der Lely, which are gratefully acknowledged.

REFERENCES

Aram, D., Ekelman, B., & Nation, J. (1984). Preschoolers with language disorders: 10 years later. *Journal of Speech and Hearing Research, 27*, 232–244.

Bates, E., & Goodman, J. (1997). On the inseparability of grammar and the lexicon. *Language and Cognitive Processes, 12*, 507–584.

Bishop, D. V. M. (1994). Grammatical errors in specific language impairment: Competence or performance limitations? *Applied Psycholinguistics, 15*, 507–550.

Bishop, D. V. M. (1997a, May 12). *Auditory and linguistic explanations to developmental language disorders.* Talk given at the Institute of Neurology. London University: London.

Bishop, D. V. M. (1997b). *Uncommon understanding: Comprehension in specific language impairment.* Hove, England: Psychology Press.

Bishop, D. V. M. (2000). Pragmatic language impairment: A correlate of SLI, a distinct subgroup, or part of the autistic continuum. In D. Bishop & L. Leonard (Eds.), *Speech and language impairments in children: Causes, characteristics, intervention and outcome* (pp. 99–114). Hove, England: Psychological Press.

Bishop, D. V. M., & Adams, C. (1991). What do referential communication tasks measure? A study of children with specific language impairment. *Applied Psycholinguistics, 12*, 199–215.

Bishop, D. V. M., & Adams, C. (1992). Comprehension problems in children with specific language impairment: Literal and inferential meaning. *Journal of Speech and Hearing Research, 35*, 119–129.

Bishop, D. V. M., Bishop, S., Bright, P., James, C., Delany, T., & Tallal, P. (1999a). Different origin of auditory and phonological processing problems in children with SLI: Evidence from a twin study. *Journal of Speech, Language & Hearing Research, 42*, 155–168.

Bishop, D. V. M., Bright, P., James, C., Bishop, S., & van der Lely, H. (2000). Grammatical SLI: A distinct subtype of developmental language disorder? *Applied Psycholinguistics, 21*, 159–181.

Bishop, D. V. M., Carlyon, R., Deeks, J., & Bishop, S. (1999). Auditory temporal information: Processing neither necessary nor sufficient for causing language impairment in children. *Journal of Speech, Language & Hearing Research, 42*, 1295–1310.

Bishop, D. V. M., North, T., & Donlan, C. (1995). Genetic basis of specific language impairment: Evidence from a twin study. *Developmental Medicine & Child Neurology, 37*, 56–71.

Bishop, D. V. M., North, T., & Donlan, C. (1996). Nonword repetition as a behavioural marker for inherited language impairment: Evidence from a twin study. *Journal of Child Psychology and Psychiatry, 37*, 391–403.

Bishop, D. V. M., & Rosenbloom, L. (1987). Classification of childhood language disorders. In W. Yule & M. Rutter (Eds.), *Language development and disorders: Clinics in developmental medicine* (pp. 101–102). London: MacKeith Press.

Bloom, P. (2000). *How children learn the meanings of words.* Cambridge, MA: MIT Press.

Bloom, P., & Markson, L. (1998). Capacities underlying word learning. *Trends in Cognitive Sciences, 2,* 39–76.

Bloom, P. (1999). Language capacities: Is grammar special? *Current Biology, 9,* 2.

Caron, C., & Rutter, M. (1991). Comorbidity in child psychopathology: Concepts, issues and research strategies. *Journal of Child Psychology and Psychiatry, 32,* 1063–1080.

Chomsky, N. (1986). *Knowledge of language: Its nature, origin and use.* New York: Praeger.

Chomsky, N. (1995). *The minimalist program.* Cambridge MA: MIT Press.

Chomsky, N. (1998). *Minimalist inquiries: The framework.* Unpublished manuscript, MIT, Cambridge, MA.

Chomsky, N. (1999). *Derivation by phase.* Unpublished manuscript, MIT, Cambridge, MA.

Clahsen, H. (1989). The grammatical characterization of developmental dysphasia. *Linguistics, 27,* 897–920.

Clahsen, H., Bartke, S., & Goellner, S. (1997). Formal features in impaired grammars: A comparison of English and German SLI children. *Journal of Neurolinguistics, 10,* 151–171.

Coltheart, M. (1999). Modularity and cognition. *Trends in Cognitive Sciences, 3,* 115–120.

Conti-Ramsden, G., Crutchley, A., & Botting, N. (1997). The extent to which psychometric tests differentiate subgroups of children with SLI. *Journal of Speech, Language and Hearing Research, 40,* 765–777.

Curtiss, S., Katz, W., & Tallal, P. (1992). Delay versus deviance in the language acquisition of language-impaired children. *Journal of Speech and Hearing Research, 35,* 373–383.

Curtiss, S., & Yamada, J. (1988). *The Curtiss-Yamada Comprehensive Language Evaluation. (CYCLE).* Unpublished test, University of California, Los Angeles.

Dalalakis, J. (1994). English adjectival comparatives and familial language impairment. In *The McGill working papers in linguistics* (Vol. 10, pp. 50–66). Montreal, Canada: McGill University.

Dalalakis, J. (1996). *Developmental language impairment: Evidence from Greek and its implications for morphological representation.* Unpublished doctoral thesis, McGill University.

Davies, L. (2001). *The nature of SLI: Optionality and principle conflict.* Unpublished doctoral thesis, University of London, England.

Davies, L., & van der Lely, H. (2000, November). *The representation of negative particles in children with SLI.* Paper presented at the 25th annual Boston University Conference on Language Development, Boston, MA.

Elman, J., Bates, E., Johnson, M., Karmiloff-Smith, A., Parisi, D., & Plunkett, K. (1996). *Rethinking innateness: A connectionist perspective on development.* Cambridge, MA: MIT Press.

Fisher, S. E., Vargha-Khadem, F., Watkins, K. E., Monaco, A. P., & Marcus, E. P. (1998). Localisation of a gene implicated in a severe speech and language disorder. *Nature Genetics, 18,* 168–170.

Frith, U., & Happé, F. (1998). Why specific developmental disorders are not specific: On-line and developmental effects in autism and dyslexica. *Developmental Science, 1,* 267–272.

Froud, K., & van der Lely, H. K. J. (2002). *Interactions between linguistic and extra-linguistic knowledge in collective noun learning: Insight from normal and SLI development.* Manuscript submitted. UCL, London.

Gallagher, A., Frith, U., & Snowling, M. (2000). Precursors of literacy-delay among children at genetic risk of dyslexia. *Journal of Child Psychology and Psychiatry, 41,* 203–213.

Gathercole, S., & Baddeley, A. (1989). Evaluation of the role of phonological STM in the development of vocabulary in children: A longitudinal study. *Journal of Memory and Language, 28,* 200–213.

Gathercole, S., & Baddeley, A. (1990). Phonological memory deficits in language disordered children: Is there a causal connection? *Journal of Memory and Language, 29,* 336–360.

Gollner, S. (1995). *Morphological deficits of children with specific language impairment: Evaluation of tense marking and agreement.* Unpublished master's thesis, University of Essex.

Gopnik, M. (1990). Feature blind grammar and dysphasia. *Nature, 344,* 715.

Gorden, P. (1985). Evaluating the semantic categories hypothesis: The case of the count/mass distinction. *Cognition, 20,* 209–242.

Hamann, C., Penner, Z., & Lindner, K. (1998). German impaired grammar: The clause structure revisited. *Language Acquisition, 7,* 193–245.

Harris, J. (1994). *English sound structure.* Oxford, England: Blackwell.

Houser, M. (1996). *The evolution of communication.* Cambridge, MA: MIT Press.

Ingham, R., Fletcher, P., Schelletter, C., & Sinka, I. (1998). Resultative VPs and specific language impairment. *Language Acquisition, 7,* 87–112.

Jakubowicz, C., Nash, L., Rigaut, C., & Gérard, C-L. (1998). Determiners and clitic pronouns in French-Speaking children with SLI. *Language Acquisition, 7,* 113–160.

Jusczyk, P. W. (1999). How infants begin to extract words from speech. *Trends in Cognitive Sciences, 3,* 323–328.

Karmiloff-Smith, A. (1998). Development itself is the key to understanding developmental disorders. *Trends in Cognitive Science, 2,* 389–398.

Leonard, L. (1998). *Children with specific language impairement.* Cambridge, MA: MIT Press.

Marcus, G. (1999). Genes, proteins and domain-specificity. *Trends in Cognitive Sciences, 3,* 367.

Neville, H., Coffey, S., Holcombe, P., & Tallal, P. (1993). The neurobiology of sensory and language processing in language-impaired children. *Journal of Cognitive Neuroscience, 5,* 235–253.

Norbury, C., Bishop, D., & Briscoe, J. (in press). Does impaired grammatical comprehension provide evidence for an innate grammar module? *Applied Psycholinguistics.*

Oetting, J., & Rice, M., (1993). Plural acquisition in children with specific language impairment. *Journal of Speech and Hearing Research, 36,* 1241–1253.

O'Hara, M., & Johnston, J. (1997). Syntactic bootstrapping in children with specific language impairment. *European Journal of Disorders of Communication, 2,* 189–205.

Peiris, D. (2000). *The influence of prosodic complexity on segmental production in specific language impairment: A case study.* Unpublished master's thesis, University of London, Department of Human Communication Science, UCL, London.

Pinker, S. (1994). *The language instinct.* London: Allen Lane.

Pinker, S. (1999). *Words and rules: The ingredients of language.* London: Weidenfeld & Nicolson.

Precious, A., & Conti-Ramsden, G. (1988). Language-impaired children's comprehension of active versus passive sentences. *British Journal of Disorders of Communication, 23,* 229–244.

Radford, A. (1990). *Syntactic theory and the acquisition of English syntax.* Oxford, England: Blackwell.

Rapin, I., & Allen, D. (1983). Developmental language disorders: Nosologic considerations. In U. Kirk (Ed.), *Neuropsychology of language, reading, and spelling* (pp. 155–184). New York: Academic Press.

Rosen, S., van der Lely, H., & Adlard, A. (1999, March). Auditory abilities in SLI. Paper presented at the third AFASIC conference, University of York.

Rosen, S., van der Lely, H., & Dry, S. (1997). Speech and non-speech auditory abilities in two children with disordered language. *Speech, Hearing & Language, 10,* 185–198.

Rice, M., & Wexler, K. (1996). Toward tense as a clinical marker of specific language impairment in English-speaking children. *Journal of Speech and Hearing Research, 39,* 1239–1257.

Rice, M., Wexler, K., & Cleave, P. (1995). Specific language impairment as a period of extended optional infinitive. *Journal of Speech and Hearing Research, 38,* 850–863.

Smith, N. (1999). *Chomsky: Ideas and ideals.* Cambridge, England: Cambridge University Press.

Snowling, M. (2000). *Dyslexia* (2nd ed.). Oxford, England: Blackwell.

Snowling, M., & Hulme, C. (1994). The development of phonological skills. *Philosophical Transactions of the Royal Society B, 346,* 21–28.

Stravrakaki, S. (2001a). Comprehension of reversible relative clauses in specifically language impaired and normal Green Children. *Brain and Language.*

Stravrakaki, S. (2001b). Sentence comprehension Greek SLI children. In N. Hewlett, L. Kelly, & F. Windsor (Eds.), *Themes in clinical linguistics and phonetics* (pp. 57–72). Hillsdale, NJ: Lawrence Erlbaum.

Tallal, P. (2000). Experimental studies of language learning impairments: From research to remediation. In D. Bishop & L. Leonard (Eds.), *Speech and language impairments in children: Causes, characteristics, intervention and outcome* (pp. 131–156). Hove, England: Psychological Press.

Tallal, P., Miller, S., Bedi, G., Byma, G., Wang, Z., Nagarajan, S., Schreiner, W., Jenkins, W., & Merzenich, M. (1996). Language comprehension in language-learning impaired children improved with acoustically modified speech. *Science, 217*, 81–84.

Tallal, P., & Piercy, M. (1973). Defects of non-verbal auditory perception in children with developmental aphasia. *Nature, 241*, 468–469.

Tomblin, J., & Pandich, J. (1999). Lessons from children with SLI. *Trends in Cognitive Sciences, 3*, 283–286.

Ullman, M., & Gopnik, M. (1999). The production of inflectional morphology in hereditary specific language impairment. *Applied Psycholinguistics, 20*, 51–117.

van der Lely, H. K. J. (1994). Canonical linking rules: Forward vs reverse linking in normally developing and specifically language impaired children. *Cognition, 51*, 29–72.

van der Lely, H. K. J. (1996). Specifically language impaired and normally developing children: Verbal passive vs adjectival passive sentence interpretation. *Lingua, 98*, 243–272.

van der Lely, H. K. J. (1997). Narrative discourse in grammatical specific language impaired children: A modular language deficit? *Journal of Child Language, 24*, 221–256.

van der Lely, H. K. J. (1998). SLI in children: Movement, economy and deficits in the computational-syntactic system. *Language Acquisition, 7*, 161–192.

van der Lely, H. K. J., & Battell, J. (1998, November). *Wh-movement in specifically language impaired children.* Paper presented at the 23rd Boston University Conference on Language Development, Boston, MA.

van der Lely, H. K. J., & Battell, J. (2001). *Wh-movement in children with Grammatical SLI: A test of the RDDR hypothesis.* Unpublished manuscript, University College, London.

van der Lely, H. K. J., & Christian, V. (2000). Lexical word formation in children with grammatical SLI: A grammar-specific versus and input-processing deficit? *Cognition, 75*, 33–63.

van der Lely, H. K. J., & Dewart, M. H. (1986). Sentence comprehension strategies in specifically language impaired children. *British Journal of Disorders of Communication, 21*, 291–306.

van der Lely, H. K. J., & Drozd, K. (1999). An investigation of quantifiers in children with SLI and normally developing children. Unpublished data, 1999, UCL, London.

van der Lely, H. K. J., & Harris, J. (1999). Repetition of novel-words of differing phonological complexity. Unpublished data, 1999.

van der Lely, H. K. J., & Harris, M. (1990). Comprehension of reversible sentences in specifically language impaired children. *Journal of Speech and Hearing Disorders, 55*, 101–117.

van der Lely, H. K. J., & Hennessey, S. (1999, November). *Linguistic determinism and theory of mind: Insight from children with SLI.* The 24th Boston University Conference on Language Development, Boston, MA.

van der Lely, H. K. J., Rosen, S., & Adlard (2002). *Evidence for a developmentally domain specific subsystem in the brain.* MS., University College, London.

van der Lely, H. K. J., Rosen, S., & McClelland, A. (1998). Evidence for a grammar-specific deficit in children. *Current Biology, 8*, 1253–1258.

van der Lely, H. K. J., & Stollwerck, L. (1996). A grammatical specific language impairment in children: An Autosomal Dominant Inheritance? *Brain & Language, 52*, 484–504.

van der Lely, H. K. J., & Stollwerck, L. (1997). Binding theory and specifically language impaired children. *Cognition, 62*, 245–290.

van der Lely, H. K. J., & Ullman, M. (1996). The computation and representation of past-tense morphology in normally developing and specifically language impaired children. In A. Stringfellow, D. Cahana-Amitay, E. Hughes, & A. Zukowski (Eds.), *Proceedings of the 20th annual Boston University conference on language development* (pp. 816–827). Somerville, MA: Cascadilla Press.

van der Lely, H. K. J., & Ullman, M. (2001). Past tense morphology in specifically language impaired children and normally developing children. *Language and Cognitive Processes, 16,* 113–336.

Vargha-Khadem, F., Watkins, K., Fletcher, P., & Passingham, R. (1995). Praxic and nonverbal cognitive deficits in a large family with a genetically transmitted speech and language disorder. *Proceedings National Academy of Science, USA. Psychology, 92,* 930–933.

Wexler, K. (1998). Very early parameter setting and the unique checking constraint: A new explanation of the optional infinitive stage. *Lingua, 106,* 23–79.

Wexler, K., Schütze, C., & Rice, M. (1998). Subject case in children with SLI and unaffected controls: Evidence for the Agr/Tns omission model. *Language Acquisition, 7,* 317–344.

Wright, B., Lombardino, L., King, W., Puranik, C., Leonard, C., & Merzenich, M. (1996). Deficits in auditory temporal and spectral resolution in language impaired children. *Nature, 387,* 176–171.

5

Pragmatics and SLI

Jeannette Schaeffer

Ben-Gurion University of the Negev

Models of cognition and grammar can help generate hypotheses about the nature of language disorders, and vice versa. Specific language impairment (SLI) is a particularly relevant field of research in this respect because the impairment is supposed to be restricted to language (i.e., no other cognitive function is disordered). Although this chapter focuses on SLI, it would be interesting to test the proposed hypotheses in other language disorders as well.

One important hypothesis, the modularity hypothesis, concerning cognition and grammar has been proposed by Fodor (1983) and Chomsky (1986). It views cognition in general and language in particular as arising from a complex interaction of various cognitive domains and, further, that these domains are autonomous in the sense that they are governed by distinct principles. This description suggests that two types of modularity, within cognition and within language, can be distinguished. The first type, within cognition, considers language to be one of the modules of cognition ("big modularity"; Levy & Kave, 1999); the second, within language, concerns the modular organization within language ("small modularity"; Levy & Kave, 1999).

Results of SLI studies showing that impairment can be isolated to language only provide support for big modularity. As for small modularity, the question arises as to what modules language itself comprises. The present discussion takes a Chomskyan view of language as a starting point, and assumes the modules of language to be as in Fig. 5.1.

I. Lexicon
II. Computational System: Grammar: - morphosyntax
                                           - semantics
                                           - phonology
                              Processor/Parser
III. Pragmatic System

FIG. 5.1. Modules of language.

This study focuses on the question of whether and how the computational system and the pragmatic system are distinct modules, and how they interact. More specifically, it concentrates on the influence of a certain type of pragmatics on (morpho-)syntax. The hypothesis is that this type of pragmatics is a distinct module separate from the computational system, and therefore from (morpho-)syntax. Hypothesizing furthermore that children with SLI have deficits in their grammar, the prediction is that, unlike normally developing children (MLU, language age matched), children with SLI will not display errors caused by the lack of certain pragmatic principles. If this turns out to be the case, there is support for the hypotheses that pragmatics is a system, and perhaps a module, distinct from (morpho-)syntax, and for the hypothesis that children with SLI do not have pragmatic deficits. If the prediction described is not borne out, it might be necessary to assume that SLI implies deficits in both (morpho-)syntax and the pragmatic system, or that (part of) the pragmatic system belongs to the grammar module.

These hypotheses are tested by comparing the spontaneous language production of Dutch children with SLI with younger Dutch normally developing children. The topic of investigation is object scrambling, a syntactic phenomenon driven by a pragmatic principle.

The next section provides some relevant background regarding adult pragmatics, speaker and hearer knowledge, object scrambling in adult Dutch, and object scrambling in child Dutch. A later section lays out the hypotheses and predictions and is followed by a methods section describing the way tests were done. Later, results are provided and then are subsequently discussed.

BACKGROUND

Different Types of Pragmatics

An investigation into the literature on the pragmatic abilities (to be specified later) of children with SLI reveals a variety of results. In some studies, children with SLI perform below the level of MLU controls (Sheppard, 1980;

Siegel, Cunningham, & van der Spuy, 1979; Snyder, 1975, 1978; Stein, 1976; Watson, 1977). In other instances, no differences are found (Prelock, Messick, Schwartz, & Terrell, 1981; Prinz, 1982; Rowan, Leonard, Chapman, & Weiss, 1983), and in still others, the children with SLI perform at higher levels (Craig & Evans, 1989; Johnston, Miller, Curtiss, & Tallal, 1993; Leonard, 1986; Leonard, Camarata, Rowan, & Chapman, 1982). Furthermore, a few studies report no differences between children with SLI and normally developing children of the same age (for more discussion on the pragmatic abilities of children with SLI, cf. van der Lely, chap. 4 in this volume). The studies reporting poorer performance on pragmatic skills by children with SLI than control children evoke the question of whether the weaker morphosyntactic abilities of the children with SLI get in these children's way, restricting their ability to exhibit pragmatic knowledge that they possess or whether they really lack certain pragmatic principles.

Most studies concern pragmatic abilities such as speech acts, conversational participation and discourse regulation (initiations, replies, topic maintenance, turn taking, utterance repair, etc.), and code switching. It is feasible that these types of pragmatic skills are shaped by morphosyntactic abilities. If, for example, there are problems with verbal inflection, then this may affect the production of a correct imperative (i.e., the speech act of a command or a request). Whether the opposite is true (linguistic pragmatic principles affecting morphosyntax) is less clear, but the possibility is not excluded.

The present study concentrates on a different type of pragmatics, which seems to have a much more immediate impact on the linguistic structure. Along the lines of Kasher (1991), it is assumed that notions such as "reference" and "presupposition" belong to this type of pragmatics, which is referred to as "interface pragmatics." For example, understanding and producing certain referential expressions, such as *she* or *there*, involves integration of the output of a language module with the output of some perception/production module, each serving as input for some central unit, which produces the integration of the linguistic structure and its context. Furthermore, in order to use referential expressions correctly, the speaker needs to be aware of the hearer's current knowledge or assumptions. A speaker cannot refer to an object that has not been mentioned in the preceding discourse or is not present in the situational context with a definite determiner, or with a pronoun.

In this sense, pragmatic principles immediately influence the realization of certain linguistic structures, such as the choice of pronominal elements versus noun phrases, the choice between definite and indefinite nominal expressions, and, in turn, their correct position in the syntactic structure. Thus, pragmatic principles such as those illustrated serve as some sort of a connector between linguistic structures and context—hence the term *interface pragmatics*.

In order to obtain an answer to the question as to whether the pragmatic system of children with SLI can be impaired in its own right, and is not the result of impaired morphosyntax, interface-pragmatic principles were investigated, because they clearly influence the realization of the (morpho-) syntax. The next section discusses a concept that is likely to be part of interface pragmatics.

SPEAKER AND HEARER KNOWLEDGE

Referential expressions such as pronouns and locative *there* are the output of interface pragmatics. The question is what exactly the interface pragmatic principles are that govern the appropriate use of such linguistic elements: one of them is the "concept of nonshared knowledge" (Schaeffer, 1997, 1999, 2000). This concept makes crucial use of the notions "speaker knowledge" and "hearer knowledge," which are explained first.

In order for a conversation not to break down, speakers need to take into account what their interlocutor, the hearer, knows. For example, if speakers start a conversation out of the blue with the sentence, "The tree fell down," in a situation in which there is no tree visible, then the interlocutor/hearer will be confused because the use of the definite determiner *the* implies that the reference of the noun *tree* is known, or familiar to the speaker as well as the hearer. The hearer does not know the reference of *tree* because it has not been introduced in the preceding discourse. Consequently, communication breakdown takes place. This phenomenon is also referred to as "presupposition failure." Similar breakdowns occur when pronouns are used out of the blue.

Breakdowns such as those described are the result of a failure in the interface pragmatics, namely, in the application of the concept of nonshared knowledge, which states that speaker and hearer knowledge are always independent. The concept of nonshared knowledge expresses an obligation for the speaker to consider the hearer's knowledge as a separate entity and therefore as something that is, in principle, different from the speaker's knowledge. However, in certain cases, speaker and hearer knowledge may coincide. Notice that if the concept of nonshared knowledge is absent, or fails to apply, speaker and hearer knowledge are not always independent, implying that there are situations in which speakers automatically attribute their own knowledge to the hearer.

Returning to SLI, investigating speaker/hearer knowledge in children with SLI can provide a better insight into the question of whether interface pragmatics is a device separate from other types of pragmatics and from the computational system, and the question of whether pragmatics, in general, and interface pragmatics, in particular, can be problematic for children with SLI in its own right, rather than being the consequence of impaired morphosyntax. Analysis is given of one of the many linguistic effects of the application of the concept of nonshared knowledge, namely, the syntactic phenomenon of "object scrambling" in the language production of Dutch children with SLI. But, before turning to SLI, first consider this phenomenon in adult Dutch, as well as some results regarding object scrambling in normally developing Dutch child language.

Object Scrambling in Adult Dutch

Schaeffer (1997, 2000) showed that speaker/hearer knowledge has an effect on the choice of certain syntactic structures, such as the position of the object in languages like Dutch and German. In these languages, the object can occupy a position either preceding or following an adverb or negation. When it precedes the adverb or negation, it is said to be "scrambled." In the literature, object scrambling is often argued to be driven by referentiality: A referential object scrambles (over adverbs and/or negation), and a nonreferential object does not. This is illustrated in Example 1 (the adverb and the object are bold-faced):

(1) a. *nonreferential object: unscrambled*
 . . . dat Saskia **waarschijnlijk een boek** gelezen heeft
 . . . that Saskia probably a book read has
 '. . . that Saskia probably read a book'
 b. *referential object: scrambled*
 . . . dat Saskia **het boek waarschijnlijk** gelezen heeft
 . . . that Saskia the book probably read has
 '. . . that Saskia read the book probably'

Referentiality can be formulated in terms of speaker and hearer knowledge: A nominal expression is referential if its referent is known to at least the speaker; it is nonreferential if the referent is not known to either the speaker or the hearer.

 Furthermore, there are two types of referentiality: referentiality that is caused by the introduction of the referent in the previous linguistic discourse, and referentiality that is due to long-term shared knowledge between speaker and hearer. An example of the former, called "discourse-related referentiality," is given in Example 2a, and an example of the latter, called "non-discourse-related referentiality," is given in Example 2b:

(2) a. *discourse-related referentiality*
 Weet je nog dat Jan vorige maand **een boek** gekocht heeft?

know you still that Jan last month a book bought has
'Do you remember that John bought a book last month?'
Hij heeft **het boek waarschijnlijk** nog steeds ongelezen in de kast staan.
he has the book probably still unread in the book case stand-INF
'The book is probably still in the book case without having been read'
???Hij heeft **waarschijnlijk het boek** nog steeds ongelezen in de kast staan.
he has probably the book still unread in the book case stand-INF

b. *non-discourse-related referentiality*
Wat heeft Jan toch al die tijd gedaan?
what has Jan yet all that time done
'What has John been doing all that time?'
Hij heeft **waarschijnlijk de bijbel** gelezen.
Hij has probably the bible read
'He has probably been reading the bible'

In Example 2a, the nominal expression *het boek* ('the book') receives its referential interpretation from the fact that it has been introduced in the preceding linguistic discourse as *een boek* ('a book'). In Example 2b, on the other hand, the nominal expression *de bijbel* ('the bible') is referential because its referent is part of the long-term shared knowledge between speaker and hearer. Therefore, it does not need to be introduced in the linguistic discourse.

Notice furthermore, that a discourse-related referential nominal expression (such as *het boek*, 'the book') must scramble over the adverb, whereas a nondiscourse related referential nominal expression can remain in a position following the adverb. Thus, the two types of referentiality render different syntactic effects in terms of word order. It may now become clear that in order to determine whether or not a nominal expression is referential, it must be possible to distinguish discourse-related from nondiscourse-related referentiality. This requires an understanding of exactly what speaker and hearer knowledge is, and a realization that they are independent of each other. If speakers realize that the referent of a nominal expression they want to use is not part of the hearer's knowledge, they must introduce it in the linguistic discourse. This turns it into a discourse-related referential expression, which must scramble. If, on the other hand, speakers know that the referent of a nominal expression they want to use is part of the hearer's knowledge (e.g., by virtue of long-term shared knowledge between speaker and hearer), they need not introduce it in the linguistic discourse, and they do not need to scramble it over the adverb.

Findings for Normally Developing Dutch Children

Schaeffer (1999, 2000) argued that normally developing children up to about age 3;0 lack the pragmatic concept of nonshared knowledge. This means that children of this age often automatically attribute their own knowledge to the hearer. If they do this, then they cannot correctly infer what referentiality is. This is the reason that Dutch 2-year-old children often fail to scramble referential objects in obligatory contexts. The findings of two studies on object scrambling carried out in 1995 and in 1997 are summarized in Tables 5.1, 5.2, 5.3, and 5.4.

Schaeffer (1995) investigated object scrambling in the spontaneous speech of two Dutch children, Laura and Niek. Laura's data were kindly

TABLE 5.1
Scrambling in Spontaneous Child Dutch (Schaeffer, 1995)

Subject	Stage I	Stage II
Laura	1;9–3;4	3;4–5;4
Niek	2;7–3;5	3;6–3;11

TABLE 5.2
Proportions of Unscrambled Referential
Objects (Pronouns) in Spontaneous Speech

Subject	Stage I	Stage II
Laura	70%	12%
Niek	29%	22%

TABLE 5.3
Scrambling Results from Elicited Production Task (Schaeffer, 1997, 2000)

Subject	Number of Subjects	Age
Dutch 2-year-olds	7	2;4–2;11
Dutch 3-year-olds	13	3;0–3;11

TABLE 5.4
Proportions of Unscrambled Referential Objects
in Elicited Production Task

Subject	Definite DP	Personal Pronoun	Demonstrative Pronoun
2-year-olds	70%	67%	83%
3-year-olds	28%	5%	22%

TABLE 5.5
Proportions of Scrambled and Unscrambled Determinerless Object Nouns
in Dutch Spontaneous Child Speech (Schaeffer, 1995)

Subject	Stage I		Stage II	
	Scrambled	Unscrambled	Scrambled	Unscrambled
Laura	0% (0)	100% (18)	0% (0)	100% (1)
Niek	18% (11)	82% (50)	23% (10)	77% (33)

TABLE 5.6
Percentage of Scrambled and Unscrambled Determinerless Object Nouns in
Elicited Production Task with Dutch Children (Schaeffer, 1997)

Subject	Scrambled	Unscrambled
2-year-olds	11% (3)	89% (24)
3-year-olds	30% (3)	70% (7)

made available by her mother and linguist, Jacqueline van Kampen, who kept track of Laura's language development from age 1;9 to 5;4 in the form of written diary notes. Niek is one of the Dutch children whose data are accessible through CHILDES (MacWhinney & Snow, 1985). He was recorded biweekly from age 2;7 to 3;11 in play situations. Neither child showed high numbers of relevant utterances, however, their speech provides an indication for the use of object scrambling by young Dutch children.

The results show that Laura fails to scramble referential objects in obligatory contexts around 70% of the time up until age 3;4. After this age, this percentage drops to 12%. Niek leaves referential objects unscrambled around 25% of the time, but for a longer period, up until age 3;11.[1]

A larger scale study using an elicited production task with 49 Dutch-speaking children between the ages of 2;4 and 3;11 (Schaeffer, 1997, 2000) shows that Dutch 2-year-olds fail to scramble referential objects in obligatory contexts around 70% of the time, a percentage that drops dramatically in the responses of the 3-year-olds.

Young Dutch children also produce a large number of determinerless object nouns (prohibited in adult Dutch), of which the majority is unscrambled. The results of both the spontaneous speech and the elicited production task studies referred to earlier are provided in Tables 5.5 and 5.6, respectively. This phenomenon is probably due to the more general syntactic phenomenon of determiner drop that has been observed crosslinguistically in the speech of young children. The reason why these determiner-

---

[1]Niek is known to be a slow developing child in terms of language.

less object nouns do not scramble is as follows: The determiner spells out an abstract referentiality feature and marks the whole nominal expression as referential. When there is no determiner, referentiality is not realized, which means the entire nominal expression is not marked for referentiality. Therefore, scrambling does not take place.

In terms of developmental stages, the syntactic phenomenon of determiner drop in child language co-occurs with the failure of object scrambling, including unscrambled objects with determiners. However, it remains to be seen whether there is a causal correlation between the two phenomena, or whether they just happen to appear at around the same age. The language development of normally developing Dutch children cannot provide much insight in this matter.

The next section turns to the language development of Dutch children with SLI and lays out the hypotheses and predictions regarding pragmatics and the syntactic phenomenon of object scrambling.

HYPOTHESES AND PREDICTIONS

As was hinted at in the start of the chapter, there are several types of hypotheses to be formulated with respect to the status of the pragmatic system and the syntactic and pragmatic competence of children with SLI. The more general hypotheses deal with the nature of pragmatics, and some additional hypotheses concern the language of children with SLI.

As for the pragmatic system, it may be hypothesized that interface pragmatics is a system, and perhaps a module in itself. Fodor (1983) and Kasher (1991) defined *module* as a cognitive system that is independent, in several significant respects: It is domain specific, is informationally encapsulated, is associated with fixed neural architecture, has specific breakdown patterns, and its ontogeny has a characteristic pace and sequencing. Kasher differed from Fodor in assuming that a module is not necessarily a system that functions as the input to other systems.

Furthermore, the hypothesis is adopted that children with SLI are impaired in their grammar only, and therefore not in their interface pragmatics. More specifically, according to this hypothesis, children with SLI older than age 3 have an intact concept of nonshared knowledge, one of the principles of interface pragmatics. If older children with SLI have the concept of nonshared knowledge, similar to their normally developing age mates, they know what speaker and hearer knowledge is, and therefore they are able to construe and interpret referentiality correctly in an adult-like fashion. Assuming that referentiality is the driving force behind object scrambling, it is predicted that children with SLI older than age 3 do not fail to scramble referential objects in obligatory contexts.

Moreover, adopting the assumption that determiner drop in normally developing child language is a syntactic phenomenon, independent of the concept of nonshared knowledge, it may be predicted that children with SLI may drop determiners. If they do, then referentiality is not realized, and therefore determinerless object nouns will remain unscrambled.

METHODS

Subjects

The study investigated the spontaneous speech of 20 Dutch children with SLI between ages 4;2 and 8;2 and an MLU range from 2.1 to 5.7. These data were collected by Bol and Kuiken (1988). The details regarding their gender, age, and MLU are provided in Table 5.7.

Materials

Each child was recorded at school for about half an hour, in the presence of one speech therapist and one investigator. This rendered representative transcripts of minimally 100 utterances each. During the recording, the

TABLE 5.7
Details Children with SLI

ID	Gender	Age	MLU
01	M	6;00.24	2.1
02	F	4;09.08	2.2
03	F	4;01.16	2.4
04	M	6;02.10	2.5
05	M	6;07.22	2.8
06	F	5;03.07	3.2
07	M	6;00.10	3.3
08	M	6;00.13	3.4
09	M	6;01.26	3.5
10	M	4;08.21	3.7
11	F	5;01.02	3.7
12	F	5;01.04	3.9
13	M	8;01.17	4.2
14	M	4;07.20	4.4
15	M	5;04.28	4.4
16	M	5;11.22	4.4
17	M	6;01.13	4.4
18	M	7;00.18	4.6
19	M	7;01.26	4.8
20	M	7;04.19	5.7

speech therapist held a conversation with the child while playing with toys or a picture book.

In order to study the phenomenon of object scrambling, the following material was selected from the transcripts: All child utterances containing a verb, an object, and negation (*niet* or nie - 'not') or one of the following adverbs: *nu* ('now'), *nou* ('now'), *gisteren* ('yesterday'), *morgen* ('tomorrow'), *altijd* ('always'), *even* ('just', 'for a moment'), *eventjes* ('just', 'for a moment'), *ook* ('also'), *maar* (?), *weer* ('again'), *zo* ('this way'), *gewoon* ('just').

Analysis

Because utterances with a verb, an object, and an adverb or negation were not abundant, the data of all children were collapsed and analyzed as one group. Furthermore, objects were divided up into five different categories, namely pronouns, proper names, definite DPs, indefinites, and determinerless object nouns.

For each category, the percentage of scrambled and unscrambled objects was calculated.

RESULTS

The results showed that children with SLI do not have many problems with scrambling of referential objects. This is shown in Table 5.8.

Referential objects, such as pronouns, in obligatory contexts are correctly scrambled at a rate of 96%. The one utterance with an incorrectly unscrambled pronoun is given in Example 3 (again, in all utterances, the negation or the adverb and the object are bold-faced):

TABLE 5.8
Object Scrambling in the Language of All 20 Dutch Children with SLI

	Pronoun		Proper Name		Definite DP		Indefinite		Determinerless	
	s	u	s	u	s	u	s	u	s	u
otal	96%	*4%	—	—	33%	67%	0%	100%	0%	*100%
	23/24	1/24			1/3	2/3	0/18	18/18	0/13	13/13
egation	92%	*8%	—	— ·	50%	*50%	0%	100%	0%	*100%
	12/13	1/13			1/2	1/2	0/1	1/1	0/5	5/5
dverbs	100%	0%	—	—	0%	0%	0%	100%	0%	*100%
	11/11	0/11			0/1	1/1	0/17	17/17	0/8	8/8

Note: s = scrambled, u = unscrambled, definite DP = noun preceded by definite determiner, indefinite = noun preceded by indefinite determiner, determinerless = bare noun
*incorrect in adult language

(3) ik wil **niet die** opeten·   (ID 12, 5;1, MLU 3.7)
    I want not that up-eat-inf
    'I don't want to eat that one'

As for the definite DPs, there were only three in total, which makes it difficult to draw any definitive conclusions from them. One definite DP was incorrectly left unscrambled. This utterance is reproduced in Example 4:

(4) je heb **niet de ziekenauto**.   (ID 19, age 7;2, MLU 4.8)
    you have not the ambulance
    'You don't have the ambulance'

The other unscrambled definite DP was correct, which is sometimes possible in Dutch, and is reproduced in Example 5:

(5) en hij Boef heb **ook een keertje**
    't badje pepot gemaakt.   (ID 20, age 7;4, MLU 5.7)
    and he Boef has also a time the bath-DIM broken made
    'And Boef broke the bath one time too'

The indefinite objects were all nonreferential, and were left correctly unscrambled. An example of a correctly scrambled referential object and of a
correctly unscrambled nonreferential object are provided in Example 6:

(6) *correctly scrambled referential full object*
    a. de leeuw weet toch **de weg niet**   (ID 15, age 5;5, MLU 4.4)
       the lion knows anyway the way not
       'The lion doesn't know the way anyway'
    correctly unscrambled indefinite full objects
    c. maar dan moet je **ook een**
       wiel maken.   (ID 13, age 8;2, MLU 4.2)
       but then must you also a wheel make-inf
       'But then you must also make a wheel'

Nonetheless, just like the younger normal children, the children with SLI
produce determinerless object nouns, none of which has scrambled. This is
illustrated in Example 7:

(7)   *nonscrambled determinerless object*
        nou is **niet kaartje** kopen, he?   (ID 15, age 5;5, MLU 4.4)
        now is not ticket buy-inf huh
        'He's not buying a ticket now, is he?'

In summary, Dutch children with SLI between ages 4;2 and 8;2 behave normally with respect to object scrambling (i.e., just like their normally developing age mates, they scramble referential objects correctly), whereas younger Dutch normally developing children often fail to scramble them. On the other hand, 4- to 8-year-old Dutch children with SLI differ from their age mates in that they produce determinerless object nouns, which remain unscrambled. This linguistic behavior resembles that of younger Dutch normally developing children.

DISCUSSION

The results presented in the previous section show that the predictions formulated earlier are borne out: Dutch children with SLI older than age 3 do not fail to scramble referential objects in obligatory contexts; children with SLI drop determiners; and determinerless object nouns remain unscrambled.

A comparison with the findings of earlier studies (Schaeffer, 1995, 1997, 2000) on object scrambling in normally developing Dutch child language render the following suggestions:

1. With respect to interface pragmatics, 4- to 8-year-old children with SLI are similar to their age mates: They do not lack the pragmatic concept of nonshared knowledge, contrary to normally developing 2/3-year-olds. This indicates that pragmatic principles such as the concept of nonshared knowledge develop as a function of age, rather than as a function of language developmental stage in both normally developing children and children with SLI.
2. Syntactically, 4- to 8-year-old children with SLI and normally developing 2/3-year-olds are in the same grammar developmental stage: Both groups often drop determiners in object nominal expressions with the consequence that the objects remain unscrambled.

The suggestion that pragmatic principles such as the concept of nonshared knowledge develop as a function of age, rather than as a function of grammar developmental stage, is consistent with findings reported by Skarakis and Greenfield (1982). They studied presuppositional ability in children with SLI and found that whereas the (younger) MLU controls showed a pattern of omitting old information at lower MLU levels and pronominalizing such information at higher levels, the (older) children with SLI showed a tendency to pronominalize at all levels of MLU.

The fact that Dutch children with SLI between ages 4;2 and 8;2 are (morpho-)syntactically similar to, but pragmatically different from, normally developing Dutch 2/3-year-olds provides support for the hypotheses that interface pragmatics is a system independent of the computational system, and that children with SLI have deficiencies in the grammar module, but not in interface pragmatics.

Consider the first hypothesis. Because the children with SLI display similar morphosyntactic anomalies as 2/3-year-old normally developing children, it can be assumed that they are in the same "grammar developmental stage," or they have the same "language age." However, they behave differently with respect to an interface pragmatic principle, namely, the concept of nonshared knowledge. This suggests that the development of interface pragmatics is not tied to the development of the computational system or the grammar. Rather, it is an independent device, developing at its own pace.

Next, look at the second hypothesis. Children with SLI make similar morphosyntactic errors to much younger normally developing children, such as determiner drop. However, such errors are no longer observed in the language of their age mates. This suggests that children with SLI are impaired, or at least delayed, in terms of their grammar. However, just like their normally developing age mates, children with SLI between ages 4;2 and 8;2 perform adultlike in areas of syntax that depend on interface pragmatic principles, such as object scrambling, indicating that their interface pragmatics is not impaired.

CONCLUSIONS

This study showed how a linguistic theoretical approach such as the one described in Fig. 5.1 can guide research in the field of SLI. Distinguishing pragmatics from the computational system allows researchers to tease apart morphosyntactic phenomena that are purely grammatical (e.g., determiner drop), on the one hand, and syntactic phenomena driven by pragmatics (e.g., object scrambling), on the other hand, and therefore to investigate them separately. The differences in results regarding the two types of morphosyntactic phenomena in children with SLI are explained by the fact that they are driven by two different language components: one by grammar only, the other by pragmatics. Thus, the findings of this study of Dutch children with SLI provide support for a model of language as in Fig. 5.1.

In addition, the results of the present study support an analysis of object scrambling based on referentiality as the driving feature. In pragmatically mature populations, such as normal adults and children with SLI between ages 4;2 and 8;2, referentiality marking is no problem, because the knowledge of the independence between speaker and hearer knowledge is in place (concept of nonshared knowledge). Therefore, object scrambling takes place correctly. However, in pragmatically immature populations, such as 2/3-year-old children, object scrambling often fails to take place, because referentiality marking is a problem, due to the absence of the concept of nonshared knowledge.

Theories of the organization of language and syntactic theory are useful guides in the research of specific language impairment, and results of SLI studies can help refine such theories. An interesting continuation of this line of research would include populations with other disorders, such as high functioning autistic children, who have difficulties with pragmatics but perhaps not with grammar. If, for instance, it is found that (Dutch-speaking) autistic children have problems with scrambling but show no errors with respect to purely grammatical phenomena, then this would provide a double dissociation between grammar and pragmatics, which is what researchers would ultimately want to see (cf. Ben Shalom, chap. 16 in this volume).

REFERENCES

Bol, G., & Kuiken, F. (1988). *Grammaticale Analyse van Taalontwikkelingsstoornissen* [Grammatical analysis of impairments in language development]. Amsterdam: Elinkwijk B.V.

Chomsky, N. (1986). *Knowledge of language: Its nature, origin and use.* New York: Praeger.

Craig, H., & Evans, J. (1989). Turn exchange characteristics of SLI children's simultaneous and non-simultaneous speech. *Journal of Speech and Hearing Disorders, 54,* 334–347.

Fodor, J. A. (1983). *The modularity of mind.* Cambridge, MA: MIT Press.

Johnston, J., Miller, J., Curtiss, S., & Tallal, P. (1993). Conversations with children who are language impaired: Asking questions. *Journal of Speech and Hearing Research, 36,* 33–38.

Kasher, A. (1991). On the pragmatic modules: A lecture. *Journal of Pragmatics, 16,* 381–397.

Leonard, L. (1986). Conversational replies of children with specific language impairment. *Journal of Speech and Hearing Research, 29,* 114–119.

Leonard, L., Camarata, S., Rowan, L., & Chapman, K. (1982). The communicative functions of lexical usage by language impaired children. *Applied Psycholinguistics, 3,* 109–125.

Levy, Y., & Kave, G. (1999). Language breakdown and linguistic theory: A tutorial overview. *Lingua, 107,* 95–143.

MacWhinney, B., & Snow, C. (1985). The Child Language Data Exchange System. *Journal of Child Language, 12,* 271–296.

Prelock, P., Messick, C., Schwartz, R., & Terrell, B. (1981). *Mother–child discourse during the one-word stage.* Paper presented at the symposium on Research in Child Language Disorders, University of Wisconsin, Madison.

Prinz, P. (1982). An investigation of the comprehension and production of requests in normal and language-disordered children. *Journal of Communication Disorders, 15,* 75–93.

Rowan, L., Leonard, L., Chapman, K., & Weiss, A. (1983). Performative and presuppositional skills in language-disordered and normal children. *Journal of Speech and Hearing Disorders, 26,* 97–106.

Schaeffer, J. (1995). On the acquisition of scrambling in Dutch. In D. MacLaughlin & S. McEwen (Eds.), *Proceedings of the 19th Annual Boston University Conference on Language Development* (Vol. 2, pp. 521–532). Somerville, MA: Cascadilla Press.

Schaeffer, J. (1997). *Direct object scrambling in Dutch and Italian child language.* Unpublished doctoral dissertation, University of California, Los Angeles.

Schaeffer, J. (1999). Articles in English child language. Linguistics Society of America (LSA) Annual Meeting. Los Angeles, CA. January, 1999.

Schaeffer, J. (2000). *The acquisition of direct object scrambling and clitic placement: Syntax and pragmatics.* Amsterdam: John Benjamins.

Sheppard, A. (1980). *Monologue and dialogue speech of language-impaired children in clinic and home settings.* Unpublished master's thesis, University of Western Ontario.

Siegel, L., Cunningham, C., & van der Spuy, H. (1979). *Interactions of language delayed and normal pre-school children with their mothers.* Paper presented at the meeting of the Society for Research in Child Development, San Francisco.

Skarakis, E., & Greenfield, P. (1982). The role of old and new information in the verbal expression of language-disordered children. *Journal of Speech and Hearing Research, 25,* 462–467.

Snyder, L. (1975). *Pragmatics in language disabled children: Their prelinguistic and early verbal performatives and presuppositions.* Unpublished doctoral dissertation, University of Colorado, Boulder.

Snyder, L. (1978). Communicative and cognitive abilities and disabilities in the sensorimotor period. *Merill-Palmer Quarterly, 24,* 161–180.

Stein, A. (1976). *A comparison of mothers' and fathers' speech to normal and language-deficient children.* Paper presented at the Boston University Conference on Language Development, Boston.

Watson, L. (1977). *Conversational participation by language deficient and normal children.* Paper presented at the Convention of the American Speech-Language-Hearing Association, Chicago.

Wexler, K., Schaeffer, J., & Bol, G. (1998). *Verbal syntax and morphology in Dutch normal and SLI children.* Proceedings of the 14th annual conference of the Israel Association for Theoretical Linguistics, 115–134. Be'er Sheva, Israel.

6

Specific Language Impairment and Linguistic Explanation

Jan de Jong
Utrecht University

This chapter discusses some issues concerning the linguistic explanation of the clinical symptoms found in children with specific language impairment (SLI). It shows that predictions about the symptoms of SLI can change depending on the descriptive framework that is adopted. Explanatory accounts themselves can also change due to new evidence about SLI from a previously unreported language.

Some positions taken in the literature are reviewed in order to clarify in what manner linguistic expertise is either applied to SLI or benefits from information on SLI. After a brief outline of an investigation into the reflexes of language impairment in Dutch children, the results are discussed with respect to their relevance for linguistic explanation.

LINGUISTIC THEORY AND SLI

Hansson (1997) studied the use of verbs in Swedish children with SLI. The subtitle of her article is "an application of recent theories." Hansson prefaced her study with the following statement: "The present work is based within the framework of research on specific language impairment in children (SLI) that mainly uses methods and concepts from linguistic science to *describe* and take the first steps towards an *explanation* of the nature of the problems that these children have" (Hansson, 1997, p. 196).

Hansson's approach is typical of much current work on SLI. The italics are added to mark the key words. The description of symptoms, in a linguistically consistent manner, has long been the primary aim of SLI research. It was thought that if the symptoms could be characterized within an agreed on linguistic framework, then linguists were in a position to add to the specificity of the diagnosis and of the goals for therapy. Over the last decade, however, linguistic interest in SLI has grown more ambitious and the focus has shifted. Several theories have been advanced that aim to explain the constellation of grammatical symptoms rather than describe them. The rationale is that coherent linguistic difficulties may have a well-defined common linguistic origin. This position strongly contradicts an alternative position that attributes a causal role to specific abilities that are conditional for language processing (exemplary processes are temporal processing and the accessing of phonological short-term memory).

The road to a linguistic explanation has been paved by a certain amount of theoretical consensus. Nowadays, perhaps more so than in previous stages of linguistic theory, linguistic terms are agreed on to some extent. It has therefore become easier to describe symptoms of SLI in terms that are shared by most researchers. Where explanation (the analysis of the symptoms) is at stake, on the other hand, researchers' views do differ.

There is also a broad consensus on the grammatical symptoms that are closely related to SLI. In particular, the serious difficulties language impaired children have in mastering grammatical morphology and freestanding functional morphemes have been documented in a number of languages (cf. Ravid, Levie, & Ben-Zvi, chap. 7 in this volume).

One example of a core symptom of SLI that has been described in a uniform fashion but can be explained in different ways is the occurrence of agreement errors. In several languages, SLI is characterized by the difficulties that language impaired children face with agreement. Obviously, the main locus of this problem is in the domain of verbal morphology (subject-verb agreement), but determiner-noun agreement has been shown to be vulnerable in language impairment as well. A language for which the latter was established is German (Clahsen, 1992), where the gender of the noun is marked on the determiner that accompanies it. Problems with determiner-noun agreement have been explained in two ways.

Clahsen followed the widely accepted view that determiners are heads of a separate phrase, the determiner phrase (DP) (Fig. 6.1a). Consequently, determiner-noun agreement is agreement between two heads, rather than between a specifier and a head. Rice (1994) argued for a deficit in Spec, head agreement in SLI. In an attempt to explain the fact that these errors are found in German but not in English SLI, she proposed that in German determiners may be in the specifier position instead (Fig. 6.1b): "These differences could be resolved if it proves to be the case that the determiners for which agreement marking is difficult for German-speaking children with SLI are located in Spec rather than in the head of DP" (Rice, 1994, p. 81).

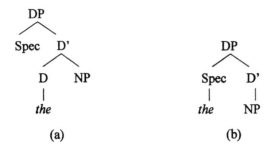

FIG. 6.1. Determiner-noun agreement represented as Head, Head agreement (a) and Spec, Head agreement (b).

The general point that this example illustrates is that linguistic theory (by virtue of the analysis proposed for a linguistic phenomenon) can alter explanatory accounts adopted for the linguistic behavior of children with SLI. Similarly, data from children with SLI in languages not previously studied can undermine existing explanatory accounts. This chapter examines data on verb forms from Dutch-speaking children with SLI, from the perspectives of available accounts of inflectional impairment in other languages, and descriptions of typically developing Dutch children.

SLI IN DUTCH: AN INTRODUCTION TO THE STUDY

The investigation of Dutch SLI excerpted in this chapter (for a full report, see de Jong, 1999) addresses *inflectional morphology*. Virtually every theory on grammatical SLI predicts that inflectional morphology is affected by language disorder (for a review of these accounts, see Leonard, 1998; cf. Ravid, Levie, & Ben-zvi, chap. 7 in this volume). The aim of this study was to describe the characteristics of tense and agreement marking in Dutch children with SLI and to compare them to accounts of SLI that are based on data from different languages.

Subjects

The Dutch subjects were specifically language impaired children between ages 6 and 9 (Table 6.1). They were recruited from special schools for language impaired children. In this study, comparatively older children were included than is often the case in research on SLI (although lately more re-

TABLE 6.1
Mean Chronological Age in Months of Subjects

	Children with SLI (n = 35)	Younger ND children (n = 20)	ND Chronological Age Matches (n = 35)
Chronological age	93.4 (11.9)[a]	59.6 (7.4)	91.4 (13.8)

Note: ND = normally developing.
[a]Standard deviations in parentheses.

search has been done on older children with SLI; e.g., Hamann, Penner, & Lindner, 1998; Rice, Wexler, & Hershberger, 1998). A consequence of choosing a relatively advanced age group is that the initial stages of morphological development cannot be monitored. Therefore, the data are not directly comparable to the results from studies of SLI that include younger children. It should be noted that the size of the group exceeds that of the average group in SLI research. This allows for a representative view of the symptoms of persistent SLI (Bishop & Edmundson, 1987) in Dutch.

For the control groups, chronological age peers were selected as well as a group of younger children. The latter group was randomly selected; however, the chronological age difference with the SLI group was similar to the difference found in most studies of SLI that match on mean length of utterance (MLU): the difference averaged 2 years. MLU was disfavored as a matching criterion because the dependent variables (number of grammatical morpheme realizations and omissions) directly translate into utterance length.

Materials

Linguistic theories on grammatical SLI differ in the symptoms they predict. For instance, there is a debate going on about whether errors concern primarily tense or rather agreement marking. In addition, it has been hypothesized that morphemes with low phonological salience are particularly vulnerable. The aim of the present inflection study was to identify the symptoms of grammatical SLI in Dutch and to test the predictions that derive from the different theories.

Data for the analysis of tense and agreement marking were collected in the following way. The children were shown a short animated video, starring Pingu, a young penguin, and his sister Pinga. The video was shown first without commentary, then with a prepared script in which a range of verbs (regular as well as irregular types) was modeled by the researcher in the present tense form. As an illustration of the diversity of the set of verbs in-

1. Daddy is telling Pingu and the baby that mummy and daddy are going out for the evening. Mummy is putting her make-up on. She puts her hat on. Mummy and daddy stroke their heads and then they wave and off they go.
2. They're crying; they're jumping on their beds.
3. The baby turns on the music and Pingu puts some wood on the fire.
4. Mummy and daddy are going to a concert to listen to music. Pingu tosses a pancake. He tosses it again and, oops!, the pancake covers his head.
5. Mummy and daddy are listening to the music. Pingu is bouncing a ball.
6. Pingu throws the ball and she heads it. They knock the picture down and they knock the shelf down.
7. Daddy has fallen asleep but mummy is listening to the music.
8. Then they dress up and Pingu pushes the baby in a box.
9. He empties the cupboard. He covers his head with a blanket and then he covers them both.
10. They look at a picture and mummy cries. The baby fills the bath.
11. Pingu jumps in. They play and the bath tips over.
12. Mummy and daddy clap. Pingu points at the clock.
13. Baby wipes up the mess. She squeezes out the water and they tidy up.
14. Baby turns off the music. Pingu tidies up and jumps on the clothes.
15. Mummy and daddy come home. Pingu and the baby pretend they are asleep and then the clothes fall out of the cupboard.
16. Mummy asks if they did it; they nod. They nod again. Mummy tidies up. Mummy and daddy cuddle them.

FIG. 6.2. Narrative script that was used in the tense and agreement task.

cluded, Figure 6.2 contains the English version of the script—the same diversity that is found here holds for the Dutch equivalent. Finally, the film was shown in 16 separate episodes; after each episode, the child was asked to tell the researcher "what happened."

The task aimed to elicit data that could be analyzed for tense and agreement features alike. The stimulus question encouraged the children to produce a past tense form (to prevent the past tense forms from being memorized, the researcher modeled the verbs in the present). The data were analyzed for past tense realizations. The past tense elicitor, however, was not always followed up by a past tense response from the child: Some children preferred the historical present when relating the narrative episodes. Therefore, not all data were available for the analysis of past tense marking.

In addition, the children's marking of subject-verb agreement (for person and number features) was investigated. More data could be included here than in the analysis of (past) tense. After all, even when the past tense node was disfavored, utterances could still be analyzed for the subject features marked on the children's verb forms. An analysis was made of tense as well as agreement marking.

Analysis and Results

Table 6.2 shows the inflectional paradigm of Dutch verbs. Clearly, there are some differences with the English verb system, most notably the marking of the number dimension in Dutch that English lacks. Apart from the morphemes that represent tense, number, and person features, Dutch (again, unlike English) has an inflectional marker, -en. Obviously, this results in *syncretism*: The infinitival form is formally identical to the present tense plural form.

The data reveal four types of errors that predominate in the results gathered from the SLI group:

1. Omission of present tense third person marker -t.
2. Substitution of plural marker by a singular marker (e.g., for a regular verb, the correct present tense marker -en is substituted by singular marker -t).
3. Omission of past tense marker or substitution of present tense marker in a past tense adverbial context.
4. Production of infinitive instead of a finite form.

All error types are illustrated underneath by utterances from language impaired subjects. Omission of an inflectional marker in Dutch typically results in a form that is identical to the first person singular and/or the stem of the verb (i.e., the 0-forms in Table 6.2). In the examples underneath, they are indicated as "stem," which should be taken as shorthand for a form that lacks an inflectional marker (either for finiteness or infinitive).

In the examples, the first line contains the child utterance, and the second shows its grammatically correct target equivalent. The third line is an English gloss for the child utterance; the fourth is a translation of the grammatical sentence.

TABLE 6.2
Inflectional Paradigm of the Dutch Verb System

Tense	Singular	Plural
Present Tense		
First person	-0[a]	-en
Second person	-t (-0 in inverted order)	-en
Third person	-t	-en
Regular Past Tense		
All persons	-de / -te	-den / -te

[a]ø indicates zero affix.

(1) a. *dan kijk mama naar kast* (boy, chronological age: 6;11)
dan kijkt mama naar de kast
then look (*stem*) mother at cupboard
'then the mother looks at the cupboard'

    b. *hem moeder klap met hem vader* (boy, 7;2)
zijn moeder klapt met zijn vader
him (*accusative form*) mother applaud (*stem*) with him (*accusative form*) father
'his mother applauds with his father'

(2) a. *boeken valt en koppie valt* (boy, 6;10)
de boeken vallen en het kopje valt
books falls (*singular form*) and little-cup falls
'the books fall and the little cup falls'

    b. *en toen viel de lakens d'r af* (boy, 8;6)
en toen vielen de lakens d'r af
and then fell (*singular past tense form*) the blankets there off
'and then the blankets fell off'

(3) a. *toen wordt ie een olifant* (boy, 8;5)
toen werd ie een olifant
then he becomes (*present tense form*) an elephant
'then he became an elephant'

    b. *en toen duwt de pinguin hem zusje weg* (boy, 9;2)
en toen duwde de pinguin zijn zusje weg
and then pushes (*present tense form*) the penguin him (*accusative form*) sister away
'and then the penguin pushed his sister away'

(4) a. *de oudste pinguin die alle kleren uit de kast halen* (boy, 9;1)
de oudste pinguin haalt alle kleren uit de kast
the oldest penguin that+one all clothes from the cupboard take (*infinitive*)
'the oldest penguin takes all the clothes from the cupboard'

    b. *en dan mama papa wakker maken* (boy, 6;5)
en dan maakt mama papa wakker
and then mother father wake (*infinitive*)
'and then mother wakes up father'

    c. *pannekoek aan e zusje hoofd plakken* (boy, 7;5)
de pannekoek plakt aan het zusje d'r hoofd
pancake to the sister head stick (*infinitive*)
'and then the pancake stuck to the sister's head'

    d. *hem z'n kindje nog aaien* (boy, 7;9)
hij aait z'n kindje nog

TABLE 6.3
Percentage of Realization of Three Morphemes in Obligatory Context

| | *% of Use in Obligatory Context* | | |
Group	*Present Tense Marker -t*	*Plural Marker -en*	*Past Tense Form*[b]
Children with SLI	0.61 (0.34)[a]	0.69 (0.30)	0.77 (0.26) (*n* = 29)
Younger ND children	0.87 (0.28)	0.95 (0.13) (*n* = 20)	0.98 (0.04)
CA Matches	0.89 (0.27)	0.97 (0.05)	0.99 (0.00) (*n* = 35)

Note: Significant group differences (Mann–Whitney *U* test): *Percentage of use of -t*–SLI < Chronological age peers, *p* = 0.0012, *z* = –3.2397; SLI < Younger children, *p* = 0.0037, *z* = –2.9040. *Percentage of use of -en*–SLI < Chronological age peers, *p* = 0.0000, *z* = –4.8199; SLI < Younger children, *p* = 0.0001, *z* = –3.8446. *Percentage of use of past tense form*–SLI < Chronological age peers, *p* = 0.0000, *z* = –6.1823; SLI < Younger children, *p* = 0.0000, *z* = –4.2563.

[a]*M(SD)* [b]Strictly taken, past tense is not always morphemic; realization of irregular past tense forms was included in the ratio.

    him (*accusative form*) his little-child still stroke
    'he still stroked his little child'
  e. *en toen 't meisje in de bad liggen met water* (boy, 9;1)
    en toen lag het meisje in het bad met water
    and then the girl in the tub lie (*infinitive*) with water
    'and then the girl lay in the tub with water'

The frequency of all but one of these error types can be recalculated as a percentage of the use of a particular grammatical morpheme in an obligatory context. The one exception are the errors exemplified by utterances (Examples 4a–4e). The next section shows that for a Dutch verb to be marked for tense and agreement features, it has to move to second position. Because in Examples 4a–4e the child produces the verb in final position, there is no obligatory context for a specific inflectional morpheme to be affixed to a verb moved to second position.

    A ratio for realization of morphemes in an obligatory context was computed (Table 6.3). Although two research groups included 35 children (the children with SLI and the age controls) and the younger group consisted of 20 children, the subject numbers in the table are different.[2] The reason is that some children did consistently use past tense forms, so there were no obligatory contexts for the present tense marker -t. The obligatory context for production of a past tense form was narrowed down to the presence of

---

[2]This resulted in differences from the chronological ages presented in Table 1. These differences, however, were marginal and are not included here.

TABLE 6.4
Number of Utterances with Nonfinite Predicates

	Absolute Numbers *M(SD)*
Children with SLI	
(n = 35)	2.85 (5.36)
Younger ND Children	
(n = 20)	0.10 (0.31)
CA Matches	0.03 (0.17)

Note: Significant group differences (Mann–Whitney U test): SLI > Chronological age peers, p = 0.0000, z = –5.2839; SLI > Younger children, p = 0.0001, z = –3.8769.

a past adverbial. Some children did not produce these adverbials and consequently had no obligatory contexts for a past tense form.

The SLI group differed significantly from both control groups on the following measures:

1. marking of third person -*t* in obligatory context was less consistent
2. marking of plural -*en* in obligatory context was less consistent
3. marking of past tense in obligatory context was less consistent
4. the use of utterance-final infinitive instead of verb second (finite) was more frequent (Table 6.4).

Interpretation of the Results

Several conclusions can be drawn from the results in the previous section. First, omission of an overt morpheme in an obligatory context is a familiar phenomenon in SLI in various languages. It is found in the language production of Dutch children with SLI as well. There is, however, an important difference with, for instance, comparable data for English: The Dutch forms lack an infinitive marker. English, on the other hand, does not have an infinitival inflection. The use of stemlike forms in second position implies that the verb is finite, because the marker for nonfiniteness is absent (the implication is that this is not an unmarked verb form).

Whereas omission has been described widely in the literature on SLI, substitution errors are not considered to be frequent, certainly not in English-speaking children. It appears that substitution of agreement markers, singular forms for plural forms, is more common in Dutch SLI than it is in English. The same is true for other languages. Leonard, Bortolini, Caselli, McGregor, and Sabbadini (1992) also found substitutions of singular forms for third person plural in Italian children with SLI. Just like in the Dutch data, these substitutions were unidirectional: Only rarely did plural forms

TABLE 6.5
Past Tense Error Types ($n = 81$) in the SLI Data

Stem Form	Infinitival Form	Present Tense Form
21	9	51

replace singular ones. The observation that SLI is characterized by omission rather than commission errors may thus originate in a bias that derives from the symptom patterns in English-speaking children, whose target language has an inflectional paradigm that is sparsely filled, leaving them with fewer opportunities for substitution.

Past tense errors most often took the form of substitutions (Table 6.5). Children with SLI substituted present tense forms for past tense forms. Alternatively, they failed to mark the verb for tense by supplying either the infinitive form or the stem form. It should be stressed that the analysis was restricted to the realization of past tense form in the context of a relevant adverbial (the adverbial *toen*, 'then' refers to past events only).

The use of infinitives in a nonelliptical context requires additional explanation. Dutch is a verb second language, which means that the proper position of the finite verb in the main clause is right after the subject. Normally developing children take some time learning that the verb should be finite and put in second position (for a review, see Wijnen & Verrips, 1998). Initially, they leave the verb in final position, with an infinitival inflection. During this stage, the infinitives are root infinitives: verbs that have a finite interpretation, but a nonfinite form. By producing the infinitives in final position, the children demonstrate that they respect the correlation between verb form and verb placement in Dutch as it holds for the infinitive. In adult Dutch, the infinitive appears in final position as well. However, an auxiliary typically premodifies it. In time, the child must learn that the verb moves from its base-generated final position to second position. In moving, it is checked for tense and agreement features (see Fig. 6.3).

Table 6.4 shows that the SLI group produced more nonfinite verbs in final position than controls. Examples 4a–4e demonstrate an important phenomenon: Nearly all infinitives co-occurred with a singular subject. This makes the possibility that the infinitive is truly a misplaced (homonymous) plural form less probable. The results confirm findings by Wexler, Schaeffer, and Bol (in press), who showed that root infinitives were still found in Dutch SLI children between ages 6 and 8.

It should be noted that there was much variability in the present data set, with some children resorting to these forms frequently, and other children hardly ever producing them. The standard deviation (that is almost

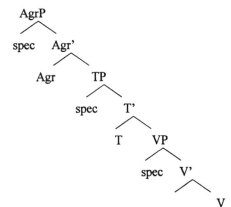

FIG. 6.3. Partial structure of the matrix sentence in Dutch.

twice the value of the mean) reflects this nonnormal distribution.[3] (Variability in the production of grammatical morphemes is often observed in groups of language impaired children; an example can be found in a study by Leonard, 1994, p. 98, in which a group of 10 children with SLI produced past tense inflection in anywhere between 0% and 72% of the obligatory contexts).

At first glance it might be inferred that, when they are frequent in individuals, such infinitive-final utterances constitute evidence for the existence of an extended optional infinitive (EOI) stage as Rice, Wexler, and Cleave (1995) proposed it. The EOI stage is an extension witnessed in children with SLI of the developmental stage during which children do not consider finiteness an obligatory feature to be marked on the verb, but a mere (optional) alternative for nonfiniteness (Wexler, 1994). In this stage, nonfinite forms are still frequent.

A straightforward optional infinitive interpretation of the data is not justified per se. Although for three of the impaired children in the present study the use of infinitives is the predominant error (in that respect they exemplify the pattern described by Rice et al., 1998), for more of the children (n = 15) this error is found next to other inflectional errors (i.e., zero marking and substitution).

If it is hypothesized that the verb forms are indeed similar to the nonfinite forms that make up the primary evidence for the optional infinitive explanation (after all, these verb forms are genuine infinitives), then what can they tell researchers about the developmental stage the child is in? This question calls for a reference to the developmental order that has been described for Dutch children.

_____

[3]Wexler et al. (in press) present only group totals. Consequently, the distribution in their data cannot be compared to ours.

According to a recent account by Wijnen (2000), during the first stage of verb acquisition, infinitives are the only verb forms and they are consistently produced in utterance-final position. This is the *infinitival* stage. There is nothing optional about it: Nonfiniteness is obligatory. These infinitives have a root infinitive interpretation. Subsequently, children enter a *lexical-finite* stage. Children now use a subset of finite forms that consists of modal auxiliaries (e.g., *kan*, 'can'), copula *is*, and a few state or nondynamic verbs (like *zit*, 'sit[s]'). At this stage, other verbs are still routinely infinitival and the two sets of verbs do not overlap: The form and position of each lexical verb are consistent. In the third stage, finiteness marking occurs with more lexical verbs. Typically, lexical verbs are now more often premodified by tense-carrying auxiliaries (most often, this concerns present and past tense forms of the pleonastic verb *gaan*, 'go'). This stage is called the optional infinitive stage and the optionality in Dutch is between root infinitives and finite verb forms and finite constructions (i.e., combinations of an auxiliary and an infinitival lexical verb). At this stage there is overlap between the two: The same lexical verbs can occur in both forms and both positions and the optional stage is resolved. In this sequence, the optional infinitive stage is preceded by a nonoptional infinitival stage and a lexical-finite stage. In the infinitival stage, children combine an infinitive with another—typically nominal—constituent (these are the infinitives that are typically found in the two- or three-word stage). In the optional infinitive stage proposed by Wijnen (2000), children produce root infinitives as well as nonroot infinitives that are part of a periphrastic predicate: Tense-carrying modals accompany the infinitival lexical verb.

The developmental sequence seen in Dutch children raises an important question about the (extended) optional infinitive account: If the extended OI stage is an explanation for SLI, and by implication for Dutch SLI, then what predictions follow from what is known about the acquisition of Dutch? And, how can a comparison between English and Dutch be made? If the utterances that contain root infinitives are compared, then it seems that there is a genuine risk of comparing data that have different contexts. The difference is that there is an optional infinitive stage that precedes a (lexical-) finite stage for English, and an optional infinitive stage that follows a lexical-finite stage for Dutch.

Rice et al. (1995; Rice et al., 1998) measured percentage of use in obligatory contexts for *-s* (third person singular present) by SLI children and compared the group mean to that of groups of normals. If Wijnen (2000) was right, then a similar comparison, when applied to Dutch data, involves the mean values for three variables—infinitives, finite forms, and (infinitival) lexical verbs that are premodified by an auxiliary marked for tense. The relative share of these categories in the data should decide on a child's stage. In addition, the degree of overlap per lexical item should be informative: Do

TABLE 6.6
Finiteness Patterns in Three Language Impaired Children

	Stem	Finite Modal Verb in Second Position[a]	Finite Lexical Verb in Second Position	Finite Auxiliary Infinitival Lexical Verb	Nonfinite Verbal Predicate
Subject A (Girl, 7;5)	2	4		2	24
Subject B (Boy, 9;1)	4	8	6	1	19
Subject C (Girl, 9;1)	1	5	12	16	10

[a]Modal verbs in Dutch can occur without a verbal complement. Instances of other verbs that are found early in a finite form—copulas and stative lexical verbs without an overt morpheme—are included in this column.

lexical verb types take one or more forms? And, finally, a crucial issue with respect to SLI is, which developmental stage is extended in Dutch children with SLI?

To illustrate the implications of these developmental stages, consider the numbers in Table 6.6. In it, relevant data are presented for three children who produced many root infinitives. After a closer look at the data, however, it is clear that the children cannot be assigned to the same developmental stage.

Subject A demonstrates scant evidence of having mastered finiteness: There are some finite forms, but they belong to the limited class of finite items that, according to Wijnen (2000), are found in the lexical-finite stage. In Subject B, the picture is slightly different, mainly because more verbs are found in second position. In Subject C, the finite constructions that contain an auxiliary outnumber the root infinitives. In addition, the child produces many lexical verbs in a finite form.

It is not easy to classify children in terms of Wijnen's sequence. Still, it seems fair to say that Subject A seems closer to obligatory nonfiniteness than to optionality and in that respect is close to the infinitival stage. Subject B shares more characteristics with children in the lexical-finite stage: The second position is more often taken by a finite verb. Subject C seems to be most representative of the Dutch optional infinitive stage.

Although the data from these children show that individual differences can be cautiously interpreted as evidence for a developmental stage, it is difficult to assign all children in the present research group to a similar stage. The reason is that many of the errors (omissions and substitutions of inflectional morphemes) concern agreement or (past) tense marking rather than finiteness. The sequence outlined by Wijnen (2000) only accounts for the acquisition of finiteness. Agreement errors, on the other hand, subsist in Dutch children long after finiteness is mastered (de Haan, 1996; Wijnen & Verrips, 1998).

The differing interpretations of determiner-noun agreement illustrated the fact that competing analyses of grammatical phenomena result in different predictions on linguistic symptoms of SLI. That observation can now be supplemented: Crosslinguistic differences in developmental order (and their linguistic interpretation) result in different predictions as well.

TOPICALIZATION VERSUS ADJUNCTION IN DUTCH SLI

The section about the infinitive-final utterances found in some children with SLI, even at a late stage, serves to introduce another example of controversy in linguistic explanation. So far, the developmental order was described in which verb placement and the marking of finiteness is acquired by Dutch children, not the linguistic analysis per se. It has become clear that the developmental order is at odds with the order that has been described for English. The stage in which finiteness and nonfiniteness are equivalent options for the child has a different context in Dutch. Here, the stage is preceded by an infinitival stage, but also by a stage in which a subset of verbs are already finite.

There is an interesting alternative to an optional infinitive explanation of the utterances in which finite forms are substituted by an infinitive. To understand this, notice that SLI children's utterances with an infinitive in final position are reminiscent of word combinations that occur quite early in Dutch child language, even in the stage in which nonfiniteness is obligatory. A notable difference is that the phrase structure of the SLI children's infinitival utterances is more elaborate than that of normal children's early output. Utterances in normal acquisition typically consist of two or three words. Utterances by SLI children are longer, demonstrating the asynchrony of semantic and morphosyntactic growth; Examples 4a–4e testify to this.

For utterances in early child German, Ingram and Thompson (1996) proposed that infinitival verb forms are not instances of a matrix verb that is neither morphologically marked nor moved. Instead, they claimed that in such utterances a modal auxiliary has been omitted.

Take a German sentence like Example 5a. In Ingram and Thompson's analysis, this utterance must be read with a modal meaning, as in Example 5b:

> (5) a. *du das haben* (you that have).
>   b. *du muss das haben* (you must that have).

Ingram and Thompson's interpretation is called the *modal drop hypothesis*. The proposal was offered in reaction to an earlier one by Poeppel and

Wexler (1993). Poeppel and Wexler considered the feasibility of an alternative to what they called the grammatical infinitive hypothesis (a precursor of the optional infinitive hypothesis). This alternative involved a reading by which early child utterances are elliptical, that is, contain a covert modal. Poeppel and Wexler claimed that this hypothesis allowed for a litmus test. The modal drop interpretation should fall through if no auxiliary omission is found in the context of a topicalized element: "Modal drop should occur wherever the modal may appear in the underlying representation. In particular, it may be dropped in syntactic contexts in which a nonsubject has been raised to Spec,C, for example a syntactic object or an adverb" (Poeppel & Wexler, 1993, p. 16). After all, topicalization (Fig. 6.4) is licensed by verb movement: This is a sentence context in which the modal must appear in the underlying representation. If no movement of the verb is assumed, then topicalization cannot be explained. Poeppel and Wexler (1993) analyzed a transcript in the CHILDES database that contains data from a German boy (the data were contributed by Wagner, 1985). In these data, they found no evidence of modal drop when a topic was raised to the specifier of the CP. Therefore, Poeppel and Wexler discarded the hypothesis that when child utterances contain an infinitival verb in final position, a modal has been dropped that precedes the infinitive.

According to Ingram and Thompson's account, utterances that have an infinitive in final position (like those illustrated earlier) have a null auxiliary. In fact, the majority of the occurrences of this error in the present data set can easily be paraphrased by inserting an auxiliary that precedes the main verb. In the following examples (present tense and past tense), forms of the pleonastic auxiliary *gaan*[4] have been added to Examples 4a–4e, rendering the verbal morphology grammatical; the remaining errors are not verb related (like the determiner omissions and the case errors).

(6) a. 'de oudste pinguin die *ging* alle kleren uit de kast halen'
b. 'en dan *gaat* mama papa wakker maken'
c. 'de pannekoek *ging* aan e zusje hoofd plakken'
d. 'hem *gaat* z'n kindje nog aaien'
e. 'en toen *ging* 't meisje in het bad liggen met water'

The paraphrases are not fully equivalent to those given by Ingram and Thompson (1996). After all, these authors introduced an omitted element that was semantically well defined by its modality. The finite forms of *gaan*, however, do not usually have a semantic weight in the present data; the verb is pleonastic and merely carries the tense marker. The paraphrases,

---

[4]*Ging* is the singular past of *gaan*; *gaat* is the present form of the third person.

(a)

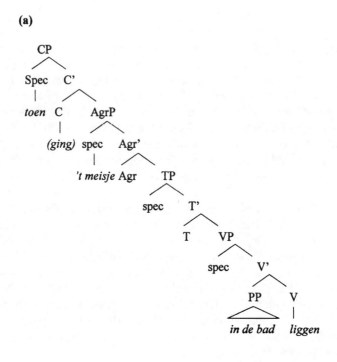

(b)

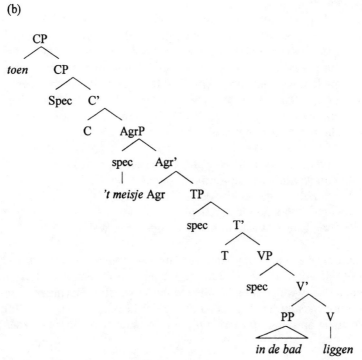

FIG. 6.4. Two readings of Example 3e, *toen 't meisje in de bad liggen*: *toen*, in topicalized (a) or adjoined (b) position.

however, follow Ingram and Thompson's proposal in that a covert element justifies the infinitive form taken by the lexical verb.

Examining the root infinitival utterances with respect to topicalization, it seems that Poeppel and Wexler's (1993) rejection of modal drop cannot be maintained in the face of the present data set. Interestingly, examples of co-occurrence of infinitives with topicalized elements were found, unlike in the data addressed by Poeppel and Wexler. Out of 78 utterances with clause-final verbs in the infinitival form, 22 had topicalized elements (importantly, these instances were divided evenly among the impaired subjects). One fronted element was a direct object; all others were temporal adverbials. Examples 4a and 4e illustrate this (*dan* and *toen* are topicalized). In Fig. 6.4a, a tree diagram is presented of Example 6e[5] (the auxiliary drop reading of Example 4e).

Ingram and Thompson (1996) did not in any way refer to specific language impairment. Their proposal involved a way of accounting for early infinitive use by normally developing children. However, because it attempted to explain precisely the (optional infinitive) stage that is protracted in children with SLI, it is a viable candidate for describing this very stage in language impaired children.

Example 4e can be interpreted in a different way. It may be claimed that the adverbial is adjoined to the clause rather than being a part of it and therefore is not an operator of movement (Fig. 6.4b). This would put *(en) toen* and *(en) dan* in the position of a sentence adverb. The interesting observation here is this one: Linguistic analyses of "surface phenomena" differ in the amount of knowledge with which they credit the child. The topicalization example is yet another instance of the way in which different analyses yield different predictions on the nature of SLI. According to one interpretation, the child is credited with the ability to move the main verb, with the topic as the operator of movement, in the other interpretation the child leaves the infinitival verb in its base position. It should be added that there is a third interpretation that does not claim full competence in the child (as in Fig. 6.4b), that contains all the relevant functional categories) but only credits the child with lexical categories (Fig. 6.5) (e.g., Radford, 1988).

These different interpretations of a single phenomenon spell out different views of the knowledge with which the (language impaired) child is credited. To take two extreme positions: Does the child have "full competence" (of functional categories) (Poeppel & Wexler, 1993) or does the child have a deficient language acquisition device (as Fletcher, 1999, labels views that propose that part of the grammar is "missing")?

---

[5]In the diagrams the ambiguous phrase 'met water' has been omitted.

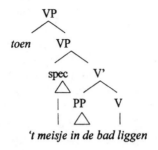

't meisje in de bad liggen

FIG. 6.5. A third reading of Example 3e: This representation contains only lexical categories.

CONCLUSIONS

This chapter has looked at the way in which linguistic explanations of SLI translate into predictions about the state of knowledge in SLI. Competing accounts of the same data were discussed. In summary, the knowledge or the lack of knowledge attributed to language impaired children appears to be partially dependent on the linguistic analysis that is adopted.

In addition, the developmental order in which finiteness is acquired—the order in Dutch is markedly different from the acquisition of finiteness in English children—has implications for the insights the child is credited with in a particular stage. The knowledge issue was illustrated by analyses of utterances like Example 4e.

One position (cf. Fig. 6.4b) is that children who persist in using infinitives know about finiteness, but reach a plateau in their acquisition of finiteness (cf. Rice et al., 1998). According to Rice et al., children know about finiteness, but they do not consistently mark it (for more discussion on this issue, see Wexler, chap. 1 in this volume).

Going by another account, the modal drop hypothesis (Ingram & Thompson, 1996), the child is credited with more knowledge: The children also know about verb movement under topicalization (Fig. 6.4a). Poeppel and Wexler (1993) rejected modal drop as a reading of the infinitives in early child language. One reason was empirical. No child utterances in the data they analyzed contained a raised topic in the absence of an auxiliary (a context in which there must be an underlying auxiliary to justify the movement of the topic). The present study found evidence to the contrary: Topics were found to co-occur with (apparent) root infinitives.

Moreover, assuming that Wijnen (2000) is correct in his observation that there is a first developmental stage with only root infinitives, it is even doubtful that children in this stage know about finiteness. The assumption that children in the initial stage of verb acquisition only have control of lexical categories (e.g., Radford, 1988) credits the child with even less knowledge.

There is an additional finding that has not been discussed so far. Dutch children with SLI produce root infinitives beyond the two- or three-word stage. In fact, these children often produced elaborate phrase (X-bar) structures. This results in asynchrony: Acquisition of X-bar develops, and acquisition of finiteness may stagnate. If this asynchrony is added to the grammatical characteristics of SLI in Dutch, it is hard to find an adequate explanation of the resulting profile. Under each account, some aspects are left unexplained. If it is assumed that the development of finiteness slows down and the language problems of children with SLI can be attributed to an immature grammar, then it is not clear why the development of phrase structure matures. If Ingram and Thompson were right and an auxiliary is dropped, then the child is credited with additional knowledge of movement. What determines the omission of (a finite form of) *gaan*, however, is not explained.

Several questions arise from the examples referred to in this chapter. One is whether increased linguistic knowledge equals increased processing abilities. This can only be done under the assumption that linguistic knowledge can be plotted in a reliable way. The question can also be mirrored: Should linguistic theories take their lead from the comparative ease or difficulty with which children with SLI master a linguistic task?

ACKNOWLEDGMENT

Thanks to Paul Fletcher and to the editors of this volume for their helpful comments.

REFERENCES

Bishop, D. V. M., & Edmundson, A. (1987). Language-impaired 4-year-olds: Distinguishing transient from persistent impairment. *Journal of Speech and Hearing Disorders*, 52, 156–173.

Clahsen, H. (1992). Linguistic perspectives on specific language impairment. *Theorie des Lexikons. Arbeiten des Sonderforschungsbereichs 282*. Düsseldorf: Universität Düsseldorf.

Fletcher, P. (1999). Specific language impairment. In M. Barrett (Ed.), *The development of language* (pp. 349–371). Hove: Psychology Press.

Haan, A. de (1996). *De verwerving van morfologische finietheid in het Nederlands* [The acquisition of morphological finiteness in Dutch]. Unpublished master's thesis, Rijksuniversiteit Groningen.

Hamann, C., Penner, Z., & Lindner, K. (1998). German impaired grammar: The clause structure revisited. *Language Acquisition*, 7, 193–246.

Hansson, K. (1997). Patterns of verb usage in Swedish children with SLI. An application of recent theories. *First Language*, 17, 195–217.

Ingram, D., & Thompson, W. (1996). Early syntactic acquisition in German: Evidence for the modal hypothesis. *Language*, 72, 97–120.

Jong, J. de (1999). *Specific language impairment in Dutch: Inflectional morphology and argument structure*. Unpublished doctoral dissertation, Rijksuniversiteit Groningen.

Leonard, L. B. (1994). Some problems facing accounts of morphological deficits in children with specific language impairment. In R. V. Watkins & M. L. Rice (Eds.), *Specific language impairments in children* (pp. 91–106). Baltimore: Brookes.

Leonard, L. B. (1998). *Children with specific language impairment*. Cambridge, MA: MIT Press.

Leonard, L. B., Bortolini, U., Caselli, M. C., McGregor, K. K., & Sabbadini, L. (1992). Morphological deficits in children with specific language impairment: the status of features in the underlying grammar. *Language Acquisition, 2*, 151–180.

Pingu 2. Building igloos (1992). BBC Children's Video.

Poeppel, D., & Wexler, K. (1993). The full competence hypothesis of clausal structure in early German. *Language, 69*, 1–33.

Radford, A. (1988). *Syntactic theory and the acquisition of English syntax*. Oxford, England: Blackwell.

Rice, M. L. (1994). Grammatical categories of children with specific language impairment. In R. V. Watkins & M. L. Rice (Eds.), *Specific language impairments in children* (pp. 69–90). Baltimore: Brookes.

Rice, M. L., Wexler, K., & Cleave, P. (1995). Specific language impairment as a period of extended optional infinitive. *Journal of Speech and Hearing Research, 38*, 850–863.

Rice, M. L., Wexler, K., & Hershberger, S. (1998). Tense over time: The longitudinal course of tense acquisition in children with specific language impairment. *Journal of Speech and Hearing Research, 41*, 1412–1431.

Wagner, K. (1985). How much do children say in a day? *Journal of Child Language, 12*, 475–487.

Wexler, K. (1994). Optional infinitives, head movement and the economy of derivations. In D. Lightfoot & N. Hornstein (Eds.), *Verb movement* (pp. 305–382). Cambridge: Cambridge University Press.

Wexler, K., Schaeffer, J. C., & Bol, G. W. (in press). Verbal syntax and morphology in Dutch normal and SLI children: How developmental data can play an important role in morphological theory. *Syntax*.

Wijnen, F. (2000). Input, intake and syntactic development. In M. Beers, B. van de Bogaerde, G. Bol, J. de Jong, & C. Rooijmans (Eds.), *From sound to sentence—studies on first language acquisition* (pp. 163–186). Groningen: Center for Language and Cognition.

Wijnen, F., & Verrips, M. (1998). The acquisition of Dutch syntax. In S. Gillis & A. De Houwer (Eds.), *The acquisition of Dutch* (pp. 223–299). Amsterdam: John Benjamins.

7

The Role of Language Typology in Linguistic Development: Implications for the Study of Language Disorders

Dorit Ravid
Ronit Levie
Galit Avivi Ben-Zvi
Tel Aviv University

In linguistics and language acquisition research there is a sometimes uneasy but always fruitful tension in the search for shared, common properties and trends defined as "universals" across languages and across children, on the one hand, and language particular or typologically determined features specific to particular languages or types of languages, on the other. This chapter intends to point out the importance of examining impaired language development as compared to nonimpaired language development in contexts sensitive to the particular typology of the language being learned.

Recent crosslinguistic research has demonstrated the powerful impact of target language typology on the process of acquisition from early preschool age in a range of domains, revealing that children are very early on sensitive to the "typological imperatives" of their language (Berman, 1986). That is, even very young children recognize "where the action is at," so to speak, in the input language—not only which categories are formally distinguished, but also how. Such studies reveal the influence of language-specific effects on speech perception and babbling in the first year of life (Jusczyk, 1997) on how children will adjust their speech output to the prosodic character of their language, as intonation or tone based (Demuth, 1993), and whether it requires vowel harmony as in Turkish (Aksu-Koc & Slobin, 1985) well before they have command of grammatical inflection; on children's construal of the underpinnings of the category of "noun" in English and Spanish as compared with Welsh and Korean (Gathercole, 1997);

on children's encoding of spatial distinctions in languages like English and Dutch as compared with Korean or Tzeltal (Bowerman, 1996); on their strategies for new word formation in English as compared with Hebrew and other languages (E. V. Clark, 1993; E. V. Clark & Berman, 1984, 1987); on children's narrative development in different languages (Berman & Slobin, 1994); as well as on children's strategies for extracting morphological information from their orthographies in Hebrew as compared with Dutch (Gillis & Ravid, 2000, 2001). Findings of research in these different domains converge to show that children are attuned to the language particular way of encoding form–meaning relations in their language. The time when this type of sensitivity finds expression will depend on shared, universal factors—linguistic, cognitive, and perceptual—which underlie developmental patternings in general. For example, the kind of spatial distinctions noted by Bowerman will precede command of derivational marking of linguistic subcategories, and these will emerge earlier than rhetorical mastery of linguistic forms in the context of extended narratives. But, in each case reported, the way children encode form–meaning relations accords with the way this is done by adult speakers of the same target language rather than by children of the same age in other languages.

Although this chapter focuses on a single language, it aims to provide further evidence for the critical impact of target-language typology on linguistic learning by investigating knowledge of Hebrew derivational morphology in grade school-age children with SLI versus nonimpaired controls.

MORPHOLOGY IN SLI

Children with SLI have impairments in inflectional morphology, a poor ability to acquire new words, and school-related problems such as persistent spelling errors and dropping morphological suffixes in writing (see Dromi, Leonard, and Blass, chap. 11 in this volume, for a study of morphology in Hebrew SLI). Although similar to their age matched peers in oral judgment, they have been found to demonstrate more difficulties in spontaneous writing (Rubin, Kantor, & Macnab, 1990; Leonard, chap. 8 in this volume). Indeed, estimates of the occurrence of SLI in the United States suggest that 5% of the preschool population may be affected, the majority of whom are at a very high risk for learning disability into the grade school years, initially with learning to read, later on in situations requiring complex language skills (Paul, 1995; Weiss, 1997).

Several studies have pointed out linguistic processing problems in children with SLI. They are slow in processing linguistic information; they do not make efficient use of sentence structure and of discourse structure in identifying the meaning of an unfamiliar word; they take more time in task of lexical retrieval; and they have difficulties in referent introduction and reference maintenance in story re-telling (de Weck, 1998; Stone & Connel, 1993). Studies have also identified metalinguistic problems in language-impaired children at a number of levels—phonology, lexicon, syntax, pragmatics—which interact and affect each other, resulting in some cases in communicative impairment (Rubin, 1988; Swisher, Restrepo, Plante, & Lowell, 1995).

The lexicon, a focus of this study, has a central role in acquisition and in language disorders. Studies have pointed out a host of lexical processing problems in children with SLI, such as taking more time in tasks of lexical retrieval and in fast mapping; a reduced tendency to extend new object names to unnamed members of the same category; and a need for phonologically and syntactically clearer and more transparent lexical input than nonimpaired children. Studies have also identified difficulties in morphological analysis typical of children with SLI, a reduced ability to manipulate morphemes and generalize morpheme meaning, and resulting problems in word learning, especially under explicit experimental conditions (Swisher & Snow, 1994; Swisher et al., 1995). The immense importance of lexical development in schoolchildren, which underlies almost every other linguistic achievement (Berman & Ravid, 1999), directs attention to words and their structure.

Derivational morphology constitutes a useful, although to date untapped, source for examining linguistic command in children with SLI. Because derivational morphology is a richer, less obligatory and more complex domain than inflectional morphology, it promises to be diagnostic of linguistic abilities in older, more linguistically sophisticated children who have already mastered the form and semantics of obligatory inflections. Moreover, it requires integrated knowledge of the interrelation between lexical convention, semantic content, and formal structure—areas that continue to develop well into school age and are related to literacy.

The degree of language syntheticity and morphological salience, transparency, and productivity has already been shown to play a crucial role in studies of inflectional morphology in English-speaking children with SLI, who did not fare as well as similar children acquiring morphologically richer languages such as Italian and Hebrew (Dromi, Leonard, & Shteiman, 1993; Leonard, Bortolini, Caselli, McGregor, & Sabbadini, 1992; Rom & Leonard, 1990). It seems that children growing up in languages with rich morphologies featuring a variety of salient, stressed morphemes find inflectional morphology tasks easier than children growing up in languages with impoverished inflection (but see Crago and Paradis, chap. 3 in this volume, for a different view based on SLI in Inuktitut). This chapter examines knowledge of derivational morphology in grade-schoolers with SLI and nonimpaired controls who are all native speakers of Hebrew, a highly synthetic language with a rich morphology.

STUDIES OF GRADE SCHOOL CHILDREN WITH SLI

It is well-accepted by now that natural language development runs its course over a long and protracted period until adolescence and beyond; and during the school years it interacts intensively with the acquisition of literacy (Berman & Ravid, 1999; Nippold, 1998). Language acquisition during the school years, or *later language development*, takes place at every linguistic level (lexical, grammatical, and pragmatic) and is accompanied by increasing metalinguistic awareness, abstractization, and explicitation of linguistic representation (Karmiloff-Smith, 1992; Scholnick, Nelson, Gelman, & Miller, 1999). Concomitantly, perception of nonliteral linguistic functions—such as figurative language, linguistic ambiguity, sarcasm, irony, and language puns—emerges and consolidates during the school-age and adolescent years (Ashkenazi & Ravid, 1998; Nippold, 1998).

By elementary school, children have acquired a large and varied vocabulary with complex hierarchical lexical and morphological connections (Anglin, 1993). Morphological and syntactic knowledge is well established beyond the level of the simple clause, and by the end of elementary school children are able, at the one extreme, to tell well-formed narratives, whereas at the other extreme, they are familiar with most morphophonological variants of words and morphemes in their language (Berman & Slobin, 1994; Ravid, 1995). Growing familiarity with written language both as a notational system and as discourse style contributes to increasing linguistic literacy (i.e., the availability of multiple linguistic resources and the ability to consciously access one's own linguistic knowledge and to view language from various perspectives) during the school years, side by side with the acquisition of new, less canonical structures typical of written language (Levin, Ravid, & Rappaport, 2001; Ravid & Avidor, 1998; Ravid & Tolchinsky, 2002).

Language in schoolchildren is thus very different from preschool linguistic knowledge, and a critical distinguishing factor is the acquisition of literacy. This has not escaped the notice of language disorders researchers, as summed up in a number of recent publications examining the relation between language disorders and literacy (Catts, Fey, Zhang, & Tomblin, 1999; Catts & Kamhi, 1999).

The ability of children with SLI to acquire new words, a critical factor in later language development, is impaired, and they demonstrate difficulty with productive application of morphological knowledge (Nagy, Anderson, Scommer, Scott, & Stellmen, 1989). Accordingly, problems in school-related abilities, such as persistent spelling errors and dropping morphological suffixes in writing, are reported. Although similar to their age matched nonimpaired peers in oral judgment, children with SLI demonstrate more difficulties in spontaneous writing (Rubin et al., 1990). The majority of children with SLI are thus at a very high risk for learning disability in elementary school, initially with learning to read, later on in situations requiring complex language skills (Paul, 1995; Weiss, 1997).

To date, most studies on derivational morphology in children with SLI have been conducted on grade school-aged English-speaking children, because rich derivational structures in English mostly require components that are not part of the mostly monomorphemic Germanic core lexicon, and are therefore acquired later. These studies have found that children with SLI are insensitive to derivational relations (Moats & Smith, 1992), storing words in isolated rather than network forms (Carlisle, 1988). They also have difficulty in applying morphological rules to unfamiliar words, and demonstrate a reduced ability for organizing and accessing words through morphological relations (Freyd & Baron, 1982; Nagy et al., 1989).

Studies in the development of Hebrew indicate the centrality of morphological knowledge in Israeli schoolchildren. Hebrew-speaking children are able to relate words by their morphological structure, they productively use semantic and structural options in morphology, and they show awareness of basic morphological components such as roots and suffixes (Ravid & Malenky, 2001). These abilities are enhanced by formal literacy instruction, which fosters metalinguistic thinking about language units (Levin et al., 2001; Olson, 1994; Ravid & Tolchinsky, 2002). For example, Hebrew spelling crucially involves phonological and morphological representation and processing (Gillis & Ravid, 2000; Ravid, 2001).

This chapter reports findings on comprehension and production of Hebrew nouns and adjectives in grade school children with SLI as compared with nonimpaired controls. In this age group, it is possible to examine morphological knowledge beyond the obligatory inflectional systems that are mastered early on, and to look for more subtle differences in formal and semantic mapping of derivational morphology, which can supply further clues on the nature of SLI.

DERIVATIONAL MORPHOLOGY IN HEBREW ACQUISITION

In view of the processing problems in children with SLI attested in the literature, Hebrew derivational morphology seems to be a particularly appropriate domain to study, because it provides its speakers with a number of structural, in many cases nontransparent, options for expressing the same notion. Hebrew word formation takes five main forms (Berman, 1987; Ravid, 1990):

1. The typically Semitic nonlinear *root-and-pattern* affixation combining consonantal roots with the necessary vocalic components of the word mostly

supplied by the pattern. For example, verb *limed* 'taught' is composed of root *l-m-d* 'teach' and verb pattern *CiCeC*, in which the actual root radicals occupy the slots signified by large *C*s. All verbs, and many noun and adjective types are constructed nonlinearly. Verb patterns are traditionally termed *binyanim*, and noun and adjective patterns are termed *miškalim*. For a discussion of root and pattern functions, see Ravid and Makenky (2001).

2. Linear suffixation of *stem and suffix*. Stems, unlike roots, contain vowels, and suffixes are attached at the end of the stem (rather than intertwining with it, as does the pattern with the root), e.g., adjective *klal-i* 'gener-al'). Suffix meanings and functions are similar to those of patterns. Many noun and adjective types employ this word formation device (Ravid, 1990).

3. N-N or A-N *compounding*, where the head often undergoes allomorphic change (e.g., *kitat limud* 'class teaching = classroom', cf. *kita* 'class'). This word formation device is almost exclusively reserved to nouns (Clark & Berman, 1987).

4. *Blending* of two noun forms (e.g., *pélefon* 'cell phone' consisting of *péle* 'miracle' and *fon* 'phone'). This word formation device is restricted to nouns and adjectives (Berman, 1987).

5. *Zero conversion* (i.e., categorical shift without structural change) deriving nouns and adjectives from present-tense verbs (e.g., *mevaker* 'criticizes = critic', *mazhir* 'shines = brilliant'). Unlike English, for example, zero conversion works only from the verbal to the nominal domain, because deriving a verb from a noun would require root and pattern formation as in (1) (Ravid, 1990).

Over the past 15 or so years, a range of studies based on both structured elicitations and naturalistic speech data has been conducted on the acquisition of derivational morphology and strategies of new word formation in Hebrew. These include work on how children derive new nouns from familiar verbs (E. V. Clark & Berman, 1984), how children produce novel compound nouns (E. V. Clark & Berman, 1987), how children derive new verbs from familiar nouns (Berman, 1999), how children learn about adjective formation (Ravid & Nir, 2000), and how children alternate verbs across the Hebrew *binyan* patterns to mark distinctions of syntactic transitivity (Berman, 1993) and voice (Berman, 1994).

The key results of these studies underline the impact of Semitically specific derivational morphology. First, across the board and from a very early age, Hebrew-speaking children construct the verbs they produce (existing verbs as well as verbs that they innovate spontaneously or under experimental conditions) according to the small set of accepted verb patterns. That is, even 2- and 3-year-olds hardly ever use other possible, but non-typically Semitic devices (e.g., zero conversion or affixation to a stem) to produce new verbs or to alternate verbs from intransitive to transitive or from active to passive. Second, and relatedly, Hebrew-speaking children form nouns and adjectives in a much wider range of morphological patterns than verbs; these include the canonically Semitic device of associating a set affixal pattern with a consonantal root (e.g., root *g-l-x* 'shave' and pattern *maCCeCa* yielding innovative *maglexa* 'shaver' for a razor); and also forms based on an existing stem plus external suffix (e.g., innovative *cmi-ut* 'thirstiness', cf. *bdid-ut* 'loneliness', both ending with the abstract suffix *-ut*). Third, in contrast to children acquiring Germanic languages like English or German, Hebrew-speaking children do not often form novel compounds for naming agent nouns, preferring the typically Semitic devices of linear and nonlinear affixation. Children's lexical innovations proceed according to universal principles of perceptual salience, structural simplicity, and semantic transparency; for example, in forming compound nouns they make fewest errors with strings that require no morphological change in the head noun, whereas it takes them until school age to make appropriate stem changes. Compare, for example, *ciporey ya'ar* 'birds-of forest,' which children form correctly by age 5, with *pirxey xag* 'flowers-of festivity,' which even 7-year-olds had a hard time with (Berman & Ravid, 2000).

Studies of Hebrew derivational morphology in older, school-age children have investigated how they understand and produce verb-derived nominals (Ravid & Avidor, 1998), how they produce adjectives of various types (Levin et al., 2001; Ravid & Nir, 2000), how they perceive roots and patterns in metalinguistic tasks (Ravid & Malenky, 2001), and how they use morphological cues in their spelling (Gillis & Ravid, 2000, 2001). These studies document a broadening perception and mastery of the diversity of morphological options in Hebrew as well as of the semantic notions encoded in them in grade school children. Moreover, by the middle of grade school, Israeli children have the same perception of the main morphological structures in their language as adults, although not the same ability of deploying them (Ravid & Kubi, 2000). Thus, from early on, Hebrew-speaking children are attuned to the typological imperatives of their language, and they follow them in undertaking complex, literacy-related morphological tasks as well.

This chapter highlights the importance of derivational morphology in testing linguistic abilities in schoolchildren and in particular language disordered populations. Berman (2000) identified lexicon size and diversity as crucial in later language development in morphology, syntax, and text production in a variety of languages. According to Anglin (1993), processes of morphological analysis and generalization underlie lexical expansion in children, and at least half of the words in a child's lexicon are acquired through morphological form-to-meaning mapping. The importance of lexical knowledge in later language acquisition and linguistic literacy is now universally acknowledged, with specific reference to language impaired children (Nippold, 1998; Scott & Windsor, 2000). For children growing up in a highly synthetic language, where spoken and written words are related through their internal components, this knowledge is critical.

TESTING WORD FORMATION IN CHILDREN WITH SLI

Given this background, this chapter reports the findings of studies in two morphological domains, nouns and adjectives, in Hebrew-speaking grade-schoolers with SLI and in nonimpaired controls.

In classical linguistic terms, *nouns* are those terms that refer, describe, or designate objects in some way, whereas *adjectives* characterize them (Lyons, 1966). This is reflected in the fact that in many languages, adjectives agree with the noun they modify in number, gender, and in other languages, also in additional values such as definiteness or case (e.g., French, Latin, Hebrew). This implies that nouns have a fixed form independent of any modifier they receive, whereas adjectives presuppose a noun and adjust their form to correspond to its inflection (Markman, 1989). The two lexical classes differ in the way people organize and retrieve information in memory. Markman (1989) presented evidence from studies of paired associate learning and semantic memory in English that suggest that nouns may have some privileged status in memory, allowing more accurate, quicker access to information, and being more effective as memory cues than adjectives and verbs. For example, nouns are better retrieval cues than adjectives, and when nouns precede adjectives, N-A pairs are learned better despite the word order mismatch in English.

The essential difference between nouns and adjectives emerges early on in development. Gelman and Markman (1985) reported an experimental study of noun and adjective interpretation in young children (ages 2;6–3;6) who were asked to "find the ball" or to "find the red one." When asked to interpret adjectives, children tended to focus on a contrast between members of the same object category, but nouns prompted children to select the more distinctive exemplar of the category.

Diary studies and surveys of natural language acquisition show that adjectives appear later in child speech than do nouns and verbs (Casseli, Bates, Casadio, & Fenson, 1995; Rice, 1990; Sommers, Kozarevich, & Michaels, 1994). Adjectives constitute a low frequency class when compared to other content words in children's early lexicons in various languages (Dromi, 1987; Marvin, Beukelman, & Bilyeu, 1994; Ravid & Nir, 2000; Valian, 1986). Nevertheless, after an early phase of acquiring predominantly common nouns, children come to acquire larger numbers of verbs and adjectives as well (Barret, 1995).

Hebrew nouns and adjectives are much richer structurally than verbs. All verbs in Hebrew are root based and take a small, restricted set of obligatory morphological patterns. Nouns and adjectives, in contrast, share a range of forms from nonderived words, loan words, blends, compounds, linear stem plus suffix forms, and roots with several dozen patterns (Ravid, 1990). For example, a hypothetical place where one dreams (based on root *x-l-m* 'dream') may be expressed as root-and-pattern *mixlama*, stem-and-suffix *xalomiya*, blend *xalomakom* (from *xalom* 'dream' and *makom* 'place'), or compound *beyt ha-xalomot* 'house of dreams'. Nouns and adjectives thus encode a wide array of structural and semantic information in different ways. Some of these forms, such as denominal adjectives, derived nominals and compound forms are later acquisitions and are still under way during grade school age (Levin et al., 2001; Ravid & Cahana-Amitay, in press).

Population

The same population was used in both studies: 14 children with SLI (9 boys, 5 girls, age range 8;7–10;3, third and fourth graders) who had been diagnosed at the municipal speech services clinic by two speech pathologists using a battery of Hebrew tests. All subjects had taken the Hebrew version of the Wexler test, indicating a discrepancy of at least 15 points between their verbal and nonverbal abilities, and with no other diagnosed problems (Stark & Tallal, 1981). The children with SLI were matched by nonimpaired children in two control groups: The *age matched* controls were 14 typically developing children (9 boys, 5 girls), age range 8;3–10;3, with no language or other problems. They were matched one to one to the children with SLI by chronological age +/– 4 months and by SES (high, middle, low). The *language matched* control group of 14 children (9 boys, 5 girls), age range 6;4–8;3, were again matched one to one to the SLI participants by language level (+/– 6 months), using a subset of the ITPA (Illinois Test of Psycholinguistic Abilities) test that examines completion of auditory analogies (which is the only normed tool in Hebrew for this age bracket, up to age 10), and by SES. All the children in the study were native monolingual speakers of Hebrew with normal hearing and no other disorders.

The Noun Study

Noun Comprehension

Procedure. The comprehension task tested children's ability to analyze nonce nouns into their components, which were extant or "real" morphemes in Hebrew—roots, stems, patterns, and suffixes. For example, nonce *takan* 'fixer' (which is often produced spontaneously by Hebrew-speaking youngsters in reference to technicians and repair persons) consists of root *t-k-n* (cf. *tiken* 'fixed') and agent pattern *CaCaC*; and nonce *re'avon* 'hunger' (which is actually an obsolete Mishnaic Hebrew word) consists of current stem *ra'av* 'hunger' and abstract suffix *–on*. Participants were presented with the stimulus nonce noun and were asked to explain it. The instructions went as follows: "I have a picture here showing a place called *baloniya* (from *balon* 'balloon'). What is this place?" The accompanying picture was not shown, and was only revealed after the item was completed. The expected response would be an analysis of the stimulus item, containing its extant root or stem and linking it with the category supplied by the investigator (e.g., *makom še-bo mafrixim balonim*, 'a place where balloons are blown').

The following 12 nouns were tested in six semantic categories. Each item is presented with a possible gloss:

1. <u>Agent</u>: *tafranit* 'sewer, Fm = a person who sews' (Stem + Suffix) *takan* 'fixer' (Root + Pattern)
2. <u>Instrument</u>: *mašbera* 'breaker' (Root + Pattern), *ta'arixon* 'dater' (Stem + Suffix)
3. <u>Place</u>: *miclama* 'camera place' (Root + Pattern), *baloniya* 'balloon place' (Stem + Suffix)
4. <u>Abstract</u>: *re'avon* 'hunger' (Root + Pattern), *cmi'ut* 'thirst' (Stem + Suffix)
5. <u>Action Nominals</u>: *hitxatnut* 'marrying' (Root + Pattern), *hišta'alut* 'coughing' (Root + Pattern), *mihur* 'hurrying' (Root + Pattern)

Results. Children's comprehension responses were scored on a scale of from 1 (no response) to 5 (full response, containing correct root or stem and correct categorical component, i.e., pattern or suffix). For example, *miclama* 'camera place' is 'a place where they sell cameras,' and *re'avon* 'hunger' is 'a feeling when you are hungry.' Intermediate response types 2–3 involved phonological and semantic associations. Response of Type 4 lacked a categorial element, for example, in explaining the collective noun *gamélet* 'camel caravan,' the child came up with singular *gamal* 'camel rather than the required plural *gmalim*. Appendix I lists actual responses and their scores.

Responses were calculated as a mean of this scale of 5. The group with SLI scored a mean of 4.7 on this scale, the language matched younger controls scored 4.79, and the age matched older controls scored the highest at 4.86. These differences, however, were not significant. All statistical details can be found in Ravid, Avivi Ben-Zvi, and Levy (1999).

Discussion. These very high comprehension scores across the board are attributable to the psycholinguistic robustness of the lexical core of the Hebrew word—the Semitic all-consonantal root and the stem. In comprehension, the actual test question (e.g., "I have a picture here of a man / a child / an instrument, a place ... who Vs) presented the child with both structural components of the word—root and pattern, or stem and suffix. The lexical core was presented in the stimulus verb or noun, whereas the categorial component of the word was explicitly identified by referring to a person, an instrument, a place, a collection, or an action. Participants' task was restricted to relating the nonce stimulus item to a real word sharing the same root or stem, with no demand for manipulating the categorial element. This ability to manipulate roots and stems has been shown time and again to be at the core of Hebrew lexical productivity, and is essential to producing an utterance with an appropriate verb, which Israeli children do well before age 3 (Berman, 1993). In the category of nouns, this ability is available to all test groups, including the group with SLI. The results of the comprehension task thus indicate that, at least for nouns, the difference between typically developing children and children with SLI does not lie in the ability to relate words through their roots/stems. This is achieved in Hebrew much earlier and seems to be a basic type of derivational process that does not pose a problem to either younger schoolchildren or learners with SLI.

Noun Production

Procedure. The production task tested children's ability to produce novel nouns from verbs or from nouns. Participants were presented with a sentence containing either a stimulus verb or noun, and were asked to derive a novel noun from it in a target category. The instructions were as follows: "I have a picture here of many *neyarot* 'papers' together. What would you call a lot of papers together?", which is a request for a collective noun. The picture was again produced after the child gave the response. The following 10 nouns were elicited in six semantic categories:

1. Agent: *le-xabek* 'to-hug' (possible target: *xabkan* 'hugger'), *le-hacik* 'to-annoy' (possible target: *mecikan* 'annoyer')
2. Instrument: *le-hadlik* 'to-light' (possible target: *madlek* 'lighter'), *li-kcoc* 'to-chop' (possible target: *makceca* 'chopper')
3. Place: *la-xalom* 'to-dream' (possible target: *xalomiya* 'dreaming place', *le-vašel* 'to-cook' (possible target: *mivšala* 'cooking place')
4. Collective: *harbe diskim* 'lots of discs' (possible target: *diskiya* 'disc collection', *harbe neyarot* 'lots of papers' (possible target: *nayéret* 'paperwork')

    5. Abstract: *le-hitragez* 'to-get mad' (possible target: *hitragzut* 'getting mad', Action Nominal: *le-saxek* 'to-play' (possible target: *sixuk* 'playing')

The scoring scale for production ranged from 1 to 11. Response types 1–5 involved, apart from no response and repetition, extant words, and phonological and semantic associations (e.g., giving *menora* 'lamp' for "an instrument whose function is to light things"). Types 6–7 were a syntactic response (e.g., *ze maxshir she-madlik*, 'it's an instrument that lights') and a response with an incorrect morphological element (e.g., instead of deriving an abstract nominal *hitragzut* from *le-hitragez* 'to get mad,' the child coined agentive *ragzan*). Responses 8–11 were all counted as "correct," and they consisted of all the morphological options described earlier. Zero-converted responses (e.g., present tense verb *mexabek* for agent noun 'hugger') received a lower correct score of 8 because they do not involve much structural work. Compounds, a semisyntactic option, received a score of 9, and suffixed forms a score of 10. The highest score of 11 was assigned to nonlinear root-and-pattern forms, as in most of the possible targets suggested earlier. Appendix I lists actual responses and their scores.

    Results. Responses were calculated as means on this scale of 11. The children with SLI scored a mean of 6.82 on the scale, the language matched controls scored 7.9, and the mean score of the age matched control group was 9.25. These differences were all significant. When analyzing the three groups' scores on the six semantic categories, the set of more basic agent-instrument-place nouns had significantly higher scores across the board (1.64 on a scale of 2) than the set of collective-abstract nouns (0.75). However, whereas both nonimpaired groups did significantly better on the agent-instrument-place set than on the collective-abstract set, in the group with SLI the agent-instrument set was better than the place nouns, which in turn was better than the collective-abstract set. In fact, the younger language matched group did better than the group with SLI on both the basic agent-instrument set as well as on the abstract nouns, whereas the age matched group did better than both the younger language matched and the SLI groups on collective nouns. All statistical details can be found in Ravid et al. (1999).

    Discussion. The production task indicated where morphological knowledge of Hebrew nouns in children with SLI crucially differs from nonimpaired children. The production results consistently show the same pattern: Age matched controls ≥ younger language matched controls ≥ children with SLI. Despite their superiority in age and level of schooling, the children with SLI fared worse in production than the language matched group, let alone the age matched group, supporting Carlisle's (1988) claim that children with SLI fail in productive application of structural knowledge in word formation.

The difference resides in the categorial component of nouns—the pattern or the suffix, which are affixes rather than roots, categorizing nouns into ontological categories (agent, instrument, abstract noun, etc.). The ability to extract and manipulate noun categories may involve higher order abstract morpholexical organization in accommodating new words into the system and creating network relations with other words. The identification of roots and stems, which convey local lexically encodable information, is easier and more basic for Hebrew speakers. These results are in line with the finding that roots and stems, the basic lexical building blocks of words, are more accessible to metalinguistic analysis than affixes, which are categorizing elements, especially in younger Hebrew-speaking participants (Ravid & Malenky, 2001). Anglin (1993) asked English grade school children to provide the meanings of inflected or derived words. Most participants manifested a "part to whole" pattern, in which they discussed the stem embedded within the target word, either a root word or an embedded derived word. Only the oldest children were occasionally able to relate to the affixes as well as to the stems (Anglin, 1993, p. 116), showing some problem-solving strategies in analyzing morphological structure.

The problems children with SLI have with noun categories also find expression in the breakdown of semantic categories. In nonimpaired development, the agent-instrument-place set scored higher than the collective-abstract set, but the children with SLI found even this basic set hard to tackle.

The correct production responses were also ranked by degree of inner syntheticity: from analytical compounding and zero conversion respectively ranked 1 and 2, through the more synthetic linear suffixation, a word-internal device ranked 3, to the typically Semitic nonlinear root-and-pattern structure ranked 4. For example, a set of possible correct collective noun responses to "a lot of discs" might be *xavilat diskim* 'pack of discs' (compound, ranked 1); linear stem + collective *-iya* suffix *diskiya*, ranked 3; and nonlinear root-and-pattern *daséket* in the collective pattern *CaCéCet* (compare *canéret* 'pipe system' from *cinor* 'pipe'), ranked 4.

An interesting finding emerged in the patterning of participants' correct responses concerning degree of syntheticity: The older age matched controls scored significantly higher—that is, used more synthetic devices (3.71 on a scale of 4) than both the younger language matched controls (2.0) and the group with SLI (1.28). On this issue of deploying more structural devices to express the variety of semantic options presented in the noun test, the older, more linguistically mature age matched controls were better able to use the less transparent and more Semitic morphological devices than the younger controls and the SLI group.

The Adjective Study

Due to the secondary, less stable nature of adjectives, and the fact that they emerge later than nouns in acquisition, this study used real rather than nonce adjectives. Modern Hebrew has three structural categories of adjectives: One is an essentially closed class of primary, synchronically structureless *CVC* adjectives that originate in biblical present tense adjectives (e.g., *tov* 'good', *kar* 'cold'). A second category consists of nonlinear root + pattern structures, almost all appropriated from either verbal or nominal patterns in the biblical spirit (e.g., resultative adjectives such as *mesukan* 'dangerous' or *šavur* 'broken,' which take present tense verbal patterns; or potential-attribute adjectives such as *axil* 'edible' and *raxic* 'washable,' which share nominal patterns). The third is the only real, productive category of adjectives in modern Hebrew, a late historical development deriving from the biblical *-i* suffixed ethnic nouns, now a full-fledged category of linearly suffixed denominal adjectives (e.g., *xašmali* 'electric' from *xašmal* 'electricity' suffixed by adjectival *-i*).

The morphologically complex second and third categories of adjectives were tested. Three types of root-and-pattern adjectives were selected from the second category: resultative adjectives (e.g., *šafux* 'spilled', root *š-p-x*, pattern *CaCuC*), agentive-attributive adjectives (e.g., *xamkan* 'slippery', root *x-m-k*, pattern *CaCCan*), and potential-attribute adjectives (e.g., *raxic* 'washable', root *r-x-c*, pattern *CaCiC*). The linearly formed items were the denominal adjectives suffixed by *-i* (e.g., *gamadi* 'dwarf-like') from base noun *gamad* 'dwarf', and *xorpi* 'wintry', from base noun *xóref* 'winter'). Denominal adjectives are typical of higher register, written Hebrew, such as literary prose, journalistic and expository texts, and their meaning is quite complex (Berman & Ravid, 1999; Levin et al., 2001). Apart from lexicalized forms, they are completely absent from child-directed speech. They are the last type of adjectives to emerge around age 6 in Hebrew child language, and they do not occur in text production before high school (Ravid & Zilberbuch, submitted; Ravid & Nir, 2000).

Adjective Comprehension

Procedure. The adjective comprehension task tested children's ability to analyze real adjectives into their morphological components—roots, stems, patterns, and suffixes—by interpreting a set of given adjective stimuli. For example, *menusar* 'sawn' consists of root *n-s-r* and resultative pattern *meCuCaC*. Participants were presented with an adjective embedded in a sentential context, and asked to explain its meaning, which entailed using a related noun or verb: for example, "I have a picture here showing a glass with some juice, and a picture of some *spilled* juice (*mic šafux* 'juice spilled'). What happened here?" A possible response to this resultative adjective was *šafxu oto* '(they) spilled, Pl it', an impersonal active verb form from the same root and in the appropriate verb pattern. The accompanying picture was not shown, and was only revealed after the item was completed.

The following 13 adjectives were tested in two main structural categories and in three semantic categories:

I Root and pattern structure

1. Resultative, *CaCuC* pattern: *šafux* 'spilled', *atufa* 'wrapped up, Fm'
      meCuCaC pattern: *menusar* 'sawn', *mexutélet* 'diapered, Fm'
      muCCaC pattern: *muram* 'elevated', *mušxal* 'threaded'
2. Attributive, *CaCCan* pattern: *caxkan* 'laughy', *acbanit* 'nervous, Fm'
      CaCiC pattern: *ra'il* 'poisonous', *raxic* 'washable'

II Stem and suffix structure: Denominal *i*-suffixed adjectives
      tinoki 'babyish', *xorpi* 'wintry', *barvazit* 'duck-like, Fm'

The comprehension responses were scored on a scale of 1–4. A score of 1 was assigned to no response and responses such as 'don't know'. A score of 2 was assigned to a semantically, but not morphologically, appropriate response, *ko'éset* 'is angry, Fm', instead of *mit'acbénet* 'becomes annoyed' as a response to the stimuli *acbanit* 'nervous, annoyed'. A score of 3 was assigned to a partial, although morphologically appropriate, response, where one structural element (stem or root, suffix or pattern) was absent. For example, the *caxkan* 'laughy' boy *macxik harbe* 'makes (you) laugh a lot' instead of *coxek harbe* 'laughs a lot', where the verb pattern is the inappropriate causative instead of the desired simple active pattern. A score of 4 was assigned to a fully correct response, for example, responding to *menusar* 'sawn' with *nisru oto* '(they) sawed it'. Appendix II lists actual responses and their scores.

Results. On this scale of 4, the children with SLI scored a mean of 3.57, which is significantly lower than those of the two nonimpaired groups: the language matched group (3.82) and the age matched group (3.9). Specific statistical details can be found in Ravid, Levie, and Avivi Ben-Zvi (in press).

Discussion. The greater difficulty experienced by the group with SLI on the adjective test, compared with the noun results, may be due to the non-canonical, semantically and structurally diverse category of adjectives. This may have been exacerbated by the fact that the comprehension task required the analysis of extant adjectives into their morphological components. Specifically, correct responses consisted of morphologically appropriate nouns and verbs with specific patterns, related to the stimulus adjective by root. Thus, although comprehension responses involved nouns and verbs rather than adjectives, the required analysis may have proved too difficult for the schoolchildren with SLI, especially on the more difficult categories of attributive and denominal adjectives. These results may reflect a weaker processing capacity for linguistic information, difficulty in using sentence structure for the analysis of word meaning, and a reduced ability of perceiving derivational relations among words (Carlisle, 1988; Moats & Smith, 1992; Swisher et al., 1995).

Adjective Production

Procedure. The adjective production task tested children's ability to produce 13 adjectives from randomly presented verb and noun stimuli. Participants were presented with a sentence containing a verb or noun, and asked to derive an adjective from it: for example, "I have a picture here of a hand that got *stuck in glue* (*nidbeka be-dévek*). What can we say now about the hand that has got glue on it?" This sentence contained the requested root *d-b-k* in the two stimuli *stuck* and *glue*. A possible response could be '*hi dvika* 'it (is) sticky', an attributive adjective in the nominal *CaCiC* pattern, with the same root. The picture again was produced only after the participant had given the response.

The following 13 adjectives were tested in two main structural categories and in three semantic categories:

I Root and pattern structure
1. Resultative, *CaCuC* pattern: *cavuá* 'painted', *banuy* 'built'
   meCuCaC pattern: *meyubaš* 'dried', *meforéket* 'taken apart, Fm'
   muCCaC pattern: *mufšal* 'turned up', *muxba* 'hidden'
2. Attributive, *CaCCan* pattern: *xamkan* 'slippery', *navranit* 'pokey, Fm'
   CaCiC pattern: *axil* 'edible', *dvika* 'sticky, Fm'

II Stem and suffix denominal *i*-suffixed adjectives
   arsi 'venomous', *gamadi* 'dwarf-like', *kalbi* 'canine'

The production responses were scored on a 1–7 scale. A score of 1 was assigned to no response and responses such as 'don't know'. A score of 2 was assigned to a repetition response. A score of 3 was assigned to analytic rather than morphological expression (e.g., 'it can kill somebody' for *arsi* 'venomous'). A score of 4 was assigned to a semantically, but not morphologically, appropriate response (e.g., wrong-root *paxdan* 'coward' for *xamkan* 'slippery', as a response to the stimuli *xomek* 'slips away'). A score of 5 was assigned to a partial response with the requested root but from another lexical category (e.g., *bniya* 'building' for *banuy* 'built', as a response to *banu oto* '(they) built Acc-it', from root *b-n-y*). A score of 6 was assigned to an unconventional adjective (e.g., *pruka* [*CaCuC* pattern] for *meforéket* [*meCuCaC* pattern] 'taken apart', as a response to *perku ota* '[they] took it apart'). A score of 7 was assigned to a fully correct response, as in the previous examples. Appendix II lists actual responses and their scores.

Results. On this scale of 7, children with SLI scored a mean of 4.81, the language matched group scored 5.4, and the age matched group scored 6.31. All differences were significant. All statistical details can be found in Ravid et al. (in press).

Discussion. To explain these results, note that although the children with SLI were older than the language matched controls and therefore officially had more schooling, it can be assumed that their level of linguistic literacy was not as advanced (Ravid & Tolchinsky, 2000). Because SLI interferes with the acquisition of reading and writing skills, children from this group may have been less familiar with written language, having had less exposure to written texts and fewer opportunities to write, and therefore were less likely to learn new words from the written language, which constitutes the main source for new vocabulary in grade school (Anglin, 1993; Rubin et al., 1990).

Moreover, this linguistic disorder is characterized by problems in morphological processing, such as difficulties in storing and retrieving linguistic information based on derivational relations. These considerations would explain why the SLI group found it difficult to interpret and create lexically linked words (Swisher & Snow, 1994).

Focusing on the three semantic adjective categories (resultative-attributive-denominal), the resultative adjectives were easiest across the board: On the scale of 7, the children with SLI scored 5.34, the language matched controls scored 6.17, and the age matched controls scored 6.86. From a structural point of view, resultatives are not harder than other root-and-pattern forms, which children acquiring Semitic languages manipulate from early on (Berman & Ravid, 2000; Ravid & Farah, 1999). They occur in early child speech as lexicalized forms, such as *meluxlax* 'dirty', but they emerge productively only in later preschool age (4–6) due to their passive-resultative semantics (Berman, 1994; Yagev, 2001). Nevertheless, even on this easiest category, the group with SLI differed significantly than the two control groups.

The attributive and denominal adjective categories were harder, and did not differ from each other: The children with SLI scored 4.22 and 4.52, respectively; the language matched controls scored 4.60 and 4.88, respectively, and the age matched controls scored 5.89 and 5.78, respectively. On these two harder categories, the older age matched controls scored significantly better than both the younger language matched controls and the group with SLI.

In both cases, semantics seems to be a more weighty factor than structure and requires more linguistic maturity to achieve. The attributive category tested consisted of two structural constructions: *CaCCan* adjectives (e.g., *xamkan* 'slippery'), an early emerging attributive-agentive class that is immensely productive in both child and child-directed speech (E. V. Clark & Berman, 1984); but also *CaCiC* potential-attribute adjectives (e.g., *axil* 'edible). The option of encoding a *potential* attribute morphologically is not available to preschoolers, and is typical mostly of formal, written Hebrew. The combination of the two attributive adjective categories with the easier and the more difficult semantics resulted in similar scores to those of the denominal category.

Focusing on denominal adjectives, it is not the formal addition of the suffix *-i* to the noun base and the consequent morphophonological stem changes that make it so difficult: The same morphophonological stem changes (as in *kélev/kalbi* 'dog/canine') occur across the board in all types of nominal operations in Hebrew, both inflectional and derivational—noun plurals, noun feminines, noun possessives, and noun compounds. Children have plenty of opportunities to learn the rules and intricacies of the system from early childhood, although radical, idiosyncratic stem changes are difficult even in grade school (Levin et al., 2001; Ravid, 1995). Rather, denominal adjectives are semantically complex entities. The appropriate property of the base noun that is carried over to the derived adjective is not always predictable, as in other cases of denominal derivation (Aronoff, 1980; E. V. Clark & H. H. Clark, 1979). Like potential-attribute *CaCiC* adjectives, denominal adjectives are typical of formal, written Hebrew, occurring mostly in expository texts. Whereas Hebrew speakers are exposed to such texts in school and school-related activities, they do not use them productively before the end of high school (Berman & Ravid, 1999; Ravid & Zilberbuch, submitted). Certainly, the younger language matched group and the group with SLI had had fewer opportunities to encounter such forms and were less able to process them.

A qualitative analysis showed that two production strategies were especially prevalent in the responses of the SLI group as compared with the two control groups. Those were the "analytic expression" (e.g., *ha-pérax ibed máyim* 'the-flower lost water' for *meyubaš* 'dried') and "associative semantic response" (e.g., *acic* 'potted plant' for *ec gamadi* 'tree dwarf-like = dwarf-like tree') on the production scale. These two nonmorphological strategies—retrieval of familiar forms from the stored mental lexicon and syntactic expression—reflect morphological processing problems in children with SLI, and were not as widely used by the younger language matched group. They point at difficulties in performing metalinguistic derivational analyses in an online experimental situation, and a failure to identify shared mor phemes, which would facilitate establishing connections between words from the same morphological family.

A third, morphological strategy, termed *unconventional adjective*, was shared by the SLI group and their language matched peers. This involved combining a correct root with an incorrect resultative pattern, resulting in an unconventional form, *nexba* (*niCCaC* pattern) for correct *xavuy* (*CaCuC*) 'hidden'. This strategy is well known from both naturalistic and experimental Hebrew child language data, and is characteristic of spontaneous expression in preschoolers (Berman, 1994). Thus, it indicates juvenile, less well-developed morphological skills, rather than deviant strategies in the SLI group.

CONCLUSIONS

The two studies reported in this chapter focused on knowledge of nominal and adjectival structure and semantics in Hebrew-speaking grade-schoolers with SLI versus nonimpaired control groups, in a series of tasks that required the ability to relate and retrieve lexical items through their internal components. On almost all measures, derivational morphology was found to be diagnostic of the impaired population. On the whole, the children with SLI did as well as their nonimpaired peers on comprehending nonce nouns, but not as well on real adjective comprehension, indicating the less stable representation of adjectives and greater difficulty in relating their components (Levin et al., 2001). Hebrew-speaking grade-schoolers with SLI did worse than their peers on nonce noun production, including the basic category of agent-instrument (E. V. Clark, 1993), and were less able to deploy the array of Semitic structural options productively. They also did worse than their peers on real adjective production, including the more basic category of resultative adjectives, which emerges in preschool age (Berman, 1994; Yagev, 2001). Taken together, these studies indicate that the morphological problems described in the literature in young children with SLI continue to challenge them in grade school age in a knowledge domain that is crucial to language development and literacy.

This study highlights the importance of *diversity* in examining the linguistic abilities of children with SLI. Diversity refers to various aspects of linguistic systems. In one sense, it refers here to the study of a wider range of languages acquired by children with SLI in order to examine the impact of linguistic typology. A synthetic language such as Hebrew, where many notions are encoded by morphological devices, and where these notions are expressed in a variety of competing structures with numerous morpho-phonological alternations, is particularly appropriate for this endeavor. On the one hand, such morphological wealth may challenge children with SLI in areas that require processing and analysis skills in order to derive mean ing; but, on the other hand, exposure to synthetic morphology from birth has been shown to attune learners to look for exactly those meaningfu components. Further studies in Hebrew and in other synthetically rich lan guages is necessary to determine the extent to which typological impera tives feature in language impairment.

From a different perspective, diversity refers to the examination of a number of linguistic systems in the same population. The study of compre hension and production of different lexical categories in Hebrew has proved fruitful in pinpointing differences between children with SLI and typ ically developing children. The inherent semantic and morphological attri butes of nouns and adjectives highlighted domains of difficulty in the study populations. Further analyses of other linguistic systems with different fea tures are called for, such as derivational morphology in the verb system optional bound inflectional morphology, and morphological aspects of the spelling system. These may reveal more subtle characteristics of the popu lation with SLI and enhance understanding of linguistic disorders.

The findings described here may be extended to other populations as well. Knowledge of derivational morphology, linked with lexical knowledge would be diagnostic in testing late emerging language skills in other im paired populations, such as children with cleft palate (Yagev, 2001), on the one hand, and in immigrant and bilingual populations, on the other.

REFERENCES

Aksu-Koc, A., & Slobin, D. I. (1985). The acquisition of Turkish. In D. I. Slobin (Ed.), *The cross linguistic study of language acquisition* (Vol. 1, pp. 839–880). Hillsdale, NJ: Lawrence Erlbaum Associates.

Anglin, J. M. (1993). Vocabulary development: A morphological analysis. *Monographs of the Soci ety for Research in Child Development, 58,* 10.

Aronoff, M. (1980). Contextuals. *Language, 56,* 744–758.

Ashkenazi, O., & Ravid, D. (1998). Children's understanding of linguistic humor: An aspect o metalinguistic awareness. *Current Psychology of Cognition, 17,* 367–387.

Barrett, M. (1995). Early lexical development. In P. Fletcher & B. MacWhinney (Eds.), *The hand book of child language* (pp. 362–392). Oxford, England: Blackwell.

Berman, R. A. (1986). A step-by-step model of language acquisition. In I. Levin (Ed.), *Stage and structure: Reopening the debate* (pp. 191–219). Norwood, NJ: Ablex.

Berman, R. A. (1987). Productivity in the lexicon: New-word formation in modern Hebrew. *Folia Linguistica, 21,* 225–254.

Berman, R. A. (1993). Marking of verb transitivity by Hebrew-speaking children. *Journal of Child Language, 20,* 641–669.

Berman, R. A. (1994). Formal, lexical, and semantic factors in the acquisition of Hebrew resulta tive participles. *Berkeley Linguistic Society, 20,* 82–92.

Berman, R. A. (1999). Children's innovative verbs versus nouns: Structured elicitations and spontaneous coinages. In L. Menn & N. Bernstein-Ratner (Eds.), *Methods in studying language production* (pp. 69–93). Mahwah, NJ: Lawrence Erlbaum Associates.

Berman, R. A. (2000, September). *Developing literacy in different contexts and in different languages.* Final report submitted to the Spencer Foundation.

Berman, R. A. (in press). From known to new: How children coin nouns compared with verbs in Hebrew. In L. Menn & N. Bernstein-Ratner (Eds.), *Festschrift for Jean Berko Gleason.*

Berman, R. A., & Ravid, D. (1999, September). *The oral/literate continuum: Developmental perspectives.* Final report submitted to the Israel Science Foundation, Tel Aviv University.

Berman, R. A., & Ravid, D. (2000). Acquisition of Israeli Hebrew and Palestinian Arabic: A review of current research. *Hebrew Studies, 41,* 7–22.

Berman, R. A., & Slobin, D. I. (1994). *Different ways of relating events in narrative: A crosslinguistic developmental study.* Hillsdale, NJ: Lawrence Erlbaum Associates.

Bowerman, M. (1996). Learning how to structure space for language: A crosslinguistic perspective. In P. Bloom, M. Peterson, L. Nadel, & M. Garrett (Eds.), *Language and space* (pp. 385–436). Cambridge, MA: MIT Press.

Carlisle, J. F. (1988). Knowledge of derivational morphology and spelling ability in fourth, sixth and eighth graders. *Applied Psycholinguistics, 9,* 247–266.

Catts, H. W., Fey, M. E., Zhang, X., & Tomblin, J. B. (1999). Language basis of reading and reading disabilities; evidence from a longitudinal investigation. *Science Studies of Reading, 3,* 331–361.

Catts, H. W., & Kamhi, A. G. (Eds.). (1999). *Language and reading disabilities.* Needham Heights, MA: Allyn & Bacon.

Casseli, M. C., Bates, E., Casadio, P., & Fenson, J. (1995). A cross-linguistic study of early lexical development. *Cognitive Development, 10,* 159–199.

Clark, E. V. (1993). *The lexicon in acquisition.* Cambridge, England: Cambridge University Press.

Clark, E. V., & Berman, R. A. (1984). Structure and use in the acquisition of word formation. *Language, 60,* 542–590.

Clark, E. V., & Berman, R. A. (1987). Types of linguistic knowledge: Interpreting and producing compound nouns. *Journal of Child Language, 14,* 547–568.

Clark, E. V., & Clark, H. H. (1979). When nouns surface as verbs. *Language, 55,* 767–811.

de Weck, G. (1998). Anaphoric cohesion in young language-impaired and normally developing children. In A. Aksu-Koc, E. Erguvanli Taylan, A. Sumru Özsoy, & A. Küntay (Eds.), *Perspectives on language acquisition: Selected papers from the VIIth International Congress for the Study of Child Language* (pp. 292–308). Istanbul: Bogazici University Press.

Demuth, K. (1993). Issues in the acquisition of the Sesotho tonal system. *Journal of Child Language, 20,* 275–302.

Dromi, E. (1987). *Early lexical development.* Cambridge, England: Cambridge University Press.

Dromi, E., Leonard, L. B., & Shteiman, M. (1993). The grammatical morphology of Hebrew-speaking children with specific language impairment: Some competing hypotheses. *Journal of Speech and Hearing Research, 36,* 760–771.

Freyd, P., & Baron, J. (1982). Individual differences in acquisition of derivational morphology. *Journal of Verbal Learning and Verbal Behavior, 21,* 282–295.

Gathercole, V. C. M. (1997). Word meaning biases or language-specific effect? Evidence from English, Spanish and Korean. *First Language, 17,* 31–56.

Gelman, S. A., & Markman, E. M. (1985). Implicit contrast in adjectives vs. nouns: Implications for word-learning in preschoolers. *Journal of Child Language, 12,* 125–143.

Gillis, S., & Ravid, D. (2000). Effects of phonology and morphology in children's orthographic systems: A cross-linguistic study of Hebrew and Dutch. In E. Clark (Ed.), *The Proceedings of the 30th Annual Child Language Research Forum* (pp. 203–210). Stanford: Center for the Study of Language and Information.

Gillis, S., & Ravid, D. (2001). Language-specific effects on the development of written morphology. In S. Bendjaballah & W. U. Dressler (Eds.), *Morphology 2000* (pp. 129–136). Amsterdam: Benjamins.

Karmiloff-Smith, A. (1992). *Beyond modularity: a developmental perspective of cognitive science.* Cambridge, MA: MIT Press.

Jucszyk, P. W. (1997). *The discovery of spoken language.* Cambridge, MA: Bradford Books.

Leonard, L. B., Bortolini, V., Caselli, M. C., McGregor, K. K., & Sabbadini, L. (1992). Morphological deficits in children with specific language impairment: The status of features in the underlying grammar. *Language Acquisition, 2,* 151–179.

Levin, I., Ravid, D., & Rappaport, S. (2001). Morphology and spelling among Hebrew-speaking children: From kindergarten to first grade. *Journal of Child Language, 28,* 741–769.

Lyons, J. (1966). Towards a "notional" theory of the "parts of speech." *Journal of Linguistics, 79,* 1–13.

Markman, E. M. (1989). *Categorization and naming in children: Problems of induction.* Cambridge, MA: MIT Press.

Marvin, C. A., Beukelman, D. R., & Bilyeu, D. (1994). Vocabulary-use patterns in preschool children: Effects of context and time sampling. *Augmentative and Alternative Communication, 10,* 224–237.

Moats, L. C., & Smith, C. (1992). Derivational morphology: Why it should be included in language assessment and instruction. *Language, Speech and Hearing Services in Schools, 23,* 312–319.

Nagy, W. E., Anderson, R. C., Scommer, M., Scott, J. A., & Stellmen, A. C. (1989). *Reading Research Quarterly, 24,* 262–283.

Nippold, M. A. (1998). *Later Language development: The school-age and adolescent years* (2nd ed.). Austin, TX: PRO-ED.

Olson, D. (1994). *The world on paper: The conceptual and cognitive implications of writing and reading.* Cambridge, England: Cambridge University Press.

Paul, R. (1995). *Language disorders from infancy through adolescence: Assessment and intervention.* St. Louis: Mosby.

Ravid, D. (1990). Internal structure constraints on new-word formation devices in modern Hebrew. *Folia Linguistica, 24,* 289–346.

Ravid, D. (1995). *Language change in child and adult Hebrew: A psycholinguistic perspective.* New York: Oxford University Press.

Ravid, D. (2001). Learning to spell in Hebrew: Phonological and morphological factors. *Reading and Writing, 14,* 459–485.

Ravid, D., & Avidor, A. (1998). Acquisition of derived nominals in Hebrew: Developmental and linguistic principles. *Journal of Child Language, 25,* 229–266.

Ravid, D., Avivi Ben-Zvi, G., & Levy, R. (1999). Derivational morphology in SLI children: Structure and semantics of Hebrew nouns. In M. Perkins & S. Howard (Eds.), *New directions in language development and disorders* (pp. 39–49). New York: Plenum.

Ravid, D., & Cahana-Amitay, D. (in press). Verbal and nominal expression in narrative conflict situations. *Journal of Pragmatics.*

Ravid, D., & Farah, R. (1999). Learning about noun plurals in early Palestinian Arabic. *First Language, 19,* 187–206.

Ravid, D., & Kobi, E. (2000, August). *What is a spelling error? The discrepancy between perception and reality.* Paper presented at the "Writing Language" Workshop, Max Planck Institute for Psycholinguistics, Nijmegen, The Netherlands.

Ravid, D., Levie, R., & Avivi Ben-Zvi, G. (in press). Hebrew adjectives in language-impaired and typically developing gradeschoolers. In L. Verhoeven & Hans van Balkom (Eds.), *Classification of developmental language disorders: Theoretical issues and clinical implications.* Hillsdale, NJ: Lawrence Erlbaum Associates.

Ravid, D., & Malenky, A. (2001). Awareness of linear and nonlinear morphology in Hebrew: A developmental study. *First Language, 21,* 25–36.

Ravid, D., & Nir, M. (2000). On the development of the category of adjective in Hebrew. In M. Beers, B. van den Bogaerde, G. Bol, J. de Jong, & C. Rooijmans (Eds.), *From sound to sentence. Studies on first language acquisition* (pp. 113–124). Groningen: Center for Language and Cognition.

Ravid, D., & Tolchinsky, L. (2002). Developing linguistic literacy: A comprehensive model. *Journal of Child Language, 29*, 419–448.

Ravid, D., & Zilberbuch, S. (Submitted). *Morpho-syntactic constructs in the development of spoken and written text production.*

Rice, M. L. (1990). Preschoolers' QUIL: Quick incidental learning of words. In G. Contini-Ramsden & C. Snow (Eds.), *Children's language* (Vol. 7, pp. 171–195). Hillsdale, NJ: Lawrence Erlbaum Associates.

Rom, A., & Leonard, L. B. (1990). Interpreting deficits in grammatical morphology in specifically language-impaired children: Preliminary evidence from Hebrew. *Clinical Linguistics and Phonetics, 4*, 93–105.

Rubin, H. (1988). Morphological knowledge and early writing ability. *Language and Speech, 31*, 337–355.

Rubin, H., Kantor, M., & Macnab, J. (1990). Grammatical awareness in the spoken and written language of language-disabled children. *Canadian Journal of Psychology, 44*, 483–500.

Scholnick, E. K., Nelson, K., Gelman, S. A., & Miller, P. H. (Eds.). (1999). *Conceptual development: Piaget's legacy.* Hillsdale, NJ: Lawrence Erlbaum Associates.

Scott, C. M., & Windsor, J. (2000). General language performance measures in spoken and written narrative and expository discourse of school-age children with language learning disabilities. *Journal of Speech, Language, and Hearing Research, 43*, 324–339.

Sommers, R. K., Kozarevich, M., & Michaels, C. (1994). Word skills of children normal and impaired in communication skills and measures of language and speech development. *Journal of Communications Disorders, 27*, 223–240.

Stark, R. F., & Tallal, P. (1981). Selection of children with specific language deficits. *Journal of Speech and Hearing Disorders, 46*, 114–122.

Stone, C. A., & Connell, P. J. (1993). Induction of a visual symbolic rule in children with specific language impairment. *Journal of Speech and Hearing Research, 36*, 599–608.

Swisher, L., Restrepo, M. A., Plante, E., & Lowell, S. (1995). Effect of implicit and explicit "rule" presentation on bound-morpheme generalization in specific language impairment. *Journal of Speech and Hearing Research, 38*, 168–173.

Swisher, L., & Snow, D. (1994). Learning and generalization components of morphological acquisition by children with SLI: Is there a functional relation? *Journal of Speech and Hearing Research, 37*, 1406–1413.

Valian, V. (1986). Syntactic categories in the speech of young children. *Developmental Psychology, 22*, 562–579.

Weiss, A. L. (1997). Planning language intervention for young children. In D. K. Bernstein & E. Tiegerman-Farber (Eds.), *Language and communication disorders in children* (pp. 272–323). Boston: Allyn & Bacon.

Yagev, I. (2001). *Morphological and discourse knowledge in cleft-palate and non-impaired preschoolers.* Unpublished master's thesis, Department of Communications Disorders, Tel Aviv University.

APPENDIX I

Noun Comprehension Scale: 1–5 with Actual Examples

Stimulus	Correct Response	Example	Score	Motivation
hišta'alut 'coughing'	ha-yéled mišta'el 'the boy is coughing'	ha-yéled mišta'el 'the boy is coughing'	5	Full and correct response
gamélet 'camel caravan'	harbe gmalim 'lots of camels'	gamal 'camel'	4	Categorial element missing (collective pattern)
ta'arixon 'dater'	mar'e ta'arixim 'something showing dates'	torxim oto '(they) (incor.) date it'	3	Morphophonological suppletion
mihur 'hurrying'	ha-pe'ula še-osim kše-memaharim 'the act of hurrying'	racim, osim taxarut '(they) run, compete'	2	Association
mašbera 'breaker'	maxšir še-šovrim ito 'a tool used for breaking'	mašbera	1	Repetition

Note: All nouns are nonce words.

Noun Production Scale: 1–11 with Actual Examples

Stimulus	Correct Response	Example	Score	Motivation
yalda še-ohévet le-xabek 'a girl who likes to <u>hug</u>'	*xabkanit* 'hugger'	*xabkanit* 'hugger'	11	Full and correct response: nonlinear formation
yéled še-ohev le-hacik 'a boy who likes to <u>annoy</u>'	*mecikan* 'annoyer'	*mecikan* 'annoyer'	10	Full and correct response: linear formation
mašehu še-tafkido le-hadlik 'something which lights up things'	*madlek, madlikan . . .* 'lighter'	*madlik* 'lighter' (P5)	9	Full and correct response: zero conversion
makom še-banu bišvil la-xalom bo 'a place built to dream in'	*xalomiya, mixlama . . .* 'dreamplace'	*mekom ha-xalomot* 'place of dreams'	8	Full and correct response: compound
ha-hargaša šel yéled še-hitragez 'the feeling of a boy who got mad'	*rógez, regizut . . .* 'being mad'	*ragzani* 'easy to get mad'	7	Incorrect categorial element (pattern or suffix)
makom še-banu bišvil le-vašel bo 'a place built to cook in'	*mavšela, bišuliya . . .* 'cooking place'	*bišulim*	6	Morphologically related extant word
makom še-banu bišvil le-vašel bo 'a place built to cook in'	*mavšela, bišuliya . . .* 'cooking place'	*kan mevašlim bišulim* 'here (they) cook'	5	Syntactic expression
mašehu še-tafkido le-hadlik 'something which lights up things'	*madlek, madlikan . . .* 'lighter'	*menora* 'lamp'	4	Semantic suppletion
mašehu še-tafkido li-kcoc 'something which cuts up things'	*makcec, kocec, kocecan . . .* 'cutter'	*kocani* 'thorny'	3	Phonological suppletion
harbe neyarot yaxad 'lots of papers together'	*nayéret* 'paperwork'; *aremat neyarot* 'paper pile' . . .	*harbe neyarot*	2	Repetition
harbe neyarot yaxad 'lots of papers together'	*nayéret* 'paperwork'; *aremat neyarot* 'paper pile' . . .	*neyarukot*	1	No comprehension

Note: Some possible nouns are extant words, e.g., *rógez* 'annoyance', *nayéret* 'paperwork', but these are always either abstract or collective nouns, which are beyond the production abilities of this age range (Ravid & Avidor, 1998). Most nouns are nonce words and . . . means a number of responses are possible.

APPENDIX II

Adjective Comprehension Scale 1–4 with Actual Examples

Stimulus	Correct Response	Example	Score	Motivation
iš tinoki 'babyish man'	mitnaheg kmo tinok 'behaves like a baby'	lihyot tinok being a baby'	4	Full and correct response
yéled caxtan 'laughy boy'	coxek harbe 'laughs a lot (P1)'	maccxik harbe 'makes-laugh' a lot, P5	3	Incorrect categorial element (pattern)
yalda acbanit 'nervous girl'	mit'acbénet be-kalut 'becomes nervous easily/	ko'éset 'is angry'	2	Semantic suppletion
xaruz mushxal 'threaded bead'	hishxilu oto '(they) threaded it'	xilelu '(they) played the flute'	1	No comprehension

Adjective Production Scale: 1–7 with Actual Examples

Stimulus	Correct Response	Example	Score	Motivation
parpar še-xomek mi-kélev 'a butterfly that's eluding a dog'	xamkan 'elusive'	xamkan 'elusive'	7	Full and correct response
šaršéret še-perku ota 'a chain that (they) have taken apart'	meforéket 'taken apart, P4'	pruka 'taken apart, P1'	6	Incorrect categorial element (pattern)
yad še-nidbeka bešdévek 'a hand that's been stuck with glue'	dvika 'sticky'	davka 'stuck'	5	Different lexical category (V instead of Adj)
pérax še-ha-šémeš yibša 'a flower that the sun has dried'	meyubaš 'dried'	navul 'withered'	4	Semantic suppletion
naxaš imšéres 'a snake with venom'	arsi 'venomous'	yaxol la-harog mišehu 'may kill someone'	3	Syntactic expression
ec katan kmo gamad 'a small tree like a dwarf'	gamadi 'dwarflike'	katan kmo gamad 'small like a dwarf'	2	Repetition
davar še-efšar le-exol 'something you can eat'	axil 'edible'	mašehu rax 'something soft'	1	No comprehension

METHODOLOGICAL CONCERNS

AN INTRODUCTION

Gina Conti-Ramsden
Human Communication and Deafness
University of Manchester

Children with communication disorders have come to play an important role in the debate surrounding the nature of language learning in humans. In particular, the assumption that children with specific language impairment (SLI) have a primary linguistic difficulty in the absence of a number of possible explanatory factors that usually accompany other types of language impairment (i.e., no frank neurological damage, no hearing impairment, no general cognitive delay) has rendered them an important key complementary source of data to that obtained from normally developing children.

This section contains three chapters focusing on the problem space when studying SLI. Although many issues are not unique to SLI, it is clear that the comparative nature of SLI brings its own set of challenges. The section begins with Leonard (chap. 8), who introduces SLI, the disorder. This is a broad, encompassing review and key orientation to the readers of this book. Leonard makes it clear that children with SLI have problems from the outset. Instead of reaching early developmental milestones on schedule and then encountering specific difficulties (e.g., in grammatical morphology or entering a period of extremely slow development), these children are indeed slow from the beginning. It is a hallmark of SLI that these children are late in acquiring their first words and their first word combinations and difficulties and protracted development are there from the emergence of language. It is the case that all children with SLI come from the population of late talkers and it is the job of researchers to try to explain why SLI unfolds in this pattern and not in others.

late talkers and it is the job of researchers to try to explain why SLI unfolds in this pattern and not in others.

The section also includes Mervis and Robinson (chap. 9), who cover cross-group comparisons of language and cognitive profiles of children with different communication difficulties. These authors criticize common practice among researchers of language disorders by which MA control groups are chosen and differences among children with different syndromes are established. In addition to arguing that mean differences among groups of children are problematic, they show how comparing children on a particular variable does not guarantee that other variables of interest can be compared and contrasted as well. Given this state of affairs, it is argued that the field would benefit from a focus on patterns of performance of individual children. Their call is more sophisticated than advocating a case study methodology. These authors suggest an approach that allows multiple measures of individual children to be aggregated across time or disability, for example. This approach, combined with signal detention theory and growth curve modeling, has the potential to determine whether individuals exhibit the characteristic profile of performance of particular specific disabilities.

The section continues with Bol (chap. 10), who takes on MLU matching, and Dromi, Leonard, and Blass (chap. 11), who discuss Hebrew SLI. These chapters focus on very particular methodological issues and their role is not to provide readers with a broad view of methodological concerns in SLI. Instead, these chapters were conceived as illustrative of the gamut of methodological challenges that the study of SLI entails. In this vein, Bol dissects the concept of MLU as an indicator of productive morphosyntax using Dutch SLI as his starting point. He questions MLU as a matching technique and raises issues of reliability, variability, and crosslinguistic applicability, among others. Dromi and colleagues continue with the crosslinguistic theme when they focus on Hebrew SLI. These researchers present the problems surrounding choice of data collection methods (spontaneous language samples vs. elicited probe data) and the differences in the types of data that such techniques afford. These authors suggest that the combined evidence provided by naturalistic and probe data provide a more accurate picture of children with SLI's abilities. It is the case that children with SLI often find probe tasks difficult because most probe tasks are designed to target areas that are known to be problematic for children with SLI. In contrast, naturalistic contexts do not always provide opportunities for children with SLI to use forms that they may find challenging. The naturalist context simply allows children with SLI to avoid using particular forms.

The rest of this chapter is divided into two parts. As such, this chapter does not follow the "usual" format of an introductory chapter. The next section examines some of the ideas presented in this methodological section of the book. This is done within a broader framework of discussion, involving the following question: Do children with communication difficulties, and children with SLI in particular, have adultlike grammars or do they "construct" their own? The following section focuses on SLI in particular. It briefly presents a cognitive-functionalist account as an alternative model within which SLI can be conceptualized. This model is constructed within the framework of the following question: Is SLI a linguistically specific deficit or is it a more general cognitive/processing difficulty? It was thought that this was appropriate, because the cognitive-functionalist account is a relatively new approach and the reader may find it interesting to begin engaging with its main ideas.

UNDERSTANDING THE GRAMMARS
OF YOUNG CHILDREN

It would seem appropriate to begin with one important issue raised by Leonard (chap. 8). This involves his assertion that a "full competence hypothesis" has become the prevailing view among scholars in normal (and SLI) language acquisition (see also Wexler, chap. 1 in this volume). That is, it is the common assumption that the grammars of young language learning children are essentially structured like those of the adult from the earliest stages of development.

There has been a long-standing debate about whether children operate with adult syntactic categories and theories or whether they develop a symbolic system that changes with time and experience (Tomasello, 1992; 2000; Wexler, 1994, chap. 1 in this volume). This debate started with Chomsky (1957, 1965) and has continued to dominate the language development and communication disorders agenda. These are interesting times, and it is the case that new approaches are available that deeply challenge the assumptions made by generative accounts and that provide alternative, plausible, and psychologically more real theories of language learning and disorders. Some of these developments and ideas are outlined in order to provide readers with some food for thought and a different perspective that may be useful when discussing the methodological implications of such differing approaches.

In generative approaches, innate syntactic categories and rules are the universal basis for language development and processing (Chomsky, 1981; Pinker, 1999). These innate formal representations are realized in language learning through a process of lexical learning (Pinker, 1989). Interestingly, children are supposed to know syntactic constraints before, or rather in parallel to the learning of the lexical items to which such constraints are applied (Landau & Gleitman, 1985).

However, alternatives to generative approaches have developed in the form of cognitive-functional linguistics (Lakoff, 1987; Langacker, 1987; 1990). An interesting theory that comes from this approach is construction grammar. This syntactic model firmly places language as a cultural product embodying both the cognitive processes employed to produce it and the communicative purpose that it serves. Like other syntactic or lexical theories, language is seen as a pairing of phonological form and meaning. All grammatical items are symbolic units of form and meaning and in the construction grammar view, the structural level (categories and rules) is an epiphenomenon that emerges from language use by schematization, categorization, and frequency effects. To the extent that children have syntactic categories, these are built, are language specific, and emerge based on language use in context. Interestingly, in this approach, the distinction between grammar and the lexicon (rules vs. words) does not play a role in the theory and the basic building blocks of language are whole constructions (Croft, 1991, 2001; Goldberg, 1995; Langacker, 1987). It is clear that constructions are symbolic units that vary in size and in the degree of abstractness.

Furthermore, in this view, children's early productions will be lexically specific in the sense that they can be "correct" without abstract, adultlike mental representations. Initially, there is no separate and abstract level of linguistic representation (Tomasello, 2000, but cf. Wexler, chap. 1 in this volume). Lexical specificity differs from the generative concept of lexical learning in important ways. In lexical learning, children are thought to have fully abstract, adultlike representations, but these representations initially become instantiated by a few lexical items. In lexical specificity, the assumption is that children's language productions do not involve, at least initially, any adultlike, abstract knowledge. Such knowledge is abstracted through induction from interactions involving language use in context and as such this account is fully usage based. Such abstractions are part of the developmental process and therefore require time and experience (as language users).

Thus, generalizations on language structure do occur and children develop abstract knowledge with time. One mechanism involved in abstraction and generalization is that of distributional learning (MacWhinney, 1999; Maratsos, 1982). Distributional learning is based on the child noticing local cues like function elements (e.g., determiners) which become entrenched because they are stable even if other lexical elements in a construction vary (Brent, 1994). With experience of language use, lexical specific learning and distributional learning come together, that is, children will store chunks around concrete lexical items and will abstract initially low-level schemas based on recurrent elements and patterns (Lieven, Pine, Julian, & Rowland, 1998). Young language learning children replace lexical material in these schemas with new ones in a recursive fashion and they develop more and more general/abstract schemas.

It is important to note that early on children extract schemas and not symbolic rules. Children extract patterns from the input but initially these are low-level regularities, not general rules that apply across the board (Dubrowska, 2001). It is also important to note that as schemas become more general with development, they eventually function very much like abstract rules.

Do children with communication disorders, and children with SLI in particular, have adultlike grammars or do they "construct" them? The previous question provokes a heated debate. More important to this discussion is the fact that these different theoretical models can profoundly affect the methodology used in the study of communication disorders. Consider these implications in more detail. But, first, there is an important caveat that needs to be specified. What is about to be discussed represents methodological practices that are more common to one school of thought versus another. Part of the message of this chapter is that researchers need to remain open-minded with respect to methodology and interpretation within their own theoretical approach as well as when considering others. It is not the case that a particular methodology is tied intrinsically or in principle to a particular theoretical approach. Therefore, the comments provided are meant to serve as illustrations of common methodological practices and, more importantly, as catalysts for thought and discussion.

Generative approaches assume an autonomous linguistic system that is largely innate and specified. This determines the types of data that researchers are interested in examining. In this approach, syntactic information takes center stage with lexical information being of much less interest. As a matter of fact, most researchers within this framework do not "go down" to the level of lexical analysis when they interpret and examine their data. Interestingly, in the study of SLI, this approach emphasizes the importance of comparisons between children with SLI and normal younger children of the same language stage. The idea is that in such comparisons further evidence of use of an adultlike, abstract system will be found. Thus, group comparative studies are important and, consequently, the use of MLU as a matching criteria.

The comments provided by Mervis and Robinson (chap. 9) are relevant here, particularly with respect to the need to look at children's individual profiles. In the same vein, Bol (chap. 10) delves into the difficulties in using MLU in comparative studies. Also of interest is Bol's question concerning children with SLI's compensation for loss of length: When children with SLI are matched on MLU with typically developing children, it is generally found that children with SLI omit more verb inflections. Therefore, researchers need to find out what children with SLI are doing in order to compensate in their language production with other aspects of language so that they come up with the same MLU as the typically developing children with which they are being compared. Without giving the punchline of Bol's chapter, the answer to this question is not that straightforward.

One more comment with respect to MLU matching. Some researchers have argued that MLU in words is a better baseline to match children with SLI, precisely because of their tendency to omit inflectional morphology. This is an interesting alternative but still leaves the issue of compensation unresolved.

Generative approaches emphasize the issue of productivity of use. These approaches are looking for across the board generalizations in children's syntactic knowledge. In this framework, researchers are looking for evidence of accurate productivity accompanied by a very low percentage of errors (error-free learning). It is not surprising then, that many researchers working within this approach have made extensive use of probe data in order to establish productivity of a particular linguistic form (e.g., Rice & Wexler, 1996; Rice, Wexler, & Cleave, 1995). Dromi, Leonard, and Blass (chap. 11) illustrate the advantages of using probe data and particularly of complementing it with naturalistic data. Indeed, within the generative paradigm, investigators have oftentimes complemented their analysis with naturalistic examination of language samples looking particularly at use in obligatory contexts.

According to Dromi, Leonard, and Blass, elicitation of spontaneous language is not always successful in providing enough exemplars of linguistic forms used in obligatory contexts that are of special interest to the researcher. But, this problem is not unique to those investigators working within the generative paradigm, but it is a general methodological limitation for anyone working with spontaneous language samples. Having said this, generative researchers are interested in quite abstract phenomena and therefore are looking to describe language learning at a rather abstract level. Consequently, details such as particular construction types that may be used or lexical-specific usage are not necessarily of interest to such researchers. Their primary focus is on syntactic factors. Perhaps an interesting example of the level at which many generativists work can be found on their analysis and interpretation of low error rates in children's productions (see Wexler, Schütze, & Rice, 1998, on SLI).

Cognitive-functional linguistics approaches draw heavily from linguistic typology research and crosslinguistic methodologies. In this approach, the level of analysis is much more detailed with "going down" to the lexical level being of particular importance. In this framework, comparisons between children with SLI and normal younger children of the same language stage are interesting but not crucial to understanding the phenomena. This approach focuses on how children construct their linguistic systems and therefore detailed case studies of children with SLI (without comparisons with normal children) are thought to be justified.

In this paradigm, sampling from rich datasets is crucial, and indeed there is an interesting development in this area based on the work of Tomasello and colleagues at the Max Planck Institute in Leipzig, with a new methodology being used to collect particularly dense datasets at particular developmental periods. These researchers are working with normal language learning children, but the principle applies equally to research with children with communication disorders. Such dense spontaneous language samples provide researchers with an opportunity to trace the development of a particular construction over time and to pay attention to lexically specific information and carry out detailed, fine-grained analyses (see, e.g., Lieven, Tomasello, & Beherens, 2001). These very detailed analyses then have to be integrated into theoretical models of linguistic development, and interestingly some researchers are beginning to do this (Tomasello, 2000).

Researchers working within cognitive-functionalist approaches are also interested in productivity, but because of the emphasis on language use, spontaneous language sample analysis is one of the prime source of data for these investigators. The emphasis on language use also motivates these researchers to look for pragmatic or semantic factors as possible explanations of observed phenomena. To take an example from Tomasello (2000), Spanish-speaking children might produce *Te amo* a thousand times correctly. But a systematic, fine-grained analysis might also suggest that the children use this verb in none of its other forms for different persons or numbers but only focuses on themselves (first person) very likely due to pragmatic reasons. Hence, these researchers would interpret the children's competence as being of a very different level and kind (i.e., lexically specific, possibly formulaic) than researchers from a generativist background would do. Another interesting example that illustrates the approach taken by researchers working within a cognitive-functionalist framework involves their very different interpretation of low error rates in child language production. For details, refer to Pine and colleagues (Pine, 2001; Rubino & Pine, 1998).

IS SLI A LINGUISTICALLY SPECIFIC DISORDER OR IS IT BASED ON MORE GENERAL COGNITIVE DIFFICULTIES?

In attempting to discuss the aforementioned question, focus is on an approach that emphasizes the relevance of lexical learning to the construction of morphological paradigms. Based on the work of Marchman and Bates (1994), Conti-Ramsden and colleagues (Conti-Ramsden & Jones, 1997; Jones & Conti-Ramsden, 1997; Windfuhr & Conti-Ramsden, 2001) built on construction grammar's continuity between lexical and grammatical development in proposing the SLI critical mass hypothesis. They suggested that children with SLI require a larger number of verb tokens in order to learn novel lexical items and they require a larger number of verb types in order for them to abstract or generalize schemas involving morphological paradigms. The reason why children with SLI require a larger critical mass has to do with their processing limitations. Specifically, a phonological short-term memory store problem is potentially a plausible explanation for the slowness in word learning as well as difficulties with morphological development observed in children with SLI. How can a processing limitation of a short-term memory store type explain the linguistic production difficulties of children with SLI?

First of all, there is the issue of developmental time and the fact that children with SLI are slower language learners. The slow process with which children with SLI acquire new lexical items means that words are not always sufficiently close together "in time" in order for children to benefit from making comparisons across lexical items. The time factor also means that lexically specific learned items are more entrenched and hence less likely to change as they have been used far longer as lexically specific items. It is harder to schematize from exemplars that are sparse across time and also from exemplars that are more entrenched items.

Second, there is the issue that phonological representations of children with SLI may not be complete or accurate due to phonological short-term memory store problems or perhaps more general processing capacity limitations. In order for the child to notice that the verb "play" is the same in both "Let me play" and "I like to play everyday," the child has to have similar phonological representations for the word "play" in both construction types. This may not be the case in children with SLI, that is, they may have two different representations of play. Why? The answer probably lies in the differences in the construction types and the surrounding phonological material around the word play in interaction with children with SLI's difficulties establishing representations in the first place. The child with SLI then misses the opportunity to notice the similarities between these two instances of the same verb and therefore is unable to make use of this information. So it is harder for children with SLI to build a critical mass of tokens and types. It has been found that given the same number of verb types, children with SLI may require as much as double the number of verb tokens as compared to normally developing children in order for them to learn a novel verb (Windflur & Conti-Ramsden, 2001). Furthermore, longitudinal work by Conti-Ramsden (Conti-Ramsden & Jones, 1997; Jones & Conti-Ramsden, 1997) suggested that children with SLI require a larger verb vocabulary than normally developing children in terms of types before they can extract patterns or schemas, with particular reference to the ability to make morphological generalizations. The precise magnitude of the increase in types required is still a matter for further study, but there is little doubt that there will be individual differences within the group of children with SLI. This double requirement to reach a critical mass involving both types and to-kens can at least partly explain the fact that children with SLI are all late talkers and they all have protracted vocabulary development. A critical mass is also crucial for generalizations and for assessing regularities in the language (distributional learning) so there are cascading effects involved.

Third, children with SLI have unstable mental representations, which make it difficult for them to move from lexical specific learning to developing low-level schemas. Children with SLI miss information that would help them detect low-level regularities because they do not always identify the same items as identical/similar. In other words, children with SLI are not able to accumulate rote-learned lexically specific exemplars that are likely to lead to schema formation as they are not always able to process items as being cases of the same exemplar. This is problematic for children with SLI because rote learning and distributional learning can facilitate schema formation. In addition, schema formation helps learning because schemas have an organizing function. They allow for more efficient storage (shared content means possible shared representations) and as such can be thought of as a "data compression device" (Dubrowska, March 2001, personal communication). Therefore, it is also important to note that schemas also facilitate learning (the influence is bidirectional). It is easier to learn structured material and schemas may also act as retrieval cues for poorly entrenched units. For example, children with SLI may be able to access a complex unit (an inflected word) by accessing its parts (e.g. stem) once a schema is established. Without the schemas, storage is quite lexically specific and not very efficient. Furthermore, difficulties with developing low-level schemas also have a secondary effect on the development of more abstract schemas and so a vicious circle is created. Therefore, children with SLI's faulty processing mechanism can bar them from the very tools that facilitate language development.

SLI processing limitations, when combined with a dynamic system that has a slow rate of development, may have major cascading effects for later development. In addition, it is possible that the factors that play a similar role in early development for both normal and children with SLI, in later development may play a more pervasive role in children with SLI. An example of this is the greater sensitivity of children with SLI to phonological-based features of verb stems in the production of past tense suffixation and zero-marking errors (Marchman, Wulfeck, & Ellis-Weismer, 1999). Thus, phonological factors that played a role on both normally developing and children with SLI continue to influence the linguistic behavior of children with SLI at later stages whereas this is no longer the case for normally developing children. Such oversensitivity may affect lexical processing and, as a consequence, the extraction of low-level regularities. If lexical learning is slower, then it will take children longer to accumulate a sufficiently large number of inflected exemplars before they can extract low-level regularities (i.e., the SLI critical mass hypothesis discussed earlier).

In summary, children with SLI are thought to have a processing capacity limitation, very likely in phonological short-term memory, that slows down their ability to accumulate a critical mass of observed regularities and form schemas. Children with SLI are also thought to be late talkers, having a protracted period of development where their language is lexically specific, item based, and where development proceeds in a piecemeal fashion (cf. Rice, chap. 2 in this volume).

CONCLUSIONS

Different theoretical positions have major and important methodological consequences in framing the questions to be answered, in the choice of method, in the types of data collected, and in the analysis and interpretation of the results. This discussion has made biases abundantly clear. Nevertheless, as a field of research, communication difficulties and SLI in particular can benefit from some level of integration of different approaches. And, indeed, there are moves for this to be the case. Based on a workshop organized at the National Institutes of Health, Tager-Flusberg and Cooper (1999) recommended that researchers interested in SLI should universally include in their methodologies both a linguistic measure of morphosyntax as well as a processing measure of short-term memory such as nonword repetition. Such an eclectic methodological approach has an important place in the study of communication disorders.

Altogether the issues raised here and those tackled in the chapters of this book remind readers of the analogy of a group of blindfolded people who were asked to guess what animal they had in front of them. Unfortunately, some were touching the animal's front, others the back, and yet others the sides. Such windows of experience did not allow them to get a full view of the phenomenon and, not surprisingly, different groups came back with different answers and a heated debate followed. Perhaps one of the key messages of this methodological section, therefore, is that researchers must be aware of the nature of their blindfolds and also be aware of how and where they are touching base with the problem space of communication disorders and SLI in particular.

ACKNOWLEDGMENTS

This work was supported by an Economic and Social Research Council grant to the author (R000 237767). Our thanks go to the editors Yonata Levy and Jeannette Schaeffer. A particular warm thank you goes to Heike Behrens, Bill Croft, Eva Dubrowska, Kate Joseph, Ludovica Serratrice, and Mike Tomasello for lively discussions and exchange of ideas. It is important to note that these colleagues should not be held responsible, nor do they necessarily share, the particular focus of this chapter.

REFERENCES

Brent, M. R. (1994). Surface cues and robust interference as a basis for the early acquisition of subcategorization frames. *Lingua, 92*, 433–470.

Chomsky, N. (1957). *Aspects of a theory of syntax*. Cambridge, MA: MIT Press.

Chomsky, N. (1965). *Essays on form and interpretation*. New York: Elsevier North-Holland.

Chomsky, N. (1981). *Lectures on government and binding*. Dordrecht: Foris.

Conti-Ramsden, G., & Jones, M. (1997). Verb use in specific language impairment. *Journal of Speech and Hearing Research, 40*, 1298–1313.

Croft, W. (1991). *Syntactic categories and grammatical relations: The cognitive organisation of information*. Chicago: University of Chicago Press.

Croft, W. (2001). *Radical construction grammar: Syntactic theory in typological perspective*. Oxford, England: Oxford University Press.

Dubrowska, E. (2001, March/April). *What's in a rule? A usage-based account of early morphological productivity*. Paper presented at the Third Child Language Development Conference, Gregynog, UK.

Goldberg, A. (1995). *Constructions: A construction grammar approach to argument structure*. Chicago: University of Chicago Press.

Jones, M., & Conti-Ramsden, G. (1997). A comparison of verb use in children with SLI and their younger siblings. *First Language, 17*, 165–193.

Lakoff, G. (1987). *Women, fire and dangerous things: What categories reveal about the mind*. Chicago: University of Chicago Press.

Landau, B., & Gleitman, L. R. (1985). *Language and experience: Evidence from the blind child*. Cambridge, MA: Harvard University Press.

Langacker, R. W. (1987). *Foundations of cognitive grammar: Vol. 1. Theoretical prerequisites*. Stanford, CA: Stanford University Press.

Langacker, R. W. (1990). The rule controversy: A cognitive grammar perspective. *Center for Research in Language Newsletter, 4*, 4–15.

Lieven, E., Pine, V. M., Julian, M., & Rowland, C. F. (1998). Comparing different models of the development of the English verb category. *Linguistics, 36*, 807–830.

Lieven, E. V. M., Tomasello, M., & Beherens, H. (2001, July). *Syntactic creativity and productivity: Where do multiword utterances come from?* Paper presented at the Child Language Seminar, Hatfield, UK.

MacWhinney, B. (Ed.). (1999). *The emergence of language*. Hillsdale, NJ: Lawrence Erlbaum Associates.

Maratsos, M. (1982). The child's construction of grammatical categories. In E. Wanner & L. R. Gleitman (Eds.), *Language acquisition: The state of the art* (pp. 240–266). Cambridge, England: Cambridge University Press.

Marchman, V., & Bates, E. (1994). Continuity in lexical and morphological development: A test of the critical mass hypothesis. *Journal of Child Language, 21*, 339–365.

Marchman, V., Wulfeck, B., & Ellis-Weismer, S. (1999). Morphogical productivity in children with normal language and SLI: A study of the English past tense. *Journal of Speech, Language and Hearing Research, 42*, 206–219.

Pine, J. (2001, July). *Testing the agreement/tense omission model: Why the data on children's use of non-nominative third person singular subjects count against ATOM.* Paper presented at the Child Language Seminar, Hatfield, UK.

Pinker, S. (1989). *Learnability and cognition: The acquisition of argument structure.* Cambridge, MA: MIT Press.

Pinker, S. (1999). *Words and rules: The ingredients of language.* New York: Basic Books.

Rice, M., & Wexler, K. (1996). Toward tense as a clinical marker of specific language impairment in English-speaking children. *Journal of Speech and Hearing Research, 39,* 1239–1257.

Rice, M., Wexler, K., & Cleave, P. L. (1995). Specific language impairment as a period of extended optional infinitive. *Journal of Speech and Hearing Research, 38,* 850–863.

Rubino, R. B., & Pine, J. (1998). Subject-verb agreement in Brazilian Portuguese: What low error rates hide. *Journal of Child Language, 25,* 35–60.

Tager-Flusberg, H., & Cooper, J. (1999). Present and future possibilities for defining a phenotype for specific language impairment. *Journal of Speech, Language and Hearing Research, 42,* 1275–1278.

Tomasello, M. (1992). *First verbs: A case of early grammatical development.* Cambridge, England: Cambridge University Press.

Tomasello, M. (2000). Do young children have adult syntactic competence? *Cognition, 74,* 209–253.

Wexler, K. (1994). Optional infinitives, head movement and the economy of derivations. In D. Lightfoot & N. Hornstein (Ed.), *Verb movement* (pp. 305–350). Cambridge, England: Cambridge University Press.

Wexler, K., Schütze, C. T., & Rice, M. (1998). Subject case in children with SLI and unaffected controls: Evidence for the Agr/Tns omission model. *Language Acquisition, 7,* 317–344.

Windfuhr, K., & Conti-Ramsden, G. (in press). Lexical learning skills in preschool children with specific language impairment (SLI). *International Journal of Language and Communication Disorders.*

8

Specific Language Impairment: Characterizing the Deficit

Laurence B. Leonard
Purdue University

Since the first half of the 19th century, there have been reports of children exhibiting inexplicable deficits in language ability. These children's language difficulties are not accompanied by the problems so often associated with language disorders. Their hearing appears to be within normal limits, their scores on nonverbal tests of intelligence are within the normal range, and examination reveals no clear evidence of neurological impairment. The labels given to these children have varied over the decades, although in recent years, these children have most often been referred to as children with specific language impairment (SLI).

The deficits experienced by children with SLI can be long-standing, and place them at risk for reading and other academic difficulties. For this reason, it is important to discover the cause or causes of this disorder, and to search for effective ways of preventing and treating the problem.

There is a second reason why the study of SLI is important. On the face of it, SLI appears to be a condition in which language alone is adversely affected. Thus, this disorder might constitute an ideal test case for the notion that language, or at least a major component of it, is autonomous of other mental faculties.

For both of these reasons, the pace of research on SLI has accelerated in the last few years. However, as in any area of investigation, obstacles can confront the SLI researcher. This chapter discusses methods for the study of specific language impairment. Ways of overcoming some of the common obstacles are presented, although it will be apparent that in many instances even great care leaves an imperfect picture of this disorder. Three major themes are struck. These deal, respectively, with issues of definition, research design, and hypothesis testing and data interpretation. A brief history is provided to give some perspective on how the study of SLI has arrived at its present state. (More detailed reviews can be found in Leonard, 1998; Johnston, 1988; and Weiner, 1986.)

Gall (1835) was probably the first to publish a report on children who came to be known as children with SLI. This and subsequent works published over the remainder of the 19th century emphasized these children's seemingly normal nonverbal intelligence and apparently good comprehension in the face of extremely limited speech output. Initially, only children whose output was restricted to single-word utterances were included in these reports. Children who produced multiword utterances were viewed quite differently, as having severe problems confined to phonology. Toward the end of the century, subtypes of children were described, even though only children producing single words (or no words at all) were considered.

From the early 1900s, children whose output had progressed well beyond single-word utterances were included in published studies. In addition, there was increasing recognition that comprehension problems accompanied problems of production in many children. The label "aphasia" appeared in the literature with growing frequency, often accompanied by modifiers to create terms such as "infantile aphasia," "congenital aphasia," and "developmental aphasia." The latter was often subdivided into "expressive developmental aphasia" and "expressive-receptive developmental aphasia" given the presence of comprehension (receptive) difficulties in some children. "Dysphasia" gradually replaced "aphasia," and clinical labels such as "developmental dysphasia" were quite prevalent through the 1970s.

Since the 1960s, two dominant trends have become apparent. First, beginning with Menyuk (1964), increasing emphasis has been placed on deficits in the area of grammar. Many studies have provided careful descriptions of these children's morphosyntactic difficulties, and, in recent years, there have been serious attempts to explain them. The second trend is the movement away from "dysphasia" toward a descriptive term such as "language disorder" or "language impairment." *Specific language impairment*, the term used here, is most frequently adopted today.

DEFINING SLI: SUBJECT SELECTION, SUBGROUPS, AND THE NEED FOR REPLICABILITY

Criteria for Inclusion: The Language Deficit

Establishing that a child possesses a language deficit usually requires two considerations. The first is that those close to the child—parents, grandparents, preschool teachers, or others—view the child as functioning more poorly in language than they expect (Tomblin, 1983, 1996). In many cultures, this criterion is not difficult to meet, because family members and teachers are the most common sources of referral when children are scheduled for language assessment.

The second consideration is performance on a comprehensive standardized language test (Tomblin, 1996; Tomblin et al., 1997). Ideally, such a test should include lexical, morphosyntactic, phonological, and pragmatic abilities in both comprehension and production. When such tests yield both an overall score and subtest scores, the overall score is required to fall below an established level, usually −1.25 standard deviations below the mean for the child's age. In addition, the researcher may require that some minimum number of subtests also show low scores. The latter is essential if the standardized test yields subtest scores but no overall score.

Standard scores are far preferable to scores in the form of language ages (e.g., Lahey, 1990; McCauley & Swisher, 1984). This is because language ages are often interpolated or extrapolated. For example, a child might receive a language age of, say, 8;6 even though no children of this age were part of the standardization sample for the test. In many studies, scores from standardized tests are supplemented by other language measures. These often include mean length of utterance in spontaneous speech and percentage correct use of particular grammatical forms in the spontaneous speech sample (e.g., Rice, Wexler, & Cleave, 1995). Of course, in some research sites, normative data for these measures also exist (Leonard, Miller, & Gerber, 1999; J. Miller & Chapman, 1981).

Although both concern of family and teachers and language testing should be included, there is no requirement that the former always precede the latter. For example, through a screening procedure, a child might be identified as in need of further testing. At that point, the family might be contacted and their views about the child's language abilities might be determined. Sole reliance on referrals from parents and especially teachers runs the risk of underidentifying girls with SLI. In an epidemiological study, Tomblin et al. (1997) determined that girls represented 41% of the SLI population. However, prevalence studies relying solely on referrals show a lower prevalence for girls, around 25%. Quite possibly, boys and girls differ in how they behave when faced with communication obstacles. If boys are more likely to act out behaviorally, then they might be more likely to be viewed as needing help with their language.

Criteria for Exclusion

The term *SLI* is reserved for those children whose language deficits appear to represent their central, and, perhaps, only problem. This means that, at a minimum, researchers must establish that the children selected for research do not resemble children falling in other established diagnostic categories. Children must pass a hearing screening, and should not have had an excessive number of bouts with chronic otitis media with effusion, because this might have adversely affected hearing for an extended period of time prior to testing. Similarly, the children should show no evidence of frank neurological impairment, such as focal lesions or traumatic brain injury, and should not be on medication for the prevention of seizures. The children's behavior should not exhibit the symptoms of impaired reciprocal social interaction and restriction of activities associated with autism, and they should not have undergone treatment for emotional problems. Oral motor abilities should also be sufficient to support the production of language.

A criterion usually regarded as essential is an age-appropriate score on a standardized test of nonverbal intelligence, usually defined as within one standard deviation of the mean, or at least 85. However, research has indicated that the basic profile of language abilities (Tomblin & Zhang, 1999) and success with language intervention (Fey, Long, & Cleave, 1994) are very similar between children with IQs above 85 and those with IQs in the 75 to 85 range. Accordingly, in a report to the U.S National Institutes of Health, Tager-Flusberg and Cooper (1999) called for additional research to determine whether the nonverbal IQ criterion is necessary and, if so, whether 85 or some other cutoff is the most appropriate.

Other Descriptive Measures to Promote Replicability

Even if researchers recruit only children meeting the previous criteria, they will find considerable heterogeneity in their sample. There will be some dominant profiles of language and other abilities, and it might be possible to describe the modal child with SLI, but differences will nevertheless exist. This heterogeneity poses a problem for replicability. It could be the case that two studies of SLI obtain somewhat different results simply because subject recruitment in the two studies resulted in a slightly different distribution of children from the larger SLI population. Tager-Flusberg and Cooper (1999) made the very useful recommendation that researchers include many of the same descriptive measures in their studies, even when these are not used as criteria for subject inclusion or exclusion.

For example, for studies focusing on English-speaking children with SLI there are three measures that should be provided for each child. One is a finite verb morphology composite. This measure represents the overall percentage with which children use morphemes such as past -ed, present third person singular -s, and copula and auxiliary be forms (see Bedore & Leonard, 1998; Leonard et al., 1999; Rice, Haney, & Wexler, 1998; Rice & Wexler 1996; Rice et al., 1995). For many children with SLI, the use of this collection of morphemes is unusually weak.

Another measure is performance on nonword repetition—the repetition of nonce syllables up to five syllables in length. Many children with SLI do extraordinarily poorly on this measure as well (Bishop, North, & Donlan, 1996; Dollaghan & Campbell, 1998; Gathercole & Baddeley, 1990). A third measure to consider is performance on the basic *ba-da* discrimination task first used by Tallal and Piercy (1974). Many studies have shown that children with SLI do poorly on this task (see review in Leonard, 1998).

Note that the recommendation to include such measures when describing the subjects in a study is for purposes of ensuring that other researchers can select children showing the same characteristics. Inclusion of these measures does not constitute endorsement of any particular theoretical position about SLI. In fact, the reasons for poor performance on these tasks may well vary from child to child. For example, poor nonword repetition might be due to prosodic deficits, poor phonological memory, or poor phonotactic skill; difficulties with the *ba-da* contrast might be caused by discrimination problems, poor attention, or difficulties with the multiple demands of the task (e.g., remembering to press the button for *ba* and not to press the button for *da*).

There are other descriptive details that can promote replicability. For example, descriptions of the specific type of intervention (therapy) received by a child, as well as the duration of this treatment, can assist researchers in the interpretation of the child's particular pattern of use. It would be less surprising if children with SLI showing relatively mild deficits in one study and those showing more serious deficits in another study also differed in the amount of intervention already received.

Characterizing Subgroups of Children with SLI

Given the heterogeneity seen in SLI, it is commonly assumed that distinct subgroups are involved. Indeed, it is easy to select a child with SLI whose profile is quite different from that of another child with SLI. Unfortunately, these individual differences have not translated into finding cohesive subgroups. There have been several large-scale projects designed to identify subgroups in a reliable manner. Examples include Aram and Nation (1975), Korkman and Häkkinen-Rihu (1994), Rapin and Allen (1983), Wilson and Risucci (1986), and Wolfus, Moscovitch, and Kinsbourne (1980). Boundaries reflecting seemingly distinct subgroups that are formed retrospectively tend to blur or change when applied to a new sample of children.

Of course, for purposes of determining whether dependent measures differ according to subject characteristics, it is quite appropriate for researchers to subdivide children with SLI into different subgroups. For example, investigators have sometimes asked whether performance on their experimental task varies according to whether or not children's language comprehension ability is as poor as their language production ability (e.g., Edwards & Lahey, 1996; Lahey & Edwards, 1996). For this question, children with SLI are subdivided according to language comprehension and production test scores. A recent example can be seen in C. Miller, Kail, Leonard, and Tomblin (2001). Nine-year-olds with SLI were divided into subgroups according to whether language testing had revealed problems with comprehension only, or comprehension and production. The children were administered a variety of response time tasks, ranging from motor tasks (e.g., pressing a computer key in response to a signal), nonlinguistic cognitive tasks (e.g., determining whether two shapes were mirror images of each other), lexical tasks (e.g., naming pictures), phonological tasks (e.g., determining whether two words contained the same initial consonant), to grammatical tasks (e.g., deciding whether a sentence matched the picture shown on the computer screen). The majority of children with SLI were slower than control children across all tasks. Although individual differences were seen, the children's patterns of performance were not distinguishable by their subgroup membership.

Even if subgroup differences are expected on an experimental task, dividing children into subgroups requires no assumption that the subgroups are dichotomous groups. Defining a subgroup does not validate a subgroup. Validation would have to be determined through research of a different sort.

Some researchers have selected subgroups on the basis of measures that are relevant to the researchers' experimental questions. For example, van der Lely (1994, 1996) was interested in examining particular hypotheses about grammatical deficits and specifically selected those children with SLI who exhibited problems with grammar. This research strategy can be very useful for understanding the nature of certain children's difficulties. However, selection of such children for study does not mean that children with these characteristics constitute a distinct subgroup. Many children with SLI have grammatical deficits (see review in Leonard, 1998). However, researchers are not yet in a position to say that children with "grammatical language impairment" are reliably separable from other children with SLI.

A comparable situation could arise if a subgroup of children with SLI were selected, whose parents or siblings had also experienced language learning problems. This strategy is perfectly appropriate in cases such as the three-generational family studied by Gopnik and her colleagues (e.g., Gopnik & Crago, 1991), because the study was confined to that family and comparisons were made between affected and unaffected family members. However, selecting children from different families on the basis of their positive family histories for language problems does not constitute selection of a distinct subgroup. First, taken as a whole, children with SLI are, on average, three to four times more likely than typically developing children to come from families in which one or more members had problems with language (e.g., Tallal, Ross, & Curtiss, 1989; Tomblin, 1989). Furthermore, twin studies suggest that this high degree of familial concentration is more likely to reflect genetic rather than environmental factors (Bishop, 1992; Tomblin & Buckwalter, 1994). Thus, these children constitute a rather large subgroup indeed. Unfortunately, children with a positive history for language impairment fall down on many of the same measures of language as their SLI peers with no family history of language problems. For example, these children have serious problems with grammatical morphology (Rice, Haney, & Wexler, 1998), but they also do poorly on speech discrimination tasks (Tallal, Townsend, Curtiss, & Wulfeck, 1991)). It may be the case that there are factors that distinguish these children from other children with SLI. For example, Bishop et al. (1996) found that performance on nonword repetition tasks shows relatively high heritability. However, researchers are a long way from having data that validates "familial language impairment" as a meaningful subgroup. At this point, it is safer to define a positive family history as a risk factor, not as a state of affairs that produces a particular kind of child with SLI.

It can be seen, then, that when researchers do adopt the strategy of selecting children showing particular language characteristics, or having particular family histories, it is especially important to provide as well the kinds of standard measures discussed previously. For example, by providing scores on common measures—such as nonword repetition, *ba-da* discrimination performance, and finite verb morphology use—other investigators will have a clearer sense of whether the children selected are similar to those they themselves have studied.

RESEARCH DESIGN

A reasonable question to ask is whether, until reliable subgroups can be identified, it would not be better to avoid group studies altogether. As an alternative, researchers could pursue case studies, being careful to describe the characteristics of each child. By piecing together many individual case profiles, a clearer sense of how different components of language interact in SLI might be developed. Depending on whether common themes emerge from this patchwork approach, this could possibly lead to subsequent studies employing more appropriate subgroups than would have otherwise been possible.

If research in SLI were to adopt the case study method as the dominant method, then it would not be without precedent. This trend is apparent in the literature on adult aphasia, influenced in no small part by Caramazza's (1984) argument that a particular symptom (e.g., lexical comprehension difficulties) might arise from disparate sources, such that a group finding of a particular deficit may not necessarily reflect identification of a single problem. Caramazza pointed out that only by studying a single case in a variety of tasks and domains can a true understanding of the problem be possible. This point can be applied to case studies in the area of SLI.

However, there seems to be one important difference between many case studies in the area of adult aphasia and those in the area of SLI. The former often describe profiles of deficits and relative sparing that do not resemble anything seen in normal language development or in normal adult language behavior. Druks and Shallice (2000) described an adult patient who had great difficulty naming drawings, photographs, or real objects, yet was much more proficient in providing the required names when given a definition auditorily. Furthermore, he was relatively accurate in answering questions about the same pictures he was unable to name. Even children with SLI with documented word-finding problems do not present performance profiles that depart so dramatically from typical development (see McGregor & Leonard, 1995, for a review). Case studies in the area of SLI usually constitute reports of discrepancies among abilities that are simply more extreme than, rather than qualitatively different from, those seen in younger normally developing children.

Because interpretation of any case study will, by definition, be based on data from a single child, it is crucial that the description of the case contains at least all of the inclusionary and exclusionary criteria that were met, as well as the other descriptive details already noted. Data from a single child who is inadvertently included due to incomplete information can potentially muddy the findings from a group study; however, the price is far greater in a case study. It is also important to obtain multiple measures of key variables, to ensure that any unusual characteristics are not sampling errors. If they are, additional scores on the measures will regress to the mean (see Tomblin & Zhang, 1999); if they are representative of the child's functioning, then these scores will remain reasonably constant.

A related risk of case studies is that they can give the impression of an unusual (and possibly theoretically interesting) profile that, in fact, is not statistically out of the range of the profile seen for children with SLI as a whole. Tomblin and Pandich (1999) illustrated this by selecting a child with SLI whose standard score on a grammatical morpheme production task was only 75 and whose standard score on a vocabulary comprehension test was 101. However, when vocabulary scores were regressed on grammatical morpheme scores for the entire group of children with SLI, this particular child's profile fell within the 95% confidence interval. Without knowledge of the performance of a larger group of children with SLI, it would be possible to assume that a unique profile is being studied when such a profile is not statistically different from those of other children.

Group studies have other virtues; indeed, even in the area of adult aphasia, these kinds of studies are commonly conducted. One advantage of group studies is that they have the potential of revealing characteristics that describe the modal child with SLI. To be sure, one needs to inspect the distribution to be sure the characteristic in question holds for the majority of children in the group. However, assuming it does, this commonly shared characteristic could prove to be an important component of the disorder. For example, studies that have shown unusually poor use of finite verb morphology in English-speaking children with SLI have included children with varying lexical comprehension ability (ranging from poor to age appropriate) and nonverbal IQ (from 86–130) (e.g., Leonard, Eyer, Bedore, & Grela, 1997; Rice et al., 1995). Inspection of the data reveals that throughout the lexical and nonverbal IQ continuum, most of the children in these studies exhibited a very limited skill in grammatical morphology.

Group Matching

When researchers want to ask whether children with SLI are deficient in some particular language area under investigation, they usually rely on a comparison group of normally developing children matched according to chronological age. In principle, this type of matching could be highly illuminating. For example, it could be that children with SLI are normal in many aspects of language, but have highly selective deficits of a particular type. Thus, when compared to age controls, group differences might be found for only one or a few details of language. In practice, however, this type of matching serves primarily as a means of documenting the presence of a below age level skill. Even though children with SLI have uneven profiles, they nevertheless perform below age level in most any area of language assessed. Therefore, findings of group differences, although useful for documentation purposes, are not usually theoretically informative.

Groups matched according to age should be matched according to other characteristics as well. For example, as a group, children with SLI earn nonverbal IQ scores slightly below those of their same-age peers. Similarly, socioeconomic status (SES) is somewhat lower in children with SLI. It is important that these potential differences be controlled in some way. Furthermore, it is not sufficient to establish the lack of a statistically significant difference on these variables. As noted by Mervis and Robinson (1999), to be confident that the two groups are not different, values of $p > .50$ or higher are needed.

The fact that children with SLI fall behind same-age peers on many different language-related measures means that researchers run the risk of misinterpreting the reason for the group differences on the language measure of interest. For example, if English-speaking children with SLI fail to use word final [*t*] and [*d*] on a consistent basis in words such as *fast* and *load*, then it would not be surprising to see them have difficulty with past tense forms such as *passed* and *mowed*. However, prerequisites may be more subtle. For example, it might be the case that all children require a certain number of verbs in their lexicons before they can use verb inflections productively. Likewise, it is reasonable to assume that many types of grammatical morphemes will not appear in the speech of children until they can produce utterances of a certain length. Therefore, researchers should try to control for such abilities, because they loom as confounding variables in research.

In some cases, it might be possible to remove the influence of these factors through statistical techniques such as the use of covariates or other procedures. For example, Restrepo, Swisher, Plante, and Vance (1992) used covariance techniques to conclude that children with SLI did not show the same pattern as normally developing children across a series of verbal and nonverbal measures. However, such techniques assume that the relations between language variables are the same at each developmental point. For example, 4-year-old typically developing children may show 80% use of regular past inflections in obligatory contexts and, at the same time, produce overregularizations such as *throwed* and *catched* with considerable frequency. Four-year-old children with SLI might show only 20% use of regular past inflections in obligatory contexts and produce no overregularizations. It is not clear how statistical techniques can correct for these differences without painting a misleading picture. It should be noted that at earlier points in normal development, when children use regular past inflections in only 20% of obligatory contexts, overregularizations are not yet seen.

One way that researchers have tried to solve this problem is to recruit additional groups of comparison groups. For example, if researchers wanted to determine the productivity of regular past inflection use by studying the rate of overregularization, they could match children with SLI with younger normally developing children according to their percentage of use of past -*ed* in obligatory contexts. Thus, if both groups used the past inflection in, for example, 50% of obligatory contexts, yet the normally developing children showed significantly greater overregularization, then it would be fair to conclude that children with SLI use past tense forms with lower degrees of productivity.

The language measure used as the basis of matching should vary according to the dependent measure of interest. Frequently, this measure is mean length of utterance (MLU), on the assumption that the language ability of interest depends on the child's ability to produce utterances of a particular length. A recent example of the use of MLU matching can be seen in a study by Hansson and Leonard (in press). These investigators suspected that Swedish-speaking children with SLI were below age level in their use of a variety of grammatical morphemes, but wished to determine whether particular verb inflections were more problematic than others. The children with SLI were compared to a group of younger normally developing children matched according to MLU as well as to a group of same-age peers. The findings for two verb inflections of interest are illustrated in Fig. 8.1. The children with SLI used both present tense inflections and regular past tense inflections with significantly lower percentages in obligatory contexts than did the children serving as age controls. However, the children with SLI differed from the younger MLU controls only in the use of regular past tense inflections. The use of MLU controls in this study served two interrelated functions. First, it revealed a distinction in the use of two types of verb inflections that was not obvious from the SLI–age control comparison alone

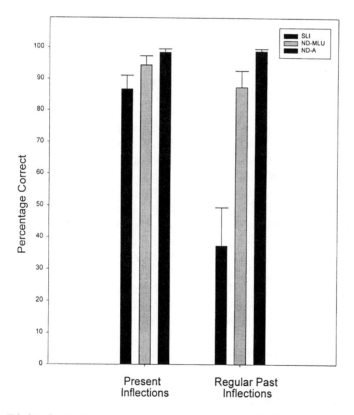

FIG. 8.1. Percentages of correct use of present tense inflections and regular past tense inflections by Swedish-speaking children with specific language impairment (SLI), younger normally developing children matched according to mean length of utterance (ND-MLU), and normally developing children matched according to chronological age (ND-A). Data are from Hansson and Leonard (in press).

(as these two groups differed on both of these inflections). Second, because both present tense inflections and regular past tense inflections in Swedish require the addition of a single morpheme to the verb stem, the MLU matching ensured that the problem with regular past tense inflections was not related to the number of morphemes the children could express in their utterances.

MLU is not the only language measure that could be used for matching; many other measures could be appropriate. For example, if children with SLI and normally developing children were compared according to their ability to include internal arguments of the verb (e.g., direct object), a researcher could include a younger group of normally developing children matched according to the number of different verbs in their lexicons that require internal arguments.

In some cases, it may be appropriate to match children according to a test score. For example, if researchers are interested in studying children's comprehension of particular grammatical morphemes, they might use the children's scores on a general test of grammatical comprehension—one that does not rely excessively on grammatical morphology—as a basis for matching. If this procedure is used, then it is important to ensure that raw scores are used for matching and the test had been normed on the entire age range covered in the study. For example, the results might be difficult to interpret if, say, 8-year-old children with SLI were matched with normally developing 5-year-olds on raw scores on a test for which there are no norms for children younger than 8 years old. It could be the case that the test is insensitive to changes in comprehension that occur below age 8. A similar problem could arise if the language ages derived for the scores of the children with SLI were extrapolated down to ages for which there are no normative data. In this case, a language age of 5 cannot be interpreted as reflecting how typically developing 5-year-olds would actually do on the same items.

One of the challenges facing the use of a younger control group is the selection of appropriate tasks. Often tasks that both children with SLI and age controls can perform (with differing degrees of accuracy) seem to require more attention and patience than younger controls can muster. If an alternative task cannot be devised and younger controls must be excluded, then researchers need to be very cautious in interpreting the data from the children with SLI. In such instances, it might be possible to conclude only that the children with SLI performed below age level, without further specification.

In some instances, exact matches between children with SLI and younger normally developing children cannot be found, but the range of scores on the matching variables are similar for the two groups. Here, regression techniques can be useful. For example, Leonard et al. (1999) used this method to inquire whether the use of finite verb morphemes increased as function of the number of verbs used by each group, whether the two groups differed in degree of finite verb morpheme use across the verb vocabulary range, and whether the rate of increase (the slope) in finite verb morpheme use as a function of increasing verb vocabulary was the same in the two groups of children. Thus, a good deal can be learned even when each child with SLI does not have a close match on vocabulary size, or whatever the important controlling variable may be.

Treatment Designs

In recent years, treatment designs have made their appearance in the literature on SLI (e.g., Clahsen & Hansen, 1997; Eyer & Leonard, 1994; Leonard et al., 1982). Studies employing such designs are especially appropriate for testing hypotheses concerning the sources of the child's difficulties. There are, of course, several considerations involved in the use of the treatment paradigm. Assume, for example, that researchers wish to determine why many Hebrew-speaking children with SLI have difficulties with the *hitpa'el binyan*, or pattern (see Dromi, Leonard, Adam, & Zadunaisky-Ehrlich, 1999). The *binyanim*, or patterns, are the phonological templates within which the consonantal roots of verbs appear. These templates take the form of predictable sequences of vowels that appear between the consonants of the root. For certain patterns, syllabic prefixes also make up part of the template. For the *hitpa'el* pattern, the template is (for present tense) *mitCaCeC*; for another pattern, the *pa'al* pattern, the corresponding template is *CoCeC*. Patterns frequently modulate the core meaning of the root, and particular semantic notions (e.g., causality, reflexiveness) are more likely to be expressed through certain patterns than through others. However, this correlation between pattern and semantic notion is quite imperfect.

A treatment design might be applied to the question about the *hitpa'el* pattern in the following way. One possible reason for the difficulty of this pattern is that its morphophonology is problematic for children with SLI. For example, verbs of this pattern (e.g., *mitlabesh*, *mitraxets*) require an unstressed initial prefix that forms a consonant cluster when affixed to the first consonant of the root (in the previous examples, [*tl*] and [*tr*]). An alternative explanation is that the semantic notions conveyed by many verbs of this pattern are difficult for these children. This pattern frequently expresses notions of reflexiveness and reciprocity. For example, *mitlabesh* is "he gets (himself) dressed"; *mitraxets* is "he washes himself."

One possible way to test these alternative explanations is to teach a different set of verbs to each of three groups of children with SLI. One group of children could learn verbs of the *hitpa'el* pattern that convey the potentially problematic semantic notions (as in *mitlabesh* and *mitraxets*). A second group could learn verbs of the *hitpa'el* pattern that convey simpler notions, such as the verb *mitgalesh* "slides." If the morphophonological explanation is correct, then this group should have considerable difficulty with these verbs, despite their simpler semantic notions. A third group could be taught verbs with simpler notions from a pattern that should be less problematic according to the morphophonological hypothesis, such as the verb *kofets* "jumps" from the *pa'al* pattern.

If the morphophonological hypothesis is correct, then learning by the first two groups of children should proceed more slowly than learning by the third group, as measured by number of treatment sessions required until mastery was reached and average percentage correct across sessions. In addition, the children in the first two groups might show poorer generalization of the new pattern to new words for which the pattern is appropriate. If, in contrast, the semantic notion hypothesis is correct, learning and generalization will be poor only for the first group. Of course, it is possible that both morphophonology and semantic notions are important and have an additive effect. In this case, each of the three groups will differ from each other, with the best performance seen by the third group, and the poorest performance seen by the first group.

Treatment designs are also ideal for testing presumed relations among components of language. For example, if it is assumed that children with SLI show difficulties with the verb-second placement of verbs in German because of their difficulty with finite features such as agreement, treatment aimed at helping these children acquire agreement should at the same time facilitate their ability with verb-second placement. Clahsen and Hansen (1997) conducted such a study. They provided children with multiple examples of verb agreement inflections in subject + verb utterances as well as in isolation. The children not only increased their use of these inflections, but also showed signs of following the verb-second rule, which they did not possess prior to the study. That is, along with producing subject + verb utterances with the appropriate agreement forms, the children began to use adverbials and objects in sentence-initial position and correctly place the appropriately inflected verb immediately after the initial element (e.g., adverbial + verb + subject).

The treatment paradigm employed by Clahsen and Hansen (1997) represented a stronger design than is seen in most studies. However, it can be strengthened further. For example, to guard against the possibility that language stimulation of any sort is sufficient to promote verb-second use, an additional group of children with SLI might be presented with multiple examples of grammatical forms that have no theoretical bearing on verb-second use (e.g., noun plural inflections).

As it turns out, there is some debate over whether the special problems with verb morphology and word order in Germanic languages is caused by agreement, or some other factor, such as tense (e.g., Rice, Noll, & Grimm, 1997). One way of testing these alternatives is to use the same treatment design with children acquiring a language such as Swedish. The finite verb inflections of this language mark tense but not agreement. Thus, if agreement is the critical factor, then treatment on Swedish tense forms should not result in the emergence of the verb-second rule in the speech of the children with SLI. Conversely, if use of this word order rule commences when improvement is seen on the verb forms, then tense would seem to be implicated as the critical factor.

Treatment designs have other advantages. The longitudinal nature of these designs means that the researcher has a much clearer record of the forms that a child has and has not yet used. This makes the determination of productivity—the creative use of grammatical forms—much easier. For example, if a language sample is obtained from an English-speaking child, and it includes forms such as *played* and *jumped*, it will not be clear if these forms reflected the child's application of the past tense rule or if they were the product of rote memory, no different from, say, *threw* and *brought*. Only by observing overregularizations, such as *catched*, or administering test items employing nonce words to elicit productions, such as *dacked*, can researchers be confident that the past form is productive. However, if in a treatment design a child receives practice on *pushed*, *walked*, and *stayed* and then once she shows significant improvement begins to produce *played* and *jumped*, then researchers can have more confidence that the latter productions were the product of rule application. Of course, this conclusion would be strengthened if a comparison group of children receiving practice on some other element of language did not begin to show past tense use at the same point in time.

Longitudinal Studies

The advantages of longitudinal designs are well known. For the study of children with SLI, they have special value. From all accounts, children with SLI have problems from the outset. Rather than hitting the early language milestones on schedule and then entering a long period of extremely slow development, these children are slow from the very beginning. They are late in acquiring first words and word combinations, and in both lexical and grammatical development they show a protracted period from emergence to mastery. This implies that all children with SLI come from the population of late talkers. In recent years, there has been a great deal of research directed at identifying the factors that predict which late talkers will catch up to peers and which will remain below age level and eventually be diagnosed as exhibiting SLI (see recent reviews in Paul, 2000; Thal & Katich, 1996).

However, longitudinal studies are also important for a clearer understanding of SLI in older children. For example, van der Lely and Stollwerk (1997) described a group of children with SLI ages 9;3 to 12;10 with unusually severe grammatical deficits for their age. The severity of their language disorder qualified them for attendance in special residential schools for children with language impairments. It would be valuable to know what the salient characteristics of these children's language deficits were when these children were preschoolers. For example, it might be that, along with a slow rate of language development, these children exhibited a particular type of error that distinguished them from other children with SLI. Alternatively, it might be the case that, early on, their severe language impairment was accompanied by other developmental problems that resolved by the time the children reached school age. Large-scale prospective longitudinal studies of SLI such as that of Tomblin and his colleagues (e.g., Tomblin et al., 1997; Tomblin & Zhang, 1999) will no doubt yield valuable information in this regard. However, it is very likely that additional studies will be needed.

One area in need of special attention is the role played by neurological maturation in the language abilities of older children with SLI. For example, if it is fair to assume that there is a period of optimal grammatical acquisition in normally developing children (e.g., Johnson & Newport, 1989), a child acquiring language very slowly might reach a point where, for maturational reasons, grammatical learning becomes less efficient independent of the disorder. This is not to say that children with SLI have no neurological dysfunction associated with, or even causing, their language disorder. However, even if their slow language growth is in large part due to this dysfunction, the children might reach an age at which the grammatical learning of any child can be expected to become labored and inefficient. If children with SLI are seen only at the older age, then it will not be clear which components of their difficulty are part of the disorder itself, and which represent the unfortunate but natural consequence of reaching a critical point in neurological maturation before the acquisition of grammar is complete. Longitudinal studies should be informative in such cases.

HYPOTHESIS TESTING AND DATA INTERPRETATION

Research on SLI comes from many different disciplines, each with its own methods and assumptions. In general, this is an advantage. Major breakthroughs have already come from different quarters, and given the current state of knowledge about this disorder, it would be risky to rely exclusively on research from a single discipline. Unfortunately, this multidisciplinary approach to the problem can lead to confusion on the part of the uninitiated.

Are the Measures Compatible with the Theory?

Data almost always boil down to numbers. Even in work within theoretical frameworks that seem to take an all-or-none view of certain language phenomena, there is usually a need to explain why a few productions that should not have occurred were actually heard. Of course, some might be routinized expressions, learned as unanalyzed wholes. Exclusion of these utterances from consideration is highly sensible. However, it is more difficult when a minority of nonroutinized utterances fail to conform to the expected pattern. The inclination in such cases is to perform a statistical test. If the test shows that the minority instances are significantly less frequent than the forms that were actually predicted, then this might be taken as support for the initial hypothesis.

But is this always appropriate? Consider two examples. It has been proposed that in English, nominative case is related to agreement (e.g., Wexler, Schütze, & Rice, 1998) such that when children fail to express agreement, a default (accusative) case form is selected for the subject position. Thus, when children do not produce an utterance such as *She is running*, they might be expected to use one such as *Her running*. Utterances such as *Her is running* are not expected. But if the latter occur, how many can be tolerated before the assumption of a relation is deemed incorrect? Assume, for example, the distribution in Example 1 for 200 utterances containing obligatory contexts for both subject pronouns and agreement. (Assume as well that all of the relevant pronouns—*he, she, him, her*—are used by the child.)

(1)   + nominative   −nominative
    + agreement   80   20
    −agreement   25   75

The numbers in the lower left refer to utterances such as *She running*. It turns out that these productions are not problematic for this hypothesis, because it is possible that the absence of *is* can be attributed to a failure to express tense not agreement (see Wexler et al., 1998). Only the numbers in the upper right represent exceptions to the predicted pattern. Statistical testing of the distribution in Example 1 will reveal support for the conclusion that agreement forms and nominative case pronouns are not distributed evenly. Rather, agreement forms are more likely to occur with nominative case pronouns and lack of agreement is more likely to occur with pronouns that fail to mark nominative case.

However, if the proposal is based on a universal principle that nominative case is an automatic consequence when agreement is represented in the utterance, then can any exceptions to the expected pattern be permitted? Can the 20 utterances in the upper right in Example 1 all be considered performance glitches that betray the child's actual grammar? If so, shouldn't some significant percentage of the child's productions of the default pronoun form in the lower right also be considered a mere performance error? How many more exceptions have to occur before the all-or-none assumption gives way to an assumption of gradual learning? The answers to such questions are not easy. However, researchers need to consider them carefully so that there is a clear fit between the theoretical framework and the measures used to test the hypotheses within that framework.

Uniformity of Null Hypotheses

One of the most difficult things about studying disorders is to resist the natural inclination to assume that low levels of ability are a direct reflection of the impairment rather than some other factor. This temptation affects both the hypotheses advanced and the way the data are interpreted.

First consider a hypothetical example that closely resembles the real situation. Two English-speaking siblings are diagnosed as exhibiting SLI. They are 4 and 5 years old. Both show highly telegraphic speech. Occasional function words and inflections appear in their speech, although they tend to occur in frequent expressions. The 5-year-old is slightly more advanced than the 4-year-old in language development. During the next year, both children make small gains. Some of the function words and inflections heard in their speech cannot be so easily characterized as routinized. However, the limited range of use of these forms suggests that the rules they reflect are of narrow scope.

Imagine that the pattern of these children's early use might be taken to reflect a grammar devoid of implicit rules (Gopnik & Goad, 1997). The children's pattern of use during the following year might be assumed to reflect the learning of rules that are narrow rather than broad in scope (Ingram & Carr, 1994; Morehead & Ingram, 1973). Such interpretations might be accurate. However, when testing these proposals, researchers must ask whether they are framing their null hypothesis in a manner that is consistent with the way it would be posed if applied to young, normally developing children.

In the late 1980s and early 1990s, it was proposed that the grammars of young normally developing children lacked functional categories such as DET, INFL, and COMP (Radford, 1988). For example, it was proposed that children's telegraphic main clauses (e.g., *Mommy eat lunch*) are akin to small nonfinite clauses in adult grammar (e.g., *I saw Mommy eat lunch*). However, two types of arguments were raised against this view. First, the occasional appearance of elements associated with functional categories had to be explained in a rather unparsimonious manner (Leonard, 1995). For example, assume a child produced forms such as *Danny played with my car* and *Danny's mom nice*. To deny functional category status to *-ed*, *my*, and *'s*, three unrelated assumptions would be needed. It would have to be assumed that *played* was learned as a participle, that is, that *Danny played* was comparable to *Danny has played* without the auxiliary. Hence, *played* did not express tense and therefore did not involve INFL. The appearance of *my* would be explained by assuming that this form was miscategorized as an adjective rather than representing a specifier of DET. Finally, it would have to be assumed that *'s* was learned by the child as a derivational suffix that serves the function of converting a noun into an adjective with possessive qualities. A more parsimonious interpretation would be that the child's grammar possessed functional categories.

The second type of argument against the *no functional category* view came from languages other than English. Both the word order and verb inflection properties of the speech of young French- and German-speaking children do not suggest a grammar without functional categories (e.g., Pierce, 1992; Poeppel & Wexler, 1993). For example, in French, negative particles follow finite verbs but precede nonfinite verbs. In German, finite verbs appear in second position but nonfinite verbs appear in final position. Young children acquiring these languages show precisely these patterns, even though their utterances are quite telegraphic in other respects.

These arguments have resulted in the *full competence hypothesis* becoming the prevailing view among scholars in normal language acquisition. That is, it is assumed that, from the earliest age, children's grammars are essentially structured like those of the adult. This means that the high frequency of functional category elements missing from young children's utterances (e.g., frequent absence of past *-ed*, third singular *-s*, determiners, possessive *'s*) are attributed to something other than a deficiency in the underlying grammar. It appears that the null hypothesis for research on typically developing children is: "In spite of their limited output, do (normally developing) children possess grammars that are largely adult-like?"

With some notable exceptions (e.g., Rice & Wexler, 1996), some research on the grammatical limitations of children with SLI seems to operate from a different perspective. Rather than assuming a normal underlying grammar until it is proven otherwise, the null hypothesis seems to be something like "Do children with SLI possess incomplete grammars"?

This is far from a trivial distinction. There are many reasons for a failure to reject a null hypothesis, including sampling error and minor design flaws. Unfortunately, although the same degree of experimental imprecision will lead to a failure to reject the null hypothesis in both the case of children with SLI and of normally developing children, the differences in the way the hypotheses are framed will lead to very different conclusions. On the one hand, it might be concluded that children with SLI have incomplete grammars (or, at least, that it cannot be proven otherwise) and, on the other hand, it might be concluded that normally developing children have adultlike grammars (or, at least, it cannot be proven that they do not).

It is interesting to note in this regard that Tomasello (2000) expressed a dissenting view concerning normal language development. His conclusions—that most of children's early linguistic competence is "item based" and development proceeds in a "piecemeal" fashion—resemble some of those that have been made about children with SLI. Yet, some advocates for this "piecemeal" view of SLI might be less persuaded by Tomasello's arguments about normal language development. If data from these two groups of children are interpreted as divergent, then it should be because the data differ and not the null hypotheses.

CONCLUSIONS

The study of SLI has both clinical and theoretical importance. Without question, research is needed from many disciplines. However, such a multidisciplinary approach requires common guidelines in terms of how groups of children are defined and how much (and which) additional descriptive information should be provided. These guidelines should enhance the ability to replicate the research of others, and will help to determine when individual differences constitute scientifically valid subgroups.

Given the heterogeneity of SLI, case studies will always have a place in this area of research. However, group studies will also play a major role, especially those involving more than one comparison group of children. Longitudinal studies and studies employing a treatment paradigm are especially needed because the designs of such studies provide a clearer picture of the relations among factors.

Steps should be taken to ensure that the scientific contribution of a discipline's perspective is not lost through a failure to communicate clearly. In particular, each discipline's basic assumptions should be spelled out, measures should be compatible with these assumptions, and null hypotheses should be framed in a uniform manner. It is unlikely that these changes will lead to immediate answers to the important questions. However, they may reduce the number of detours on the path toward finding them.

REFERENCES

Aram, D., & Nation, J. (1975). Patterns of language behavior in children with developmental language disorders. *Journal of Speech and Hearing Research, 18,* 229–241.

Bedore, L., & Leonard, L. (1998). Specific language impairment and grammatical morphology: A discriminant function analysis. *Journal of Speech, Language, and Hearing Research, 41,* 1185–1192.

Bishop, D. (1992). The biological basis of specific language impairment. In P. Fletcher & D. Hall (Eds.), *Specific speech and language disorders in children* (pp. 2–17). London: Whurr.

Bishop, D., North, T., & Donlan, C. (1996). Nonword repetition as a behavioural marker for inherited language impairment: Evidence from a twin study. *Journal of Child Psychology and Psychiatry, 36,* 1–13.

Caramazza, A. (1984). The logic of neuropsychological research and the problem of patient classification in aphasia. *Brain and Language, 21,* 9–20.

Clahsen, H., & Hansen, D. (1997). The grammatical agreement deficit in specific language impairment: Evidence from therapy experiments. In M. Gopnik (Ed.), *The biological basis of language* (pp. 148–168). Oxford, England: Oxford University Press.

Dollaghan, C., & Campbell, T. (1998). Nonword repetition and child language impairment. *Journal of Speech, Language, and Hearing Research, 41,* 1136–1146.

Dromi, E., Leonard, L., Adam, G., & Zadunaisky-Ehrlich, S. (1999). Verb agreement morphology in Hebrew-speaking children with specific language impairment. *Journal of Speech, Language, and Hearing Research, 42,* 1414–1431.

Druks, J., & Shallice, T. (2000). Selective preservation of naming from description and the "restricted preverbal message." *Brain and Language, 72,* 100–128.

Edwards, J., & Lahey, M. (1996). Auditory lexical decisions of children with specific language impairment. *Journal of Speech and Hearing Research, 39,* 1263–1273.

Eyer, J., & Leonard, L. (1994). Learning past tense morphology with specific language impairment: A case study. *Child Language Teaching and Therapy, 10,* 127–138.

Fey, M., Long, S., & Cleave, P. (1994). Reconsideration of IQ criteria in the definition of specific language impairment. In R. Watkins & M. Rice (Eds.), *Specific language impairments in children* (pp. 161–178). Baltimore: Brookes.

Gall, F. (1835). *The function of the brain and each of its parts. 5, Oganology.* Boston: Marsh, Capen, & Lyon.

Gathercole, S., & Baddeley, A. (1990). Phonological memory deficits in language disordered children: Is there a causal connection? *Journal of Memory and Language, 29,* 336–360.

Gopnik, M., & Crago, M. (1991). Familial aggregation of a developmental language disorder. *Cognition, 39,* 1–50.

Gopnik, M., & Goad, H. (1997). What underlies inflectional error patterns in genetic dysphasia? *Journal of Neurolinguistics, 10,* 109–137.

Hansson, K., & Leonard, L. (in press). The use and productivity of verb morphology in specific language impairment: An examination of Swedish. *Linguistics.*

Ingram, D., & Carr, L. (1994, November). *When morphology ability exceeds syntactic ability: A case study.* Paper presented at the convention of the American Speech-Language-Hearing Association, New Orleans.

Johnson, J., & Newport, E. (1989). Critical period effects in second language learning: The influence of maturational state on the acquisition of English as a second language. *Cognitive Psychology, 21,* 60–99.

Johnston, J. (1988). Specific language disorders in the child. In N. Lass, L. McReynolds, J. Northern, & D. Yoder (Eds.), *Handbook of speech-language pathology and audiology* (pp. 685–715). Toronto: Decker.

Korkman, M., & Häkkinen-Rihu, P. (1994). A new classification of developmental language disorders. *Brain and Language, 47*, 96–116.

Lahey, M. (1990). Who shall be called language disordered? Some reflections and one perspective. *Journal of Speech and Hearing Disorders, 55*, 612–620.

Lahey, M., & Edwards, J. (1996). Why do children with specific language impairment name pictures more slowly than their peers? *Journal of Speech and Hearing Research, 39*, 1081–1098.

Leonard, L. (1995). Functional categories in the grammars of children with specific language impairment. *Journal of Speech and Hearing Research, 38*, 1270–1283.

Leonard, L. (1998). *Children with specific language impairment.* Cambridge, MA: MIT Press.

Leonard, L., Eyer, J., Bedore, L., & Grela, B. (1997). Three accounts of the grammatical morpheme difficulties of English-speaking children with specific language impairment. *Journal of Speech, Language, and Hearing Research, 40*, 741–753.

Leonard, L., Miller, C., & Gerber, E. (1999). Grammatical morphology and the lexicon in children with specific language impairment. *Journal of Speech, Language, and Hearing Research, 42*, 678–689.

Leonard, L., Schwartz, R., Chapman, K., Rowan, L., Prelock, P., Terrell, B., Weiss, A., & Messick, C. (1982). Early lexical acquisition in children with specific language impairment. *Journal of Speech and Hearing Research, 25*, 554–564.

McGregor, K., & Leonard, L. (1995). Intervention for word-finding deficits in children. In M. Fey, J. Windsor, & S. Warren (Eds.), *Language intervention* (pp. 85–105). Baltimore: Brookes.

McCauley, R., & Swisher, L. (1984). Use and misuse of norm-referenced tests in clinical assessment: A hypothetical case. *Journal of Speech and Hearing Disorders, 49*, 338–348.

Menyuk, P. (1964). Comparison of grammar of children with functionally deviant and normal speech. *Journal of Speech and Hearing Research, 7*, 109–121.

Mervis, C., & Robinson, B, (1999). Methodological issues in cross-syndrome comparisons: Matching procedures, sensitivity (*Se*), and specificity (*Sp*). Commentary in M. Sigman & E. Ruskin, Continuity and change in the social competence of children with autism, Down syndrome, and developmental delays. *Monographs of the Society for Research in Child Development, 64*(1, Serial No. 256).

Miller, C., Kail, R., Leonard, L., & Tomblin, J. B. (2001). Speed of processing in children with specific language impairment. *Journal of Speech, Language, and Hearing Research, 44*, 416–433.

Miller, J., & Chapman, R. (1981). The relation between age and mean length of utterance in morphemes. *Journal of Speech and Hearing Research, 24*, 154–161.

Morehead, D., & Ingram, D. (1973). The development of base syntax in normal and linguistically deviant children. *Journal of Speech and Hearing Research, 16*, 330–352.

Paul, R. (2000). Predicting outcomes of early expressive language delay: Ethical implications. In D. Bishop & L. Leonard (Eds.), *Speech and language impairments in children: Causes, characteristics, intervention, and outcome* (pp. 195–209). Hove: Psychology Press.

Pierce, A. (1992). *Language acquisition and syntactic theory.* Dordrecht, The Netherlands: Kluwer.

Poeppel, D., & Wexler, K. (1993). The full competence hypothesis. *Language, 69*, 1–33.

Radford, A. (1988). Small children's small clauses. *Transactions of the Philological Society, 86*, 1–46.

Rapin, I., & Allen, D. (1983). Developmental language disorders: Nosologic considerations. In U. Kirk (Ed.), *Neuropsychology of language, reading, and spelling* (pp. 155–184). New York: Academic Press.

Restrepo, M. A., Swisher, L., Plante, E., & Vance, R. (1992). Relations among verbal and nonverbal cognitive skills in normal language and specifically language impaired children. *Journal of Communication Disorders, 25*, 205–219.

Rice, M., Haney, K., & Wexler, K. (1998). Family histories of children with SLI who show extended optional infinitives. *Journal of Speech, Language, and Hearing Research, 41*, 419–432.

Rice, M., Noll, K., & Grimm, H. (1997). An extended optional infinitive stage in German-speaking children with specific language impairment. *Language Acquisition, 6*, 255–295.

Rice, M., & Wexler, K. (1996). Toward tense as a clinical marker of specific language impairment in English-speaking children. *Journal of Speech and Hearing Research, 39,* 239–257.

Rice, M., Wexler, K., & Cleave, P. (1995). Specific language impairment as a period of extended optional infinitive. *Journal of Speech and Hearing Research, 38,* 850–863.

Tager-Flusberg, H., & Cooper, J. (1999). Present and future possibilities for defining a phenotype for specific language impairment. *Journal of Speech, Language, and Hearing Research, 42,* 1275–1278.

Tallal, P., & Piercy, M. (1974). Developmental aphasia: Rate of auditory processing and selective impairment of consonant perception. *Neuropsychologia, 12,* 83–93.

Tallal, P., Ross, R., & Curtiss, S. (1989). Familial aggregation in specific language impairment. *Journal of Speech and Hearing Disorders, 54,* 167–173.

Tallal, P., Townsend, J., Curtiss, S., & Wulfeck, B. (1991). Phenotypic profiles of language-impaired children based on genetic/family history. *Brain and Language, 41,* 81–95.

Thal, D., & Katich, J. (1996). Predicaments in early identification of specific language impairment. In K. Cole, P. Dale, & D. Thal (Eds.), *Assessment of communication and language* (pp. 1–28). Baltimore: Brookes.

Tomasello, M. (2000). Do young children have adult syntactic competence? *Cognition, 74,* 209–253.

Tomblin, J. B. (1983). An examination of the concept of disorder in the study of language variation. In *Proceedings from the Symposium on Research in Child Language Disorders* (Vol. 4, pp. 81–109). Madison: University of Wisconsin, Madison.

Tomblin, J. B. (1989). Familial concentration of developmental language impairment. *Journal of Speech and Hearing Disorders, 54,* 287–295.

Tomblin, J. B. (1996). Genetic and environmental contributions to the risk for specific language impairment. In M. Rice (Ed.), *Towards genetics of language* (pp. 191–210). Hillsdale, NJ: Lawrence Erlbaum Associates.

Tomblin, J. B., & Buckwalter, P. (1994). Studies of genetics of specific language impairment. In R. Watkins & M. Rice (Eds.), *Specific language impairments in children* (pp. 17–35). Baltimore: Brookes.

Tomblin, J. B., & Pandich, J. (1999). Lessons from children with specific language impairment. *Trends in Cognitive Science, 3,* 283–285.

Tomblin, J. B., Records, N., Buckwalter, P., Zhang, X., Smith, E., & O'Brien, M. (1997). Prevalence of specific language impairment in kindergarten children. *Journal of Speech, Language, and Hearing Research, 40,* 1245–1260.

Tomblin, J. B., & Zhang, X. (1999). Are children with SLI a unique group of language learners? In H. Tager-Flusberg (Ed.), *Neurodevelopmental disorders* (pp. 361–382). Cambridge, MA: MIT Press.

Van der Lely, H. (1994). Canonical linking rules: Forward vs reverse linking in normally developing and specifically language impaired children. *Cognition, 51,* 29–72.

Van der Lely, H. (1996). Specifically language impaired and normally developing children: Verbal passive vs adjectival passive sentence interpretation. *Lingua, 98,* 243–272.

Van der Lely, H., & Stollwerck, L. (1997). Binding theory and grammatical specific language impairment in children. *Cognition, 62,* 245–290.

Weiner, P. (1986). The study of childhood language disorders: Nineteenth century perspectives. *Journal of Communication Disorders, 19,* 1–47.

Wexler, K., Schütze, C., & Rice, M. (1998). Subject case in children with SLI and unaffected controls: Evidence for the Agr/Tns omission model. *Language Acquisition, 7,* 317–344.

Wilson, B., & Risucci, D. (1986). A model for clinical-quantitative classification. Generation I: Application to language-disordered preschool children. *Brain and Language, 27,* 281–309.

Wolfus, B., Moscovitch, M., & Kinsbourne, M. (1980). Subgroups of developmental language impairment. *Brain and Language, 10,* 152–171.

9

Methodological Issues in Cross-Group Comparisons of Language and Cognitive Development

Carolyn B. Mervis
University of Louisville

Byron F. Robinson
Georgia State University

Researchers concerned with theoretical or applied aspects of language ability and disability typically ask questions of the form, "Do children with a particular developmental disability and children who are developing normally show the same or different developmental relations between particular aspects of language and/or cognitive development?" This question is then tested by matching the two groups on one aspect (control variable) and testing for group mean differences on the variable of interest (target variable). If the two groups do not differ significantly on the control variable, but do differ significantly on the target variable, then it is typically concluded that the group with the disability does not show the normal relation between the target and control variables. In most cases, the group with the disability performs significantly worse than the control group, leading the researchers to conclude that the disability group shows a deficit on the target variable. For example, suppose a researcher wishes to determine if children with specific language impairment (SLI) have more difficulty with grammar than typically developing children at the same nonverbal cognitive level. The standard way to address this question has been to conduct a t test comparing the scores of the two groups of children on the measure of nonverbal cognitive ability (e.g., Columbia Mental Maturity Scale; Burgemeister, Blum, & Lorge, 1972), confirm that the two groups do not differ significantly on this measure ($p > .05$), and then conduct another t test comparing the grammar scores (e.g., mean length of utterance, MLU) of the two groups. If the grammar scores are significantly different, then the typical conclusion would be that children with SLI have a deficit in grammatical ability.

This type of matching strategy is sometimes expanded to include control groups of children with other forms of developmental disabilities (e.g., particular syndromes, mental retardation of unknown or mixed etiology) in addition to a normal control group. If it is found that the children with the disability of interest differ significantly not only from the normal control group but also from children with other forms of developmental disability, then it often is concluded that the nonnormal relation between the target and control variables is universal for and specific to the disability of interest. For example, a group of children with Williams syndrome (who typically have mild mental retardation but a relative strength in language ability) could be added to the hypothetical study of the relation between nonverbal cognitive ability and grammatical ability. If the three groups of children did not differ significantly on nonverbal cognitive ability, but the SLI group performed significantly worse than either the Williams syndrome group or the typical control group, then a common conclusion would be that a grammatical deficit relative to nonverbal cognitive ability was universal among children with SLI and specific to this disability. Theoretical arguments or models of development may then be built on these results and their interpretations.

Unfortunately, the foundation provided by findings based on these types of designs is often weak. This chapter argues that there are serious flaws in group matching designs as they typically are used and therefore in the conclusions that can be drawn from them. The problems with group-matching designs include difficulties with the matching procedure, chronological age (CA) confounds, and the inability of the cross-group design to address issues concerning individual variability and syndrome heterogeneity. Suggestions for improving group designs, including pair-wise matching, are offered. It is then argued that many important questions for researchers and theoreticians interested in these issues focus not on mean differences among groups of children, but rather on patterns of performance of individual children. This does not mean advocating a simple case study methodology, however. Instead, a method is proposed that focuses on the performance of individual children across multiple measures, but allows the performance of these individuals to be aggregated by disability (or any other variable of interest). Signal-detection theory can then be used to determine the extent to which a particular profile of performance on the dependent variables is characteristic of and/or specific to that disability—a question to which an answer is needed, if the data from individuals with developmental disabilities are to be used to address theoretical issues in language acquisition.

DIFFICULTIES WITH GROUP-MATCHING DESIGNS

The simplest way to explore the characteristics of an atypical population (e.g., those with a known disability, syndrome, or unusual genotype) is to compare a sample of those individuals to a comparison group of normally developing individuals (perhaps matched for CA) on a specific characteristic or target variable. If the two groups differ on mean levels of the target variable, then researchers may conclude that the characteristic is central to the atypical group. Imagine, for instance, a sample from a group (e.g., individuals with Williams syndrome) that scores significantly below a comparison group of individuals who are developing normally on a test of grammatical ability. Based on such a difference, one might consider the possibility that the population of interest has a specific deficit in grammatical ability. This conclusion, however, would be immediately called into question if there was a factor that covaried with the target variable and differed between the two groups. Suppose the population of interest also had some level of deficit in vocabulary knowledge. Because lexical knowledge is related to grammatical ability (e.g., Bates & Goodman, 1999), it would be expected that a group with a smaller mean vocabulary would also score below other groups on a test of grammatical ability. There is no need to invoke a specific deficit in grammatical ability to explain this finding. Accordingly, in order to determine if the population of interest displayed a specific deficit in grammatical ability, vocabulary size and any other factor that covaried with grammatical ability and differed between the groups would need to be controlled.

The cross-group matching design is commonly used to provide this control for covariates that may explain group differences on the variable of interest. Typically, two groups, one from the population of interest and one comparison group, are matched on a characteristic (the control variable) and then the two groups are tested for mean differences on a variable of interest (target variable). If the two groups do not differ significantly on the matching variable, but the individuals from the population of interest score significantly lower on the target variable, then it is generally considered that the population of interest evidences a deficit on the target variable. As in the example at the start of this chapter, the population of interest is often a group that is developing atypically (e.g., children with SLI, individuals with Down syndrome) and the comparison group is often a group of normally developing individuals who are matched to the atypical group on one or more variables that are measured on an interval scale: CA, nonverbal IQ, overall IQ, and so on. In some cases, the groups are matched based on variables that are measured on an ordinal scale, such as "mental age" or "language age." Use of the latter type of variable, which creates special difficulties in matching groups, is discussed later in this chapter.

Recently, it has become common to compare two or more atypical groups to each other after matching on a control variable, as in the second example provided at the beginning of the chapter. For instance, if little is known about a syndrome, then researchers may compare that syndrome to "reference groups," about whom more is known (or who are more readily available than other groups). Children with Down syndrome, children with mental retardation of unknown etiology, and children with mental retardation of mixed etiology are three common de facto reference groups. Finally, if the researcher is interested in determining the specificity of a characteristic, then multiple comparison groups may be used. If only one group differs from the other groups on the target variable, after controls are in place, then the characteristic assumed to be represented by that variable is considered to be unique, or specific, to the standout group.

ACCEPTING THE NULL HYPOTHESIS

The logic underlying group-matching designs requires that the two (or more) groups do not differ on the control variables. Determination that the groups do not differ usually is made based on the results of a test of the difference between group means on the control variable (e.g., a t test). The group-matching design requires the acceptance of the null hypothesis that the two groups do not differ on the control variable. That is, if researchers cannot reject the null hypothesis of no group differences on the control variable, then they tacitly accept the null hypothesis and assume that the groups are equivalent. However, based on what is taught in undergraduate statistics books, rejecting the null hypothesis because it is improbable under the theoretical sampling distribution should be a very different decision from accepting the null hypothesis because it is likely to be true.

As Cohen (1990) pointed out, the null hypothesis is almost never literally true. Therefore, the question, "How close is close enough?" must be considered. Researchers must determine how to index the equivalence of the two groups on the control variable. Usually, they set alpha to the traditional .05 level. Thus, in the case of the matching design, if the probability that the groups differ on that variable is greater than .05, then the groups are considered to be matched. In most studies, the actual p value for the test for the control variable is not reported; it is simply stated as being "> .05." If the means and standard deviations for the control variable for the two groups are reported, however, the p value may be determined by the reader. In many studies, p values for comparisons involving control variables are only slightly higher than .05. Nevertheless, these values are accepted as evidence that the groups are appropriately matched. Harcum (1990, p. 404) described this response as "casual acceptance of the null hypothesis."

In terms of the matching design, it is not so much the alpha level but rather the probability of making a Type II error (accepting the hypothesis that the groups do not differ even though they do) that is of primary concern. For practical purposes, it can be very difficult to estimate accurately the probability of making a Type II error. However, it is known that the larger the alpha level, the less likely the researcher is to make a Type II error. The question then becomes: How high should alpha be in order for the researcher to accept the null hypothesis that the groups do not differ on the matching variable? Frick (1995) proposed the following guidelines: Any p value less than .20 is too low to accept the null hypothesis. A p value greater than .50 is large enough to accept the null hypothesis. Finally, p values between .20 and .50 are ambiguous. Thus, at a minimum, p values of at least .50 should be obtained before the groups are considered "matched."

The consequences of accepting the null hypothesis when the p value for the test of mean differences for the control variable is low can be illustrated with an example drawn from actual data. As part of a study examining intellectual strengths and weaknesses of 9- and 10-year-olds with Williams syndrome or Down syndrome (Klein & Mervis, 1999), a cohort of 18 children with Williams syndrome and 23 children with Down syndrome was tested on the McCarthy Scales of Children's Abilities (McCarthy, 1972) and the Peabody Picture Vocabulary Test–Revised (PPVT–R; Dunn & Dunn, 1981). The two groups were well matched on CA (p = .502). Here, these samples are used to address the question of whether children with Williams syndrome have significantly larger vocabularies than children with Down syndrome, even when the groups are matched for overall level of cognitive ability (in this case, raw score on the McCarthy). First consider the full sample of 18 children with Williams syndrome and 23 children with Down syndrome. As indicated in Table 9.1, receptive vocabulary size was significantly larger for the Williams syndrome group. However, overall cognitive ability was also significantly higher for the Williams syndrome group. The distributions for

TABLE 9.1

Significance of Difference in PPVT–R Raw Scores for Children with Williams Syndrome and Children with Down Syndrome, as a Function of p Level for Group Match on Overall Cognitive Ability (McCarthy Raw Score)

N		McCarthy Raw Score Mean			PPVT–R Raw Score Mean		
DS	WS	DS	WS	p Level	DS	WS	p Level
23	18	105.87	142.89	<.001	50.52	76.61	<.001
15	16	121.67	137.50	.106	60.33	74.50	.030
14	15	123.71	134.73	.254	60.86	72.40	.074
12	14	128.00	132.50	.650	64.00	72.57	.204

PPVT–R raw score and McCarthy raw score are shown in Fig. 9.1. Because the two groups were not matched on the control variable, there is a reasonable possibility that the apparent weakness of children with Down syndrome on receptive vocabulary reflected not a specific difficulty with receptive vocabulary, but rather a general weakness in overall cognitive ability.

A more considered test of vocabulary differences should take into account general cognitive ability. In order to better match the two groups on this variable, the standard policy was followed (e.g., Sigman & Ruskin, 1999): The children with the lowest McCarthy raw scores from the Down

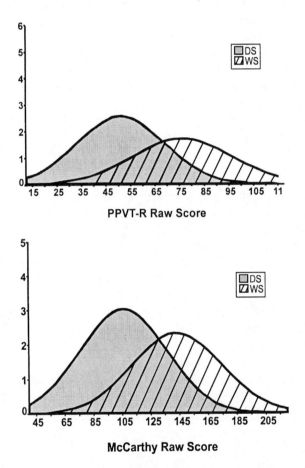

FIG. 9.1. Raw score distributions for the Peabody Picture Vocabulary Test–Revised and the McCarthy Scales of Children's Abilities for the original samples of children with Down syndrome ($N = 23$) and children with Williams syndrome ($N = 18$). The two groups are not matched for McCarthy raw score ($p < .001$). The Williams syndrome group performed significantly better than the Down syndrome group on the PPVT–R ($p < .001$).

syndrome group and the children with the highest McCarthy raw scores from the Williams syndrome group were gradually removed until the difference between the two groups on McCarthy raw score was no longer significant ($p = .106$). These groups would then be considered by many researchers to be matched. The distributions for PPVT–R raw score and McCarthy raw score are shown in Fig. 9.2. As indicated in Table 9.1, the two groups continued to differ significantly on PPVT–R raw score, a finding that typically would be interpreted as indicating that children with Down syndrome have smaller receptive vocabularies than would be expected for their overall level of cognitive ability (or perhaps that children with Williams syn-

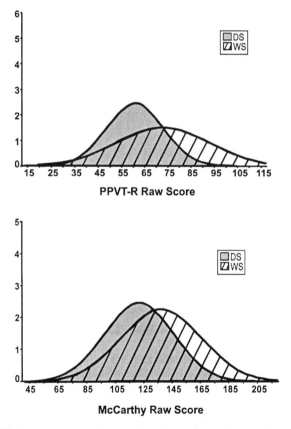

FIG. 9.2. Raw score distributions for the Peabody Picture Vocabulary Test–Revised and the McCarthy Scales of Children's Abilities for the samples of children with Down syndrome ($N = 15$) and children with Williams syndrome ($N = 16$) "matched" for McCarthy raw score at $p = .106$. By Frick's criteria, these groups should not be considered matched. The Williams syndrome group performed significantly better than the Down syndrome group on the PPVT–R ($p = .030$).

drome have larger receptive vocabularies than would be expected for over-all level of cognitive ability).

Based on Frick's (1995) guidelines, however, the McCarthy raw score p value (.106) is too low to accept the null hypothesis that the two groups are matched on general cognitive ability. Thus, by his criteria, the researchers still were not in a position to address the question of relative receptive vo-cabulary sizes for a given level of overall cognitive ability. Accordingly, the process of removing children from both groups was continued, following the same rule as previously, until the groups were matched on McCarthy raw score at the $p = .254$ level. This p level falls in Frick's "ambiguous" range: It is not clear whether or not the groups are matched. Distributions are illustrated in Fig. 9.3. Now, as indicated in Table 9.1, the difference be-tween the two groups on receptive vocabulary is no longer significant ($p = .074$). Some researchers would interpret a p value at this level as indicating a trend for a difference in receptive vocabulary ability between the Down syndrome group and the Williams syndrome group.

A final analysis was conducted using a p value that met Frick's criterion for considering it appropriate to accept the null hypothesis that the two groups are matched on overall cognitive ability. Following the same proce-dure as the previous two analyses for limiting the samples, the two groups were matched for McCarthy raw score at the $p = .650$ level. Distributions are illustrated in Fig. 9.4. As indicated in Table 9.1, the difference between the two groups on receptive language is definitely not significant ($p = .204$). This exercise clearly illustrates that depending on how well two groups are matched on the control variable, drastically different conclusions about whether the two groups differ significantly on the target variable may be made.

Another point that is illustrated by the previous example is the increas-ing effect of matching at different p values. That is, even if Frick's guidelines are followed, hard and fast rules concerning acceptable p value cut points for matching cannot be provided. The reason is that the dichotomous ques-tion of whether the groups are exactly equal on the control variable is not really the important question. Instead, given that in all likelihood there will be some group difference on the control variable, the effect a difference of a given magnitude (i.e., effect size) will have on the assessment of group dif-ferences on the target variable of interest must be considered. The impact of groups that are not matched can only be determined by considering the relation between the control variable and the target variable for the popula-tions of interest. In the previous example, for instance, McCarthy raw scores and PPVT–R raw scores are correlated at the $r = .799$ level. If the cor-relation had been lower, then the effect of the McCarthy raw score mis-match would have had less of an impact on the PPVT–R raw score group

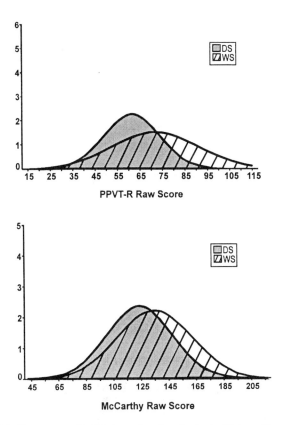

FIG. 9.3. Raw score distributions for the Peabody Picture Vocabulary Test–Revised and the McCarthy Scales of Children's Abilities for the samples of children with Down syndrome (N = 14) and children with Williams syndrome (N = 15) "matched" for McCarthy raw score at p = .254. By Frick's criteria, it is ambiguous whether these groups should be considered matched. The difference between the two groups on the PPVT–R was not significant (p = .074). However, this p value would be interpreted by some researchers as indicating a trend for the Down syndrome group to have a smaller receptive vocabulary than the Williams syndrome group.

differences. Of course, if the control variable and the target variable are not correlated, then it probably is not necessary to use the matching design to begin with. A series of simulation studies is currently being conducted in order to provide more specific guidelines for matching based on the strength of the correlation between the target and control variables. In the meantime, a researcher can reduce the likelihood of making invalid inferences from the matching design by accepting two groups as being matched on the control variable only if alpha is set at an acceptable level.

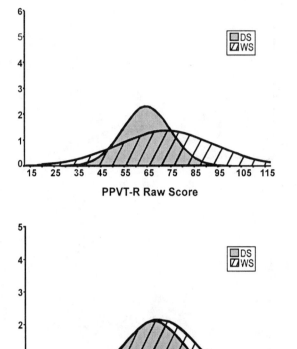

FIG. 9.4. Raw score distributions for the Peabody Picture Vocabulary Test–Revised and the McCarthy Scales of Children's Abilities for the samples of children with Down syndrome ($N = 12$) and children with Williams syndrome ($N = 14$) matched for McCarthy raw score at $p = .650$. By Frick's criteria, these groups are well matched. The difference between the two groups on the PPVT–R was not significant ($p = .204$).

STANDARD SCORES BASED ON NONEQUIVALENT NORMING SAMPLES

Researchers sometimes compare performance across two or more standardized measures that were normed on different samples. For example, vocabulary performance on the PPVT might be compared with nonverbal IQ from Raven's Progressive Matrices (Raven, 1960). Such comparisons are problematic when based on standard scores; they are even more problematic when based on mental age. A standard score is simply an individual's raw score relative to the distribution of raw scores for a group of similarly aged peers in a norming sample. Thus, if two different norming samples are used, then the two standard scores are not directly comparable. If both tests used large norming samples based on similar stratification variables, then the two norming groups may be considered roughly equivalent. However, this is frequently not the case, especially where specialized language tests are concerned. Because such tests do not have the wide marketability of more general IQ tests, publishers often do not provide the resources to obtain large comprehensive norming samples. For example, the Sequenced Inventory of Communication Development–Revised (SICD–R; Hedrick, Prather, & Tobin, 1984) has a norming sample of only 252 children between ages 4 and 48 months. Furthermore, all children were Caucasian and from the Seattle, Washington, area. As another example, although the Carrow Elicited Language Inventory (CELI; Carrow-Woolfolk, 1974) included more children (475 between ages 3;0 and 7;11) in the norming sample, all were from Caucasian middle-class families and attended day-care centers or church schools in Houston, Texas. Both measures have limited sample sizes and neither sample is representative of the U.S. population. Furthermore, although both tests are norm referenced, neither provides standard scores. The SICD–R provides only age equivalents, the CELI only percentile ranks. Thus, although these assessments and others like them may be useful for clinical purposes, their psychometric properties are problematic for research purposes.

Even when tests are based on otherwise appropriate norming procedures, it is important to consider potential cohort differences based on the time frame during which the test was developed. Consider the Columbia Mental Maturity Scale (CMMS; Burgemeister et al., 1972), a commonly used test for measuring nonverbal intelligence. This test has good psychometric properties (Sattler, 1992) and an excellent stratified norming sample of 2,600 children from ages 3;6 through 9;11. However, the CMMS was last normed in 1972. Given that intelligence is generally assumed to be on the rise when time is measured in increments of decades—the Flynn effect (1987)—it would be expected that a test normed in recent years would yield lower standard scores for the same level of absolute performance than a test normed many years ago. Flynn found that over the past 50 years, nonverbal IQ has increased by an average of 5.7 points per decade and verbal IQ has increased an average of 3.7 points per decade. Thus, the common practice of using measures such as the CMMS and Raven's Progressive Matrices, which were normed 30 or more years ago, as screening measures to ensure that children with SLI have "normal" nonverbal intelligence is problematic. In fact, a study of 4- to 11-year-old children with Williams syndrome reported a mean standard score of 79 for the CMMS (Gosch, Stading, & Pankau, 1994), even though most children with Williams syndrome have mental retardation. Direct comparisons of standard scores on tests that were normed recently (e.g., the PPVT–III; Dunn & Dunn, 1997) to those on tests that were normed 30 or more years ago (e.g., CMMS, Raven's Progressive Matrices) are highly problematic, for the same reasons.

The ultimate solution to the problem of nonequivalent norming samples across tests is to restrict the control and target variable measures to tests that were adequately normed on the same sample. This would limit research to comparisons of subtests across the same instrument, such as typical IQ tests (e.g., WISC–III; Wechsler, 1991), the Clinical Evaluation of Language Fundamentals (CELF–III; Semel, Wiig, & Secord, 1995), or tests with a similar structure. Of course, many research questions cannot be answered using extant standardized tests. In such situations, if sufficient resources are available, then joint norms could be developed for the comparison tests. This may seem to be an extravagant solution, but it is important to remember that the norming of the comparison tests could be tailored to the study at hand. For instance, the CA ranges and stratification variables could be restricted in such a way to generalize only to the populations of interest. This strategy has been followed by the Center for Research on Language at the University of California, San Diego, for their studies of the language and cognitive development of children with SLI, focal lesions, and Williams syndrome (Appelbaum, personal communication, April 1996). It is important to make sure that the normally developing participants used to create the norms are truly representative of the general population in terms of cognitive ability (e.g., have a mean IQ of approximately 100).

LANGUAGE AGE AND MENTAL AGE CONFOUNDS

Researchers sometimes attempt to match individuals using language age (LA) or mental age (MA). Typically, this strategy is used when standard scores cannot be obtained for some or all of the participants because their CA exceeds the oldest CA of the norming sample. Therefore, raw scores are converted to LAs or MAs before matching. At first blush, this seems to be a reasonable strategy. After all, if both groups score at the same age level on the control variable, then they are likely functioning at the same ability levels. The problem with this logic is due to the likelihood of nonlinear growth patterns in language and other areas of development. For instance, it is well known that the rate of language development changes repeatedly throughout early development (Robinson & Mervis, 1998). A 2-month difference in the LA of 5-year-old children would equate to only slight differences in language ability. A 2-month LA difference between 16 and 20 months, however, represents a large difference in language ability. At 16 months, children would be expected to have very small vocabularies and to be speaking in single words. At 18 months, children would likely be beginning their vocal ulary spurt and starting to produce multiword utterances. At 20 months, children would be expected to be in the midst of their vocabulary spurt and to be producing a large proportion of multiword utterances (Fenson et al., 1994). Thus, slight differences in a LA measure, despite large p values in a test of mean differences, could equate to large and meaningful differences in the true language abilities of the two groups. Similar nonlinear growth patterns undoubtedly occur in most domains of development. Therefore, it is necessary to understand the typical growth patterns of a control factor before one can truly evaluate the question, "How close is close enough?", when trying to match groups on that factor.

DIFFERENTIAL RATES OF DEVELOPMENT AND CA DIFFERENCE CONFOUNDS

Even if groups are well matched on the control variable, differences in CA may confound the group matching design. If the control and target variables develop at different rates, then the differences between the raw scores (and therefore the age equivalents) will not be stable across CA. In such situations, one cannot predict that two groups (or two individuals) with identical age equivalents on the control variable, but differing CAs should be expected to have similar scores on the target variable. The situation in which two or more variables are developing at different rates is not unusual. To illustrate this issue, the relations between age equivalents on different subtests from the Differential Ability Scales (DAS; Elliott, 1990) as a function of CA (Mervis & Robinson, 1999) were examined. An age equivalent of 8;3 on the Similarities subtest (corresponding to an ability score of 83) was selected and then compared to the expected age equivalents for the Definitions, Matrices, Pattern Construction, and Recall of Digits subtests, for different CAs, based on the test norms. Thus, Similarities age equivalent was treated as the control variable and the age equivalents for the other subtests as target variables. That is, the question was asked, if children have an age equivalent of 8;3 on the Similarities subtest, and all of their abilities are at the same level (i.e., they earn the same standard score on each subtest), then what are their predicted age equivalents for each of these other subtests? As expected, if children's CA is 8;3 and their age equivalent on Similarities is also 8;3, then age equivalents for each of the other subtests would be 8;3 as well. (See Fig. 9.5.) These hypothetical children are performing at the median level for their CA on Similarities, and would therefore be expected to perform at the median level on each of the other subtests, assuming they have equivalent abilities in each of the domains tested. But what happens when their performance on Similarities is either above or below the median for their CA? As illustrated in Fig. 9.5, this rela-

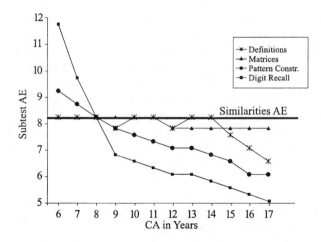

FIG. 9.5. Variability in expected age equivalents as a function of CA for four subtests of the Differential Ability Scales, given a constant age equivalent of 8;3 on the Similarities subtest and the assumption that the child has earned the same standard score on each of the five subtests. From "Methodological Issues in Cross-Syndrome Comparisons: Matching Procedures, Sensitivity (*Se*), and Specificity (*Sp*)," by C. B. Mervis and B. F. Robinson, 1999, *Monographs of the Society for Research in Child Development, 64(1*, Serial No. 256), p. 120. Copyright 1999 by the Society for Research in Child Development. Reprinted with permission.

tion varies as a function of which subtest is the target variable. The relation between Similarities and Matrices age equivalents remains reasonably stable across the entire CA range from 6 to 17 years. Therefore, if Similarities age equivalent was the matching variable and Matrices age equivalent was the target variable, then the researcher could sample from a large CA range without invalidating group comparisons. On the other hand, matching on Similarities with Recall of Digits as the target variable would be quite problematic if participants varied in CA. In this case, there is actually a crossover in the relation from 6 to 17 years CA. A 6-year-old who earned an age equivalent of 8;3 on the Similarities subtest would be expected to earn an age equivalent of 11;9 on the Recall of Digits subtest. In contrast, a 12-year-old who earned the same age equivalent as the 6-year-old on the Similarities subtest would be expected to earn an age equivalent of 6;1 on the Recall of Digits subtest; this is much lower than the age equivalent predicted for the younger child on that subtest. Thus, a significant difference between groups of 6- and 12-year-olds on Recall of Digits would be predicted, assuming the groups had been well matched for age equivalent on the Similarities subtest and the participants had the same level of ability (same standard score) for the constructs measured by the two subtests.

Even two relatively similar abilities may develop at different rates, especially for children at the extremes of the distribution (who either are gifted or have developmental delay or mental retardation). Thus, children of the same CA who have identical standard scores on two measures normed on the same sample may still have very different age equivalent scores on these measures. As an example, consider performance on two language measures normed on the same extensive and carefully stratified sample. The Peabody Picture Vocabulary Test–III (PPVT–III; Dunn & Dunn, 1997) measures receptive vocabulary and the Expressive Vocabulary Test (EVT; Williams, 1997) assesses expressive vocabulary. A 7-year-old child with standard scores of 55 on both the PPVT–III and the EVT will have a receptive vocabulary age equivalent of 36 months but an expressive vocabulary age equivalent of 49 months. Examples such as this one illustrate the problem of using age equivalent scores even when children are the same CA and the measures are normed on the same sample. These problems are due to the fact that age equivalents do not constitute an interval scale and are subject to distortion due to patterns of developmental trajectories, especially across measures or subtests within measures. (Note that standard scores are not susceptible to these problems.) Thus, the use of age equivalents violates the standard assumptions underlying statistical analysis. Unfortunately, statistical comparisons often are made based on age equivalent scores.

NONEQUIVALENT NORMING SAMPLES AND AGE EQUIVALENTS

Another problem with comparisons across nonequivalent norming samples arises when the comparisons are based on age equivalents. In the example derived from the DAS, differential rates of growth between measures can be identified because each of the DAS subtests was individually normed on the same group of children. Similarly, because the PPVT–III and the EVT were normed on the same sample of children, differential rates of growth can be identified in receptive and expressive vocabulary. When comparing across tests normed on different samples, however, it is difficult to compare norming samples within the same age range, and it is impossible to evaluate if there are any differences across groups in CA that would confound the group comparisons. That is, the impact of CA could be minimal, as in the DAS example of Similarities age equivalent as the control variable and Matrices age equivalent as the target variable, or it could be substantial, as occurs with the same control variable but with Recall of Digits as the target variable. Without norming on the same sample, however, it is impossible to assess the impact of the differential growth rates problem.

A PARTIAL SOLUTION: PAIR-WISE MATCHING

It is possible to reduce the problem of CA confounds by restricting the age range of the samples to a point where there are no important differences in the rate of development of the target and control variables. However, this type of restriction often is not realistic. In such cases, it may be possible to alleviate the CA confound by using pair-wise matching on both CA and the control variable. If the match is close enough, then the researcher may be confident that differential rates of development of the control and target variables will not confound group differences on the target variable.

However, pair-wise matching introduces additional difficulties. Foremost among these is the reduction in generalizability of the findings that is likely to result, due to the necessity of excluding many children ascertained with each disability, because of lack of a child in the other group who matches on both CA and the control variable. The sample of children for whom matches are available may be atypical of one or both of the original ascertainment samples. In such cases, generalizability of findings may be limited. Reconsider the example comparing children with Williams syndrome to children with Down syndrome on the PPVT–R raw score after controlling for McCarthy raw score (see Fig. 9.1). The sample of 18 children with Williams syndrome comprised, to our knowledge, all of the 9- and 10-year-old children with Williams syndrome within a 6-hour radius of Atlanta during a 2-year data collection period. The 23 children with Down syndrome came from a database of children with Down syndrome in the metropolitan Atlanta area. Moreover, the sample included all of the 9- and 10-year-olds in the area during the same 2-year data collection period, who did not have significant hearing loss. In the original full sample, there were 18 children with Williams syndrome with a mean McCarthy raw score of 142.89 and 23 children with Down syndrome with a mean McCarthy raw score of 105.87. In order to match the two groups to the $p = .650$ level, it was necessary to exclude the 4 highest functioning children from the Williams syndrome group and the 11 lowest functioning children from the Down syndrome group. The mean of the smaller Williams syndrome group is now 10 points lower than the mean for the original sample. The mean for the Down syndrome group, on the other hand, is now 23 points above the original mean. If it is assumed that the original means represented reasonable approximations of true population means, then the analysis is no longer a comparison of individuals with Williams syndrome to individuals with Down syndrome. Instead, it is a comparison of moderate to low functioning individuals with Williams syndrome to moderate to high functioning individuals with Down syndrome. The problem of generalizability may often be an issue with the group-matching procedure. Given the additional constraint of pair-wise matching on both a control variable and CA, generalizability is especially likely to be problematic in pair-wise matching designs.

CONCEPTUAL DIFFICULTY WITH GROUP- AND PAIR-WISE MATCHING DESIGNS

Even if it was possible to be sure that all necessary assumptions are met to produce valid group tests of syndrome differences, there is a deeper conceptual concern with the use of group designs to test many questions that are important for researchers concerned with theoretical issues involving potential differences between syndromes and their implications for developmental or linguistic theory. Significant findings on a test of mean differences indicate (assuming the requirements for matching have been met) that one group performs significantly worse than the other group on the target variable. This finding often is treated as though it implies that the former group may be characterized as having a deficit on the target variable. In fact, a significant group difference often results even when there is a large overlap in the distributions, with a substantial proportion of the children in the "deficit group" earning scores above the mean for the other group. In such cases, it is clear that the deficit is not characteristic of the entire group, or perhaps not even most of that group.

In a recent monograph concerning core deficits in autism, Sigman and Ruskin (1999) described one study in which they examined differences among four groups on responses to adult bids for joint attention: children with autism, children with Down syndrome, children with a variety of other forms of developmental delay, and children who were developing normally using a group-matching design. The four groups were matched on LA (although only at the $p > .17$ level) and then compared on the rate of responding to joint attention overtures. The children with autism had a significantly lower rate of responding ($p < .00001$), leading the authors to conclude that children with autism have a specific and unique deficit in joint attention" Sigman & Ruskin, 1999, p. 34). The mean response level to bids for joint attention for the children with autism, however, is less than one standard deviation below the mean level of responding for the children who were developing normally. Therefore, if the distributions of scores for level of responding are not skewed, then there should be substantial overlap in the distributions of the two groups. (See Fig. 9.6.) In fact, more than 20% of the children with autism would be expected to respond to joint attention initiations more frequently than the average typically developing child. Given the present example, it is possible that a substantial proportion of individuals with autism responded to joint attention at relatively high levels, which

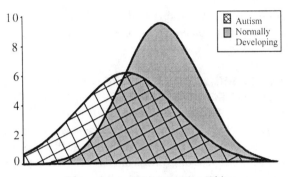

Responses to Joint Attention Bids

FIG. 9.6. Distributions of percent of bids for joint attention responded to by children with autism and children who are developing normally, based on means and standard deviations from Sigman and Ruskin (1999). Note the extensive overlap between the two distributions, despite a significant difference between groups at the $p < .00001$ level. Groups were matched for language age at the $p < .17$ level.

leads to the question of whether responses to joint attention should be considered a deficit of autism in general, or if there are subtypes of autism that do not involve such problems. It may be the case that only a small proportion of children with autism respond so infrequently to joint attention initiation that they would be categorized below low normal levels. It should be noted that such conclusions are based on the present example where the two groups were matched on LA. This is not necessarily to suggest that children with autism do not have deficits of joint attention. Appropriate matching based on general cognitive ability likely would lead to different results. Based on LA matching, however, the universality of a deficit in responses to joint attention overtures is not apparent.

The primary concern with matching designs based on tests of mean differences is that they cannot be used to address some of the most important questions—those regarding the possibility of differential patterns of language and/or cognitive development as a function of disability group. Consider the generally accepted finding that individuals with Down syndrome typically have much lower levels of expressive language ability than children with Williams syndrome. Almost any test of group mean differences will confirm this finding (e.g., Bellugi, Wang, & Jernigan, 1994). Indeed, findings from our own laboratories indicate that this is the case (Klein & Mervis, 1999; Mervis & Robinson, 2000). Note, however, that there is large variability in the language abilities of both groups. At 30 months, there is significant mean difference in expressive vocabulary size as measured by the Words and Sentences form of the MacArthur Communicative Develo ment Inventory (Fenson et al., 1993) between children with Williams syndrome and children with Down syndrome (Mervis & Robinson, 2000). Examples of individual children's expressive vocabulary growth patterns are shown in Fig. 9.7. The typical Williams syndrome growth pattern is logistic in form and results in a large vocabulary size approximately 12 to 14 months after growth begins (WS1 to WS4). For the Down syndrome group, growth is more variable. Two of the children with Down syndrome (DS1 and DS2) evidenced a linear pattern of growth characterized by a protracted period of slow growth. One child with Williams syndrome (WS6) clearly exhibited the same type of pattern and level of lexical growth. Similarly, some children with Down syndrome display logistic vocabulary growth (DS3 and DS4). Moreover, one child with Williams syndrome displayed a growth pattern unlike any child in the study. This boy had slow linear growth for almost 3 years after he began to talk. Unlike the other children with linear growth, however, he later experienced a period of rapid linear growth. In a group design, those individuals who displayed atypical patterns of development for their respective syndromes would not be identified as potential subgroups within the syndromes. They would simply be counted as statistical noise that reduced the effect size of group differences.

Although the majority of individuals with Down syndrome do appear to have a specific deficit in expressive language (e.g., Chapman, 1997), there also is ample evidence in the literature of individuals with Down syndrome who have excellent expressive language (e.g., Rondal, 1995; Vallar & Papagno, 1993). A consistent finding emerging from these studies is that individuals with Down syndrome who have good language abilities also have good auditory memory ability. For example, the young woman studied by Rondal had a backward digit span of 4, which is well within the normal range for adults without disabilities. Vallar and Papagno (1993) considered both digit span and phonological memory (memory for nonsense syllables), and found that the participant with Down syndrome who had excellent language, had both digit span and phonological memory ability within the normal range. In contrast, the other participants with Down syndrome, who had limited language abilities, also had short digit spans and very poor phonological memory. It is important to determine why some individuals with Down syndrome have good language abilities. In fact, one could argue that studying those individuals with Down syndrome who have extraordinary characteristics provides more information concerning the mechanisms underlying development than studying only those individuals with more typical Down syndrome profiles. Clearly then, portraying the universality of a characteristic as all or none, and thereby ignoring individual differences within a syndrome, may stymie further research into understanding the etiology and mechanisms underlying a developmental disorder.

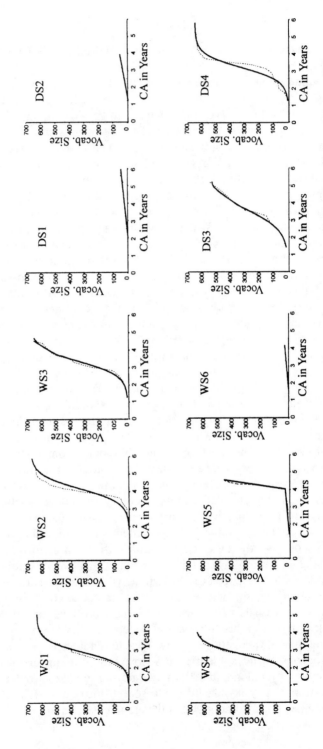

FIG. 9.7. Vocabulary growth curves for six children with Williams syndrome and four children with Down syndrome, illustrating logistic (WS1-4, DS3-4), linear (DS1-2, WS 6), and double-linear growth patterns (WS5). Solid lines indicate fitted curves; dotted lines indicate raw data.

AN ALTERNATIVE METHOD: FOCUSING ON SENSITIVITY AND SPECIFICITY OF DEVELOPMENTAL PROFILES AS A FUNCTION OF DISABILITY

The remainder of this chapter describes a two-step method for determining if there is a particular pattern of language and/or cognitive strengths or weaknesses that is characteristic of, and relatively specific to, a particular disability group. The first step involves determining if a particular profile is characteristic of a particular child. The second step involves determining how characteristic that profile is of the other participants in the child's group (the proportion of children in the target group who fit the profile) and how uncharacteristic that profile is of the children who are not in the target group (the proportion of children in the contrast group who do not fit the profile). This approach provides a methodological parallel to the idea that a specific characteristic is a quality of an individual, not a group of individuals. Rather than a group approach, specific deficits may be defined as abilities that are below the level expected given an individual's other skill levels, regardless of the syndrome group to which that person belongs. This is achieved by assessing a number of skills for all participants, and then, instead of comparing group means, examining the profile of each individual. For instance, one could measure language variables (e.g., receptive vocabulary, expressive vocabulary), nonverbal skills (e.g., performance on matrices, drawing ability), and joint attention. If a particular child's joint attention skills are worse than would be predicted based on that child's other abilities, then joint attention is a likely candidate for a specific deficit for that particular individual (Step 1). If this same pattern is shown by a large proportion of the children with autism and is not shown by most children who do not have autism, then joint attention may be argued to be a specific deficit for autism (Step 2). The use of signal detection analysis (Siegel, Vukicevic, Elliott, & Kraemer, 1989) to quantify the strength of a potential specific deficit for a particular target group is discussed below.

The Williams Syndrome Cognitive Profile (WSCP), which was recently proposed and validated (Mervis et al., 2000), is an example of the two-step profiling method. The WSCP is based on both relative and absolute level of performance on subtests of the DAS. Four criteria were included; in order to be considered to fit the WSCP, an individual had to meet all four. Criteria involve relative strength in auditory rote memory, both relative and absolute weakness in visuospatial construction, and performance above floor levels on either auditory rote memory or one of the language subtests. The DAS provides separate standard scores for each of the subtests. Moreover, the subtest standard scores are based on the same norming sample, thereby allowing a valid comparison of a single individual's subtest scores (Step

1). The WSCP was fit by 88% of the individuals with Williams syndrome but only 7% of the individuals in the mixed etiology contrast group (Step 2).

ADVANTAGES OF THE PROFILING METHOD

An important advantage of the profiling method is that aspects of a profile are identified relative to the other skills of the individual rather than in comparison to another syndrome group. The profiling approach decreases the likelihood that a characteristic will appear unique simply because the opposite characteristic is evidenced by the contrast syndrome. For instance, Bellugi and her colleagues (e.g., Bellugi, Marks, Bihrle, & Sabo, 1988; Bellugi et al., 1994) argued that individuals with Williams syndrome, despite having significant mental retardation, have extraordinary or intact language abilities. This claim is based on comparisons of people with Williams syndrome to one contrast group, Down syndrome. In actuality, however, rather than people with Williams syndrome having better language abilities than would be expected, individuals with Down syndrome have weaker expressive language abilities than would be expected for overall level of cognitive abilities (e.g., Morris & Mervis, 1999). When compared to groups of children with mental retardation (of mixed or unknown etiology) matched for IQ and CA, the language abilities of the Williams syndrome group are generally consistent with those of the contrast group (e.g., Gosch et al., 1994; Udwin & Yule, 1990).

Another advantage of the profiling method is that it allows the researcher to control for a large number of variables without the difficulties of matching. As long as a common metric (i.e., norms developed with a single sample of individuals) exists for all of the variables that the researcher wishes to control, there is no need to attempt multivariate matching with other syndrome groups. Thus, the researcher is not exposed to the aforementioned problems with generalizability.

SENSITIVITY AND SPECIFICITY

Once individual profiles and specific characteristics have been identified, systematic examination of the sensitivity (Se) and specificity (Sp) of the profile for a particular group (e.g., syndrome) can be conducted. Borrowing from signal detection and epidemiological methods (Siegel et al., 1989), Se is defined as the percent of individuals within the group who fit the predicted pattern for that group; Sp is defined as the percent of individuals who do not belong to the group and who do not fit the pattern. Given samples of two groups, those with the syndrome of interest (target group) and those without the syndrome (contrast group), Se is defined as the proportion of individuals in the target group who display the characteristic. For instance, in a sample of 50 children with SLI, if 46 displayed deficits of phonological memory relative to nonverbal ability, then the Se of phonological memory weakness as a characteristic of SLI would be 0.92. On the other hand, Sp is defined as the proportion of individuals without the syndrome who do not possess the characteristic. Therefore, if 85 individuals in a group of 150 children with heterogeneous developmental delays or normal development did not display a deficit in phonological working memory relative to nonverbal ability, then the characteristic would possess a Sp of 0.57.

Rather than simply stating that a characteristic is or is not unique or universal, reporting levels of Se and Sp gives readers a sense of how well the characteristic represents individuals with a particular syndrome. For instance, in the SLI example, a Se of 0.92 indicates that most, but not all, of the children with SLI have phonological memory deficits relative to nonverbal ability. A Sp of only 0.57, on the other hand, implies that deficits of phonological memory relative to nonverbal ability are not unique to children with SLI. Because Se and Sp range from 0 to 1.00, they provide a metric by which to measure just how unique and/or universal a characteristic is. Obviously, this is vital information for both researchers interested in identifying the etiology and typologies of SLI or other developmental disabilities and for clinicians attempting to design intervention programs.

Additionally, Se and Sp allow a comparison of the efficiency of different characteristics of a syndrome for diagnostic and/or research purposes. For instance, the Se and Sp for mental retardation (MR) could be measured for individuals with Down syndrome relative to a contrast group of individuals with other neurodevelopmental disorders. The likely result is that MR would have a high Se (i.e., most individuals with Down syndrome would have MR), but very low Sp. (Many of the individuals in the neurodevelopmental disorders contrast group would also have MR.) A characteristic profile (which may include both strengths and weaknesses) for a syndrome would be one that most individuals with the syndrome fit and most other individuals do not. In other words, one goal of a profile is to maximize Se and Sp. Receiver Operator Curve (ROC) analysis may be used to find characteristics that maximize Se and Sp values (Kraemer, 1988). The profile method also can take into account more than one characteristic at a time, as described earlier for the Williams syndrome cognitive profile.

The two-step profiling method described alleviates many problems with the group-matching design. First, because there is no matching procedure, there are no problems with generalizability as long as the ascertainment strategy was valid. Furthermore, this method allows researchers to consider as many variables as they desire to include in the profile. Because individuals act as their own control, there also are no difficulties in interpreting findings due to lack of match between groups. CA confounds are not a problem if CA-based standard scores are used in the profiling. Finally, the profiling method is conceptually more satisfying than group-matching designs in that profiling defines specific deficits (or strengths, or patterns of strengths and weaknesses) at the level of the individual (Step 1) and only then contrasts syndromes at the group level to determine Se and Sp (Step 2). It is important to remember, however, that Sp levels can differ dramatically, depending on the makeup of the contrast group. For instance, if the target group was Down syndrome and the contrast group was males with fragile X syndrome, then the Sp for MR would be very low. If the contrast group was typically developing children, however, then Sp would be very high. Therefore, Sp can only be appropriately determined if a large contrast group (or groups) is used, which includes adequate representation of those groups most likely to be similar to the target group on the variables of interest.

CONCLUSIONS

The present chapter outlined some of the difficulties with the cross-group matching design, suggested some possible improvements to the design, and then presented a method that is better suited to identifying central characteristics of a syndrome. Despite our affinity for the profiling alternative to the group-matching design, we recognize that the matching design frequently is used in research with children with language disorders, and may be useful for attempting to create equivalence for quasi-experimental designs.

As highlighted in this chapter, however, conducting a study using the matching design is fraught with potential pitfalls. Many problems may be avoided if the investigator is aware of difficulties with accepting the null hypothesis, understands the expected paths of development for both the control and target variables, and avoids using age equivalents for measuring either the control or target variables. It is important also that the investigator be cognizant of the limitations on the conclusions that are possible from studies using group-matching designs. In particular, a significant difference between well-matched groups on a target variable does not provide sufficient grounds for concluding that the lower scoring group is, in general, appropriately characterized as having a specific deficit on the target ability (recall Fig. 9.6). Before accepting findings from published studies using matched-group designs at face value, the reader should critically evaluate each study in terms of the adequacy of group matching, the expected paths of development for both the control and target variables, and the use of an interval scale for measuring performance on all variables. Findings from studies that are problematic on any of these grounds should be interpreted very cautiously.

The two-step profiling method avoids most limitations associated with the group-matching design by using individuals as their own control and providing an explicit measure of homogeneity and/or heterogeneity both within and across syndrome groups. Because of these characteristics, the two-step profiling method provides a strong basis from which researchers may address critical theoretical questions involving the relations between various aspects of language and cognition.

ACKNOWLEDGMENTS

Preparation of this chapter and the research described herein was supported by a grant (NS35102) from the National Institute of Neurological Disorders and Stroke and by a grant (HD29957) from the National Institute of Child Health and Human Development. Portions of this chapter are based on Mervis and Robinson (1999). We thank the participants and their families for their commitment to our research. Joanie Robertson created the figures for this chapter.

REFERENCES

Bates, E., & Goodman, J. C. (1999). On the emergence of grammar from the lexicon. In B. MacWhinney (Ed.), *The emergence of language* (pp. 29–79). Hillsdale, NJ: Lawrence Erlbaum Associates.

Bellugi, U., Marks, S., Bihrle, A., & Sabo, H. (1988). Dissociation between language and cognitive functions in Williams syndrome. In D. Bishop & K. Mogford (Eds.), *Language development in exceptional circumstances* (pp. 177–189). Edinburgh: Churchill Livingstone.

Bellugi, U., Wang, P. P., & Jernigan, T. L. (1994). Williams syndrome: An unusual neuropsychological profile. In S. H. Broman & J. Grafman, J. (Eds.), *Atypical cognitive deficits in developmental disorders: Implications for brain function* (pp. 23–56). Hillsdale, NJ: Lawrence Erlbaum Associates.

Burgemeister, B. B., Blum, L. H., & Lorge, I. (1972). *Columbia Mental Maturity Scale* (3rd ed.). San Antonio, TX: The Psychological Corporation.

Carrow-Woolfolk, E. (1974). *Carrow Elicited Language Inventory*. Austin, TX: Pro-Ed.

Chapman, R. S. (1997). Language development in children and adolescents with Down syndrome. *Mental Retardation and Developmental Disabilities Research Reviews, 3*, 307–312.

Cohen, J. (1990). Things I have learned (so far). *American Psychologist, 45*, 1304–1312.

Dunn, L. E., & Dunn, L. E. (1981). *Peabody Picture Vocabulary Test–Revised*. Circle Pines, MN: American Guidance Service.

Dunn, L. E., & Dunn, L. E. (1997). *Peabody Picture Vocabulary Test* (3rd ed.). Circle Pines, MN: American Guidance Service.

Elliott, C. D. (1990). *Differential Ability Scales*. San Diego: Harcourt Brace Jovanovich.

Fenson, L., Dale, P. S., Reznick, J. S., Thal, D., Bates, E., Hartung, J. P., Pethick, S., & Reilly, J. S. (1993). *MacArthur Communicative Development Inventories: User's guide and technical manual*. San Diego, CA: Singular Press.

Fenson, L., Dale, P. S., Reznick, J. S., Bates, E., Thal, D. J., & Pethick, S. J. (1994). Variability in early communicative development. *Monographs of the Society for Research in Child Development, 59* (Serial No. 242), 1–173.

Flynn, J. R. (1987). Massive IQ gains in 14 nations: What IQ tests really measure. *Psychological Bulletin, 101,* 171–191.

Frick, R. W. (1995). Accepting the null hypothesis. *Memory & Cognition, 23,* 132–138.

Gosch, A., Stading, G., & Pankau, R. (1994). Linguistic abilities in children with Williams–Beuren syndrome. *American Journal of Medical Genetics, 52,* 291–296.

Harcum, E. R. (1990). Methodological vs. empirical literature: Two views on the acceptance of the null hypothesis. *American Psychologist, 45,* 404–405.

Hedrick, D., Prather, E., & Tobin, A. (1984). *Sequenced Inventory of Communication Development–Revised.* Seattle, WA: University of Washington Press.

Klein, B. P., & Mervis, C. B. (1999). Cognitive strengths and weaknesses of 9- and 10-year-olds with Williams syndrome or Down syndrome. *Developmental Neuropsychology, 16,* 177–196.

Kraemer, H. C. (1988). Assessment of 2 X 2 associations: Generalization of signal-detection methodology. *The American Statistician, 42,* 37–49.

McCarthy, D. (1972). *McCarthy Scales of Children's Abilities.* New York: The Psychological Corporation.

Mervis, C. B., & Robinson, B. F. (1999). Methodological issues in cross-syndrome comparisons: Matching procedures, sensitivity *(Se),* and specificity *(Sp).* Commentary on M. Sigman & E. Ruskin, Continuity and change in the social competence of children with autism, Down syndrome, and developmental delays. *Monographs of the Society for Research in Child Development, 64* (Serial No. 256), 115–130.

Mervis, C. B., & Robinson, B. F. (2000). Expressive vocabulary of toddlers with Williams syndrome or Down syndrome: A comparison. *Developmental Neuropsychology, 17,* 111–126.

Mervis, C. B., Robinson, B. F., Bertrand, J., Morris, C. A., Klein-Tasman, B. P., & Armstrong, S. C. (2000). The Williams Syndrome Cognitive Profile. *Brain and Cognition, 44,* 604–628.

Morris, C. A., & Mervis, C. B. (1999). Williams syndrome. In S. Goldstein & C. Reynolds (Eds.), *Handbook of neurodevelopmental and genetic disorders in children* (pp. 555–590). New York: Guilford.

Raven, J. C. (1960). *Guide to the Standard Progressive Matrices.* London: H. K. Lewis.

Robinson, B. F., & Mervis, C. B. (1998). Disentangling early language development: Modeling lexical and grammatical acquisition using an extension of case-study methodology. *Developmental Psychology, 34,* 363–375.

Rondal, J. (1995). *Exceptional language development in Down syndrome.* Cambridge, England: Cambridge University Press.

Sattler, J. R. (1992). *Assessment of children (revised and updated 3rd ed.).* San Diego: Jerome M. Sattler.

Semel, E., Wiig, E. H., & Secord, W. A. (1995). *Clinical Evaluation of Language Fundamentals* (3rd ed.). Columbus, OH: Merrill.

Siegel, B., Vukicevic, J., Elliott, G. R., & Kraemer, H. C. (1989). The use of signal detection theory to assess DSM–IIIR criteria for autistic disorder. *Journal of the American Academy of Child & Adolescent Psychiatry, 28,* 542–548.

Sigman, M., & Ruskin, E. (1999). Continuity and change in the social competence of children with autism, Down syndrome, and developmental delays. *Monographs of the Society for Research in Child Development, 64* (Serial No. 256), 1–114.

Udwin, O., & Yule, W. (1990). Expressive language of children with Williams syndrome. *American Journal of Medical Genetics Supplement, 6,* 108–114.

Vallar, G., & Papagno, C. (1993). Preserved vocabulary acquisition in Down's syndrome: The role of phonological short-term memory. *Cortex, 29,* 467–483.

Wechsler, D. (1991). *Wechsler Intelligence Scale for Children* (3rd ed.). San Antonio, TX: The Psychological Corporation.

Williams, K. T. (1997). *Expressive Vocabulary Test.* Circle Pines, MN: American Guidance Service.

10

MLU—Matching and the Production of Morphosyntax in Dutch Children with Specific Language Impairment

Gerard W. Bol
University of Groningen

The use of mean length of utterance (MLU) is a frequently applied measure in research of involving children with specific language impairment (SLI). MLU is used to indicate children's productive grammatical complexity, to determine the stage of their grammatical development, and to compare children with language problems with typically developing children or other subgroups of children with language problems. These comparisons may involve a single language or a number of languages.

Brown (1973) stated that "the mean length of utterance is an excellent simple index of grammatical development because almost every new kind of knowledge increases length" and "two children matched for MLU are much more likely to have speech that is on internal grounds at the same level of constructional complexity than are two children of the same age" (p. 77). Brown described five developmental stages, motivated by the order of use of morphemes in obligatory contexts and defined by MLU values.

QUANTIFICATION VERSUS QUALIFICATION

Calculating MLU is part of the quantification process in language acquisition research. Van Ierland (1983) was one of the first researchers to argue in favor of a quantitative approach in linguistics. Van Ierland picked up the idea of profiling children's language production developed by Crystal, Fletcher, and Garman (1976) and decided to use a quantitative approach in her own research with Dutch children from 4 to 8 years old. At that time, an emphasis on quantity instead of quality was not obviously clear. In fact, the Language Assessment, Remediation, and Screening Procedure (LARSP) by Crystal et al. (1976) did not involve quantification. Yet, the procedure had been designed to measure early morphosyntactic development at clause, phrase, and word level. In addition, at that time, theoretical linguists were more interested in the quality of linguistic phenomena and, indeed, many still are.

Before exploring the relation between quantity and quality in linguistics, the terms must be defined. *Quantification* can be seen as the assignment of numbers to empirical phenomena. On the one hand, linguistic phenomena have a stochastic character, which means that a number can be assigned to the phenomena that are observed. To put it simply, linguistic phenomena can be counted. *Qualification*, on the other hand, deals with questions like: Which linguistic elements and categories exist and what is the relation between them? And, which linguistic phenomena are universal? The relation between quantification and qualification is that qualification can do without quantification, but quantification cannot do without qualification, because it is first necessary to determine what will be counted, which is in fact a qualitative decision.

In modern SLI research, it is desirable to use statistical analyses, which consequently must be quantified first. As a result, it is possible to show what is typical and atypical in terms of observed linguistic phenomena, and to see variation, systematicity, and possible taxonomies. Moreover, quantification in particular offers the possibility to test hypotheses, which opens the door to further formulations of new hypotheses.

There are arguments in favor of a quantitative approach to linguistics and following the previous recommendations a researcher may be forgiven for thinking that nothing is as simple as counting. However, in many cases, this is not the case. Sometimes, it may not be clear exactly what is being measured or compared based on quantitative measures. To illustrate this point, the chapter continues by illustrating problems that arise with a well known and often used quantitative measure, namely, mean length of utterance.

THE USE OF MLU

MLU as an Indicator of Productive Morphosyntax

MLU is used in research with developmental language disorders in different ways and for several purposes. MLU tells something (albeit roughly) about the development of productive morphosyntax in the early years of language development.

MLU can be counted in words, syllables, or morphemes, although MLU counted in syllables is hardly ever used. Butt (1999) gave a short overview of the high correlations found between counting MLU in words and in morphemes for several languages, except for Hebrew. Dutch research by Arlman-Rupp, Van Niekerk-De Haan, and Van de Sandt-Koenderman (1976) showed that it does not matter how a researcher counts MLU because as long as the children are not older than 2;6 years old, the results will be similar.

Although it is clear that MLU increases with age, the increase of MLU is subject to further discussion. Some researchers state that MLU is rather reliable up to a value of 3 (e.g., Klee & Fitzgerald, 1985), but after that value there is leveling off. Blake, Quartaro, and Onorati (1993) found that MLU is a valid measure of clausal complexity up to the value of 4.5, at least as an index of clausal complexity.

Dutch longitudinal data of a normally developing boy (see Fig. 10.1) seem to indicate a plateau at MLU values between 3.5 and 4.0 (Bol, 1996). This would suggest that increase in morphosyntactic complexity is not well reflected in MLU values beyond 3.5. It is important to notice that the leveling off in the Dutch research could possibly be attributed to the definition of the utterance, defined by the notion of the T-unit by Hunt (1970, p. 4): one main clause plus any subordinate clause or nonclausal structure that is attached or embedded in it. In Fig. 10.1, the MLU is counted in words, whereas the definition of utterance is based on the notion of the T-unit.

Research involving the spontaneous speech of normally developing Dutch children from 1 to 4 years (Bol & Kuiken, 1988) also showed a kind of leveling off between the ages of 3;6 and 4;0, at a MLU value somewhat higher than 4 (see Fig. 10.2). In Fig. 10.2, the MLU is counted in morphemes. The definition of utterance is based again on the notion of the T-unit.

Research on the spontaneous speech of normally developing Dutch children from 4 to 8 years old showed hardly any increase in MLU (Van den

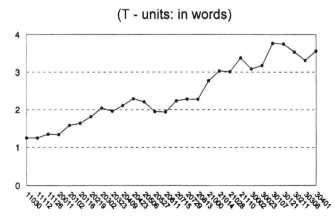

(T - units: in words)

FIG. 10.1. Increase in MLU Dutch boy. Ages of the child are given on *x*-axis in years, months, days.

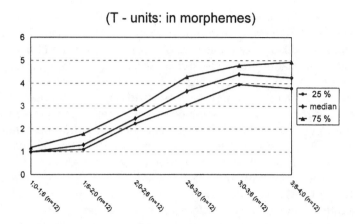

FIG. 10.2. Increase in MLU from 1–4. Ages and number of subjects in each group are given on x-axis.

Dungen & Verbeek, 1994). This in illustrated in Fig. 10.3, where the MLU is counted in words and an utterance is defined by the notion of the T-unit.

In terms of later ages, little is known. Miller (1991) stated that MLU increases over the years up to age 13, although the author does not present the MLU values for the different age groups in this particular study.

Apart from leveling off, some researchers have discovered a decrease in MLU. Klee (1992) reported on the development of a girl whose MLU decreased 0.8 morpheme per utterance between ages 2;9 and 3;2. In contrast

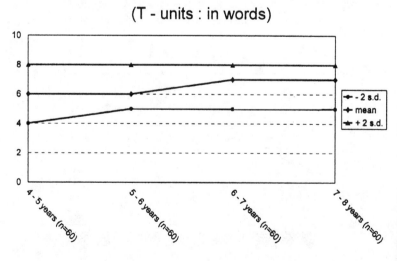

FIG. 10.3. Increase in MLU from 4–8. Ages and number of subjects in each group are given on x-axis.

her linguistic advancements were reflected in the analysis of the clause, phrase, and word structure of the LARSP profiles (Crystal et al., 1976). Klee stated that "one reason for this was that more single-word utterances were produced during the later transcript that during the earlier" (p. 325). There is no doubt that contextual influences are present (e.g., who is talking with the child and the way the conversation partner asks questions to the child; Bates, 1999).

Klee (1992) also reported a comparison of transcripts from the same tape made by 12 students. They had to calculate, among other measures, the MLU of the spontaneous speech of a girl aged 3;7 years. The range of MLU in the 12 transcripts was from 3.66 to 4.09, nearly half a morpheme per utterance difference was found. It appears, therefore, that the reliability of MLU may be questioned.

Lahey (1994) showed that the acquisition of morphemes within certain MLU ranges in normal children demonstrate a high degree of variability. She also argued that the acquisition of morphemes by children with language problems reported by Paul and Alforde (1993) falls within normal MLU ranges, whereas the authors concluded that these children still had difficulties with grammatical morphemes.

MLU is designed to provide an indication of the level of morphosyntactic development children undergo in their language learning. However, this aim does not always seem to be fulfilled. This questions both the validity and the reliability of the MLU measure.

MLU as a Matching Technique

MLU is also used to match different groups, mainly when the researcher wants to compare a group of language disordered children and a group of typically developing children. The mean MLU of each group is calculated and then the researcher is able to compare groups with the same mean MLU. The reason for doing this is so that matching for chronological age yields very big differences in linguistic proficiency between normal children and children with language disorders and, as a consequence, the actual phenomena underlying the deficit might become opaque.

The idea is to keep the group MLUs similar and compare the linguistic abilities assuming overall language level similarities. Using this matching technique, children with specific language impairment (SLI) most commonly have problems with verb morphology, tend to omit grammatical subjects, and omit copulas and modals in their sentences. Moreover, children with SLI have problems using functional categories in general (see, for an overview, Leonard, 2000).

MLU is used crosslinguistically as well to match children with SLI with a different mother tongue, as did Bortolini, Leonard, and Caselli (1998). These authors used MLU in words to match two research groups of children with language problems, namely, English children with SLI and Italian children with SLI. Plante (1996) discussed this methodology and stated "it might be argued the MLU morphology associations themselves should not be assumed to be standard across languages. Therefore, the MLU-morphology dissociations that characterise SLI in English may not be indicative of non-normal processes in all languages" (p. 258). Snow (1999) stated that "it seems that the value of MLU as a very general index of language development may reflect, to some extent, its insensitivity to various component processes" (p.). Furthermore, Peters (1999) added that she found it useful to compute MLU in two ways, comparing different languages: just open-class lexical items (excluding free grammatical morphemes); and all morphemes, whether bound or free.

Another problem arises when using MLU as a matching criterion to compare normal and language disordered children, namely, that the latter are much older. It can be argued that it may not be possible to obtain good insight into children's linguistic abilities, because the language disordered children have additional nonlinguistic experience due to their increased age. These nonlinguistic skills may influence linguistic skills and so a clear picture for children with language disorders is unlikely to emerge.

A possible solution for these problems is suggested by Plante, Swisher, Kiernan, and Restrepo (1993), who argued that it is not right to compare groups on the basis of one matching criterion at one particular cross-sectional point in time. Indeed, they suggested that groups are to be compared longitudinally. The method would then involve following the groups for some time and comparing the course of their language development. However, such research is scarce because this approach is time consuming and expensive.

Another solution brought forward by Plante et al. (1993) is the use of statistical techniques, like correlation and regression analysis, using a set of variables that is theoretically motivated. The variables are not only linguistic, but also include aspects such as age and cognition. These techniques should be used with both groups, and after that it would be possible to compare the results. Language is, according to Plante and colleagues, built on interrelations of different human skills.

Interestingly, despite the known drawbacks, and despite possible solutions brought forward, many researchers use MLU traditionally, mostly as a measure of morphosyntactic development and as a means to compare groups of language learning children.

There is another question that needs to be asked concerning the use of MLU. When children with SLI are matched on MLU with typically developing children and the result of the comparison of both groups concerning the use of, for instance, verbal inflections is such that children with language problems omit more verb inflections, then these children have to compensate in their language production with other aspects in order to have the same MLU as the typically developing children. What is it that compensates for the loss of length in the utterances of children with language problems?

COMPENSATION FOR LOSS OF UTTERANCE LENGTH

Johnston and Kamhi (1984) investigated the syntactic and semantic characteristics of a group of 10 children with SLI matched on MLU with 10 normally developing children and they asked themselves the question: "How can the same be less," because "all significant group differences are of the sort which would seem to yield shorter utterances, yet MLU for the two groups is equivalent" (p. 75). Therefore, the children with SLI had to compensate for their loss of sentence length. Johnston and Kamhi designed a series of post-hoc analyses to identify those characteristics of the language of the children with SLI that yielded length despite their omission of grammatical markers and their relative low propositionality. It appeared that children with language impairment used significantly more predicates with two arguments and twice as many verbs expressing movement, like *fly* or *run* and more verbs with a progressive aspect.

Bol and Steensma (2000) took up this question with respect to Dutch. Bol and Kuiken (1988, 1990) found that Dutch children with SLI produce, among others, significantly fewer personal and possessive pronouns, less verb inflections, and less sentence subjects than typically MLU-matched developing children. Bol and Steensma (2000) designed research into the linguistic characteristics of the same Dutch children with SLI, in particular those characteristics that these children use in their spontaneous speech to compensate for the phenomena just mentioned (i.e., phenomena that are responsible for shorter utterances).

The research question was formulated as follows: Which morphosyntactic phenomena do Dutch children with SLI produce more frequently than normally developing Dutch children with the same mean length of utterance? The authors looked at discourse variables that could contribute to shorter utterances (e.g., ellipsis) and did not concentrate on semantic aspects (i.e., number of propositions in an utterance).

Both the children with language problems and the normally developing children come from the GRAMAT research by Bol and Kuiken (1990). The data in both groups consist of spontaneous speech samples for 10 children with SLI (6 boys, 4 girls) and 10 MLU-matched normally developing children (7 boys, 3 girls). It needs to be noted that the children were matched very

TABLE 10.1
Subjects

SLI	Normally Developing Children
n = 10 (6 boys, 4 girls)	n = 10 (7 boys, 3 girls)
Age range: 4;09–6;07	Age range: 2;03–3;06
MLUm range: 2.2–3.9	MLUm range: 2.2–3.9

closely in MLU morphemes with no pair of matched children exceeding an MLU value of 0.10. Moreover, none of the values of MLU was higher than 4.0, to avoid the discussion of not being representative for morphosyntactic development. The MLU values range from 2.2 to 3.9. The age range of the children with SLI was from 4;9 to 6;7. The typically developing children's ages ranged from 2;3 to 3;6 (see Table 10.1).

The speech of the children with SLI was recorded at their schools, while they were playing with their speech therapist. The normally developing children were audio recorded for 1 hour in everyday situations at their homes in the presence of at least one of the parents and one of the observers.

For the transcripts, the utterances were defined by the notion of the T unit as defined by Hunt (1970), mentioned earlier. Each transcript contained 100 analyzable utterances.

To answer the research question, Bol and Steensma set up the following seven hypotheses concerning aspects of spoken language that could contribute to the increase in the number of morphemes in an utterance:

Hypothesis 1: There is an effect of intra-subject variation in utterance length (i.e., Dutch children with SLI produce a few utterances that are extremely long). To test this hypothesis, the authors looked at the MLU of the 10 longest utterances in both groups.

Hypothesis 2: There is an effect of discourse (i.e., the use of imperatives, ellipsis, and pronouns reduces utterance length). To test this hypothesis, Bol and Steensma compared the use of these structures in both groups. could be the case that typically developing children may use more of these structures, which can result in them having shorter utterances.

Hypothesis 3: Dutch children with SLI produce more utterances in which bound morphemes are used (with the exception of verb inflections), like diminutives, plurals, and compound nouns. The frequencies of all these phenomena were determined and Bol and Steensma looked at possible differences for each separate variable and for all the variables pulled together.

Hypothesis 4: Dutch children with SLI produce more conjunctions, prepositions, or adverbials. Again, the frequencies of all these elements were determined and the authors looked at possible differences for each separate element and for all the elements pulled together.

Before describing Hypotheses 5 and 6, there is a need for clarification as to the way the MLU was calculated. Table 10.2 gives a comparison of the Dutch verb system and the English verb system. Each verb ending is counted as a separate morpheme. So *werk-t* yields two morphemes. Notice that the Dutch inflectional morphology is slightly richer in English: Dutch distinguishes number in both the present and the past, and person in the present singular.

If in Dutch the stem of the verb ends in the phoneme /t/, the second and third person singular do not get an extra /t/, for example, *jij/hij vergeet* (you forget/he forgets). So *vergeet* yields one morpheme. The plural, however, is inflected the same way as in verbs that do not have a *t* ending, namely, *vergeten* (forget). As the production of verb endings are researched, this has consequences for the counting of the morphemes.

Hypothesis 5 is aimed at the use of these kinds of verbs, namely, verbs whose stems end in /t/. It could be the case that Dutch children with SLI use more plural forms of these kind of verbs. This would give them an extra morpheme compared to the singular forms of this kind of verbs, producing the second and third person singular.

Hypothesis 5: Dutch children with SLI use more plural forms of verbs with a /t/ phoneme stem ending. This hypothesis concerns the use of past tense and past participles. It could be the case that the Dutch children with SLI produce more of these verb forms than typically develop-

TABLE 10.2
A Comparison of Dutch and English Verb Morphology

Dutch			English	
esent				
k	werk	1sg	I	work
ij	werk-t	2sg	you	work
ij/zij/het	werk-t	3sg	he/she/it	work-s
ij	werk-en	1pl	we	work
ullie	werk-en	2pl	you	work
ij	werk-en	3pl	they	work
st				
;	werk-te	1sg	I	work-ed
;	werk-te	2sg	you	work-ed
ij/zij/het	werk-te	3sg	he/she/it	work-ed
ij	werk-ten	1pl	we	work-ed
ullie	werk-ten	2pl	you	work-ed
j	werk-ten	3pl	they	work-ed

TABLE 10.3
Dutch Verb Paradigm: Verbs Ending in /t/

Dutch			English		
ik	vergeet	*1sg*	I	forget
jij	vergeet-0	*2sg*	you	forget
hij/zij/het	vergeet-0	*3sg*	he/she/it	forget-s
wij	verge(e)t-en	*1pl*	we	forget
jullie	verge(e)t-en	*2pl*	you	forget
zij	verge(e)t-en	*3pl*	they	forget

ing children. These verb forms yield more morphemes than present tense forms.

Hypothesis 6: Dutch children with SLI produce more verb forms indicating past tense and more past participles. It needs to be noted that the way the Dutch morphemes were counted can be criticized. MLU counted in words, like in CHILDES (MacWhinney, 2000) could have been an alternative. However, the relation between MLU and morphosyntactic development in Dutch is better reflected if MLU is counted in morphemes.

The final hypothesis is about a well-known phenomenon in SLI: the use of general all-purpose (GAP) verbs. For Dutch, de Jong (1999) investigated the use of troponyms (i.e., semantically specific verbs) and hypernyms (i.e., GAP verbs) in Dutch children with SLI. He concluded that children with SLI "produced fewer troponyms than normal controls and that they produced more hypernyms, mismatches and other error types in their use of verbs" (p. 182).

Bol and Steensma (2000) looked only at particular, very frequently used GAP verb in Dutch, the verb *gaan* (to go). In Dutch, if a child is asked *What has happened?*, the child's answer could be in the past tense of the lexical verb, but often it will be the case that a child uses a construction with the verb *gaan* as the inflected verb, in order to maintain the lexical verb in the infinitival form. In fact, the use of *gaan* can be seen as the avoidance of verb placement. This is seen in both typically developing children and in children with SLI. The present tense of the verb *gaan* plus the lexical verb the infinitival form indicates a future aspect of the sentence. If children with SLI use constructions with the verb *gaan*, then this could yield more morphemes than the inflection of the lexical verb, which leads to Hypothesis 7.

Hypothesis 7: Dutch children with SLI produce more utterances with construction like gaan + infinitival form of the lexical verb (to go + infinitive), mainly in the past tense.

RESULTS

Each hypothesis was tested statistically using the Mann–Whitney U Test with a significance value of $p < 0.05$. The results of these comparisons revealed thought-provoking results. None of the hypotheses were supported. There were no statistically significant differences found between the groups.

Children with SLI did not use more long utterances in their speech than typically developing children matched on MLU. Typically developing children did not use more ellipsis and imperatives, and although they used more pronouns, this difference was not statistically significant. Furthermore, the word formation processes that children with SLI showed did not yield significant differences in the use of morphemes. The children with SLI produced more conjunctions but fewer prepositions and adverbs than typically developing children, but these differences were not statistically significant. In addition, there was no difference between the two groups in the use of verbs ending in a /t/ phoneme.

Regarding the use of past tenses and past participles, it was evident that these verb forms were rarely used. Although children with SLI used past tenses and past participles more frequently, the differences were not significant. A striking observation is that all past tense forms included irregular verbs.

The verb *gaan* appeared to be used only once in the past tense. Recall that a total of 1,000 utterances in each group have been investigated. The frequency of present tense of *gaan* + *infinitive* in the group with SLI was 31 and the frequency in the normal group was 35. In four pairs of children, the child with SLI had a higher frequency, in four pairs of children the normal child used more *gaan* + *infinitive* and in two pairs the frequency was the same. These individual differences, as well as the group differences, were not significant.

CONCLUSIONS

None of the seven aspects studied in the present investigation appeared to be responsible for the compensation in length. Therefore, unlike the children in Johnston and Kamhi (1984), it is not clear what Dutch children with SLI do to compensate for their loss of length. The question remains concerning why the MLU remains the same?

The underlying, and perhaps more important, question involves how much loss of length has to be explained in studies that make such comparisons between groups. In other words, what is the contribution of the omission of pronouns and sentence subjects and problems with verb inflection to MLU? Despite the fact that Bol and Kuiken (1990) found statistically significant differences on pronoun omission, verb inflection, and sentence subject, it is not clear what amount of omitted sentence length has to be explained. It could be the case that these statistically significant differences do not contribute that much to sentence length.

Therefore, not only are there critical comments to be made regarding the use of MLU, but in fact, child language researchers do not know what it is exactly that MLU measures. In other words, the validity of MLU can not be determined, at least for Dutch. Having said this, alternatives for MLU as a matching criterion are hard to find. This problem has been well described by Johnston and Kamhi (1984): "Creating specific indices for various domains of language-performance to replace MLU as the independent variable will be a demanding task, but one which should eventually enrich our picture of both language-disordered and normal children" (p. 82).

As an alternative to MLU, de Jong (1999; chap. 6 in this volume) used productive vocabulary age in his comparison of the use of argument structure by Dutch children with SLI and normal controls. This is an interesting avenue that future research can explore.

In the same area, Caselli, Casadio, and Bates (1999) looked at grammatical development in English versus Italian children from 1;6 to 2;6 years of age. They found a similar nonlinear relation between grammatical complexity and vocabulary size in both languages, indicating that vocabulary size could serve as an alternative for MLU.

Future research may be able to inform researchers as to whether vocabulary size is really a good alternative for MLU. Not enough is known about the relation between vocabulary size and grammar in other languages to justify using vocabulary size instead of MLU from now on as a matching criterion. As with many important methodological issues, only more research will shed light on possible solutions.

ACKNOWLEDGMENTS

The author offers thanks to Gina Conti-Ramsden, Yonata Levy, and Jeannette Schaeffer for comments on earlier versions of this chapter.

REFERENCES

Arlman-Rupp, A., Van Niekerk-De Haan, D., & Sandt-Koenderman, M. van de (1976). Brown's early stages: Some evidence from Dutch. *Journal of Child Language, 3,* 267–274.

Bates, E. (1999). Letter to the Info-Childes. *Child Language Bulletin, 19*(1), 9.

ake, J., Quartaro, G., & Onorati, S. (1991). Evaluating quantitative measures of grammatical complexity in spontaneous speech samples. *Journal of Child Language, 20,* 139–152.

l, G., & Kuiken, F. (1990). Grammatical analysis of developmental language disorders: A study of the morphosyntax of children with specific language disorders, with hearing impairment and with Down's syndrome. *Clinical Linguistics and Phonetics, 4,* 77–86.

l, G. W. (1996). Optional subjects in Dutch child language. In Ch. Koster & F. Wijnen (Eds.), *Proceedings of the Groningen Assembly on Language Acquisition* (pp. 125–133).

l, G. W., & Kuiken, F. (1988). *Grammaticale analyse van taalontwikkelingsstoornissen.* Unpublished doctoral dissertation, University of Amsterdam.

l, G. W., & Steensma, N. (2000, March). *The production of morphosyntax in Dutch children with SLI in the light of MLU-matching.* Paper presented at the international research workshop on Theoretical and Methodological Issues in the Study of Developmental Language Disorders, Jerusalem.

rtolini, U., Leonard, L. B., & Caselli, M. C. (1998). Specific language impairment in Italian and English: Evaluating alternative accounts of grammatical deficits. *Language and Cognitive Processes,* 1–19.

own, R. (1973). *A first language: The early stages.* Cambridge, MA: Harvard University Press.

tt, C. (1999). Letter to the Info-Childes. *Child Language Bulletin, 19*(1), 9.

selli, C., Casadio, P., & Bates, E. (1999). A comparison of the transition from first words to grammar in English and Italian. *Journal of Child Language, 26,* 69–111.

ystal, D., Fletcher, P., & Garman, M. (1976). *The grammatical analysis of language disability: A procedure for assessment and remediation.* London, Edward Arnold.

ngen, H. P. L. R. van den, & Verbeek, J. (1994). *STAP-handleiding: STAP-instrument, gebaseerd op Spontane-Taal Analyse Procedure ontwikkeld door Margreet van Ierland,* Publikaties van het Instituut voor ATW-UvA, nr. 63.

nt, K. W. (1970). Syntactic maturity in school children and adults. *Monograph of the Society for Research in Child Development, 35*(1, Serial No. 134).

land, M. S. van (1983). Loont tellen in taal? Een pleidooi voor een meer kwantitatieve taalkunde vanuit taalverwervingsonderzoek, *Gramma, 7*(2/3), 269–280.

ng, J. de (1999). *Specific language impairment in Dutch: Inflectional morphology and argument structure.* Unpublished doctoral dissertation, University of Groningen.

hnston, J. R., & Kamhi, A. (1984). Syntactic and semantic aspects of the utterances of language impaired children: The same can be less. *Merrill-Palmer Quarterly, 30,* 65–85.

ee, Th. (1992). Measuring children's conversational language. In S. F. Warren & J. Reichle (Eds.), *Causes and effects in communication and language intervention* (pp. 315–330). Baltimore: Brookes.

ee, Th., & Fitzgerald, M. D. (1985). The relation between grammatical development and mean length of utterance in morphemes. *Journal of Child Language, 12,* 251–269.

hey, M. (1994). Grammatical morpheme acquisition: Do norms exist? *Journal of Speech and Hearing Research, 37,* 1192–1194.

onard, L. B. (2000). *Children with specific language impairment.* Cambridge, MA: MIT Press.

acWhinney, B. (2000). CD *"The CHILDES Project"* with the CHILDES project: Computational tools for analyzing talk. Hillsdale, NJ: Lawrence Erlbaum Associates.

iller, J. F. (1991). Research on language disorders in children: A progress report. In J. F. Miller (Ed.), *Research on child language disorders: A decade of progress* (pp.). Austin, TX: Pro-Ed.

ul, R., & Alforde, S. (1993). Grammatical morpheme acquisition in 4-year-olds with normal, impaired, and late-developing language. *Journal of Speech and Hearing Research, 36,* 1271–1275.

ters, A. (1999). Letter to the Info-Childes. *Child Language Bulletin, 19*(1), 10–11.

ante, E. (1996). Commentary on chapter 9. In M. L. Rice (Ed.), *Toward a genetics of language* (pp. 257–260). Hillsdale, NJ: Lawrence Erlbaum Associates.

ante, E., Swisher, L., Kiernan, G., & Restrepo, M. A. (1993). Language matches: Illuminating or confounding? *Journal of Speech and Hearing Research, 36,* 772–776.

ow, C. (1999). Letter to the Info-Childes. *Child Language Bulletin, 19*(1), 10.

11

Different Methodologies Yield Incongruous Results: A Study of the Spontaneous Use of Verb Forms in Hebrew

Esther Dromi
Tel Aviv University

Laurence B. Leonard
Purdue University

Anat Blass
Tel Aviv University

Brown (1973) was among the first researchers to advocate the view that the relative frequency in which a morpheme is supplied in obligatory contexts is a solid measure for determining the level of its mastery by young children (see also Cazden, 1968). Throughout the years, the practice of collecting and analyzing spontaneous language samples that document natural conversations between children and adults has become one of the most common research practices in the study of language development by normally developing (ND) children and by children with specific language impairments (SLI). A methodological alternative to that of recording spontaneous language samples is that of designing a probe that directs the child to the retrieval of a certain target form. In probed data, as in natural language samples, the metric used to gauge ability is the percentage of correct use in obligatory contexts. This chapter provides an overview of published findings on the use of Hebrew verb forms during elicited tasks, as well as a report of new results on the spontaneous use of morphological inflections by Hebrew-speaking children with SLI (HSLI children).

The use of grammatical morphemes for tense and agreement represents a significant obstacle for many children with SLI in several different languages (Leonard, 1998) (see also de Villiers, chap. 17; De Jong, chap. 6; Rice, chap. 2; and Wexler, chap. 1 in this volume). This is especially true for children acquiring English. Many studies have revealed that in spontaneous language samples, as well as in more systematic probes, English-speaking children with SLI use morphemes with significantly lower percentages in obligatory contexts than typically developing children with similar mean lengths of utterance (MLU) (e.g., Cleave & Rice, 1997; Loeb & Leonard, 1991; Oetting & Horohov, 1997; Rice, Wexler, & Cleave, 1995). During the last decade, we have investigated the use of inflectional morphology by children with SLI who are acquiring Hebrew. Our research indicated that the differences between HSLI and younger normally developing children do not seem to follow the pattern described for English. HSLI children's use of grammatical morphemes resembles that of younger normally developing controls and their morphological abilities look much stronger than that of English-speaking children with SLI at similar MLU levels.

This chapter presents recent findings on the spontaneous use of verb forms in obligatory contexts by HSLI children and compares these data with results of a systematic evaluation of the morphological abilities of the same cohort of participants that employed experimental probes. Before summarizing the published results on HSLI children's use of agreement and tense, a brief description of the unique morphological characteristics of the Hebrew verb system is provided. The chapter concludes with the proposal that because different methodologies yield incongruous results, it is highly recommended to always combine research methods for studying SLI children's productive morphological abilities. This is especially true in languages that utilize rich morphology and furnish more than one option for expressing such notions as tense, person, number, and gender.

HEBREW VERB MORPHOLOGY: A SHORT DESCRIPTION

Hebrew, like other Semitic languages, possesses a rich inflectional morphology that is heavily interwoven with word formation. All Hebrew verbs are formed by consonantal roots that are cast in regular morphophonological templates, the patterns or "BINYANIM" (see also Levy, chap. 14, and Ravid, Levie, & Ben-Zvi, chap. 7 in this volume). The verb patterns defined by these morphophonological templates constitute a part of Hebrew morphology that is separate from agreement morphology. These templates take the form of predictable sequences of vowels that appear between the consonants of the root and sometimes also syllabic prefixes. The consonantal roots convey the core meaning of the verb even though they can never be pronounced outside of the patterns in which they appear. The following example (from Berman, 1985) illustrates the consonantal root *g-d-l* across four different patterns: *godel* 'grows' (Pattern 1), *magdil* 'enlarges' (Pattern 3), *megadel* 'grows something' (Pattern 4), and *mitgadel* 'becomes honorable' (Pattern 5).

As the example shows, patterns often modulate the core meaning of the root. The correspondence between a given pattern and a particular semantic notion is imperfect. For example, many causative verbs in Hebrew take the template of Pattern 3, but this pattern also accommodates verbs that convey the notion of inchoativeness (e.g., *mashmin* 'has gotten fat'). In the same way, Pattern 5 is associated with the semantic notion of reflexivity (e.g., *mitraxets* 'washes oneself'), but Pattern 5 also has verbs that convey basic meanings (e.g., *mitstalem* 'takes a picture', *mitgalesh* 'slides'). Furthermore, in some cases, when the root appears in a particular pattern, its meaning is quite different from the meanings of the same root in other patterns. As a case in point, *mitgadel* refers to becoming honorable—a psychological state—whereas the other forms containing the root *g-d-l* (*godel*, *magdil*, *megadel*) pertain to physical growth.

There are five productive and two derivative verb patterns in Hebrew. The derivative verb patterns are rarely used in everyday speech and therefore are not included in this description. Patterns 1 and 4 convey a wide range of basic meanings. Pattern 1 is the most common pattern, and verbs with this template emerge early in children's speech and are used most frequently (Berman, 1985; Berman & Armon-Lotem, 1996). However, most new verb forms that appear in the language employ the template of Pattern 4. Pattern 2 is less common and the least productive in the language. This pattern is typically used to express passive notions (e.g., *nishmar* 'was guarded').

Verbs in each pattern can be infinitival or finite in form. Finite verbs mark tense and agreement. For tense, present, past, and future forms are employed, although present forms differ from past and future forms in their participial character, which allows them to serve adjectival as well as verb functions (Berman, 1978). Tense is marked in each pattern by vocalic alternations that are intrinsic to the pattern's phonological template, as well as by regular prefixes. Table 11.1 presents the phonological templates for present, past, and infinitives for Patterns 1, 3, 4, and 5, which are the active patterns in Hebrew. In this table, "C" represents a consonant that varies depending on the root of the verb. The forms that appear in the table are the morphologically simplest form in each tense (third person masculine singular in past and future tense, masculine singular in present tense) and hence are regarded as basic forms.

The categories of agreement in the verb system are gender, number, and person. The marking of agreement is represented by a set of syllabic suffixes and prefixes that are identical for all of the patterns. These affixes merge with the basic forms in each tense and modify their phonological structure. Al-

TABLE 11.1
The Phonological Templates for Present Tense, Past Tense, and Infinitives
for the Active Patterns 1, 3, 4, and 5

Infinitive	Past	Present	Pattern
*li*CCoC	CaCaC	CoCeC	1
*leha*CCiC	*hi*CCiC	*ma*CCiC	3
*le*CaCeC	CiCeC	*me*CaCeC	4
*lehit*CaCeC	*hit*CaCeC	*mit*CaCeC	5

though the agreement paradigms are rich, not all distinctions are marked in all tenses. In present tense, only gender and number distinctions are marked. In past and future tense, only person and number distinctions are marked in first person singular and plural and third person plural, whereas gender distinctions are also required for second person and third person singular. It is important to note that agreement morphology is fusional in Hebrew. Thus, the suffix -*im* simultaneously marks both number and gender in present tense, and the suffix *ta* simultaneously marks person, number, and gender in past tense. Tables 11.2 and 11.3 list the inflections for verbs in the four commonly used patterns in present and past tense, respectively.

TABLE 11.2
Agreement Inflections in Present Tense for the Active Patterns 1, 3, 4 and 5

	Pattern 1 CoCeC	Pattern 3 maCCiC	Pattern 4 meCaCeC	Pattern 3 mitCaCeC
	go	dress somebody	climb	slide
Masc Sing	*holex*	*malbish*	*metapes*	*mitgalesh*
Fem Sing	*holexet*	*malbisha*	*metapeset*	*mitgaleshet*
Masc Plur	*holxim*	*malbishim*	*metapsim*	*mitgalshim*
Fem Plur	*holxot*	*malbishot*	*metapsot*	*mitgalshot*

TABLE 11.3
Agreement Inflections in Past Tense for the Active Patterns 1, 3, 4, and 5

	Pattern 1 CaCaC	Pattern 3 hiCCiC	Pattern 4 CiCeC	Pattern 5 hitCaCeC
First Sing	*Halaxti*	*hilbashti*	*tipasti*	*hitgalashti*
First Plur	*Halaxnu*	*hilbashnu*	*tipasnu*	*hitgalashnu*
Second Masc Sing	*Halaxta*	*hilbashta*	*tipasta*	*hitgalashta*
Second Fem Sing	*Halaxt*	*hilbasht*	*tipast*	*hitgalasht*
Second Plur	*Halaxtem*	*hilbashtem*	*tipastem*	*hitgalashtem*
Third Masc Sing	*Halax*	*hilbish*	*tipes*	*hitgalesh*
Third Fem Sing	Halxa	hilbisha	tipsa	hitgalsha
Third Plur	*Halxu*	*hilbishu*	*tipsu*	*hitgalshu*

Infinitives are also used in Hebrew. However, unlike the case for English, Hebrew infinitives are not the simplest morphological forms. They are phonologically distinct from the (finite) basic forms and, for certain patterns, they employ more syllables (e.g., *lehalbish* 'to dress somebody' *lehistarek* 'to comb one's hair').

VERB MORPHOLOGY IN HSLI CHILDREN: AN OVERVIEW OF PUBLISHED RESULTS

Similar to SLI children who learn other languages, HSLI children show the familiar early pattern of slow lexical development and late emergence of grammar with considerable phonological difficulties and recognizable pragmatic deficits in the area of discourse coherence (see Beni-Noked, 1985; Leonard, 1998; Rom & Bliss, 1981, 1983). In the first study on morphology in HSLI children, Rom and Leonard (1990) found that the range of inflections used by such children in 50 utterance language samples was as wide as the range found for a group of young normally developing Hebrew-speaking children who had similar scores according to the measure morphemes per utterance (MPU). These researchers calculated MPU scores according to the model proposed by Dromi and Berman (1982) and matched the two groups of children on this measure. The two groups ranged in MPU from 2.3 to 4.4 morphemes per utterance (a value that corresponds to an MLU of 2–3 words per utterance). Due to the relatively small sample size, all present and past tense inflections were collapsed in their analysis. The mean percentage of use for all inflections in obligatory contexts was surprisingly high, reaching an average of 90%.

In a subsequent study, Dromi, Leonard, and Shteiman (1993) examined the use of a wide range of noun and verb morphemes in a sample of 15 HSLI children who ranged in age from 4;1 to 5;11 years and had MLUs in words of 3.0 to 3.14. These children were compared to a group of 15 ND age matched children and a group of 15 normally developing children matched for MLU (ND-MLU children). The data were collected via probes resembling those used by Leonard and his colleagues for studying English- and Italian-speaking children with SLI. In these probes, pictures were presented along with sentences the children were asked to complete. The sentence contexts created obligatory contexts for the morphemes of interest. For example, for the elicitation of present tense feminine singular forms, each participant was presented with a picture of a boy and a girl cooking. The experimenter said: *hayeled mevashel vegam hayalda ___ (mevashelet)* 'the boy is cooking [present, masculine singular] and the girl ___ (is cooking) [present feminine singular].

The results indicated that the percentages of correct use of the different morphemes in obligatory contexts were considerably lower than the percentages reported by Rom and Leonard (1990). However, no significant differences were found between the HSLI and ND-MLU children in the verb and noun-related morphemes. The HSLI and ND-MLU children averaged 76% and 78% correct, respectively, for verbs in present tense. For past tense, mean percentages were 56% and 30%. Noun plural inflections averaged 76% and 75% for the two groups, whereas adjective inflections showed means of 70% and 78%. The use of the definite marker *ha-* in the nominative case and the corresponding marker *et-* in the accusative case reached extremely high values of over 90% correct in obligatory contexts for both groups. On the basis of these results, it might be argued that in Hebrew, unlike in English, grammatical morphology does not represent an area of extraordinary difficulty for SLI children. It is likely that there is a direct correspondence between the structure of the input language and the degree and pattern o morphological difficulty that is observed in SLI children.

It has been hypothesized that HSLI children are stronger than English speaking SLI children in the area of morphology, mainly because the two languages differ so widely in this domain. Specifically, the Hebrew data led to the proposal of the "rich morphology account," namely: When grammati cal morphology is pervasive and its use is mandatory in a language, chi' dren with SLI devote their limited linguistic processing resources to this as pect of the language and therefore their command of morphology seem relatively high.

The rationale for the follow-up study (Dromi, Leonard, Adam, & Zaduna isky-Ehrlich, 1999) was related to the assumption that there might be limit to the advantages that a language with rich morphology offers to HSLI chi dren. This study compared HSLI children's use of verb agreement in pre ent and in past tense and also examined the use of agreement in verbs b longing to different verb patterns (B1, B3, B4, and B5). Agreement wa manipulated while tense remained unchanged. The rationale for controllir tense when manipulating agreement only was motivated by the theoretic proposal that agreement marking and marking of tense differ radically, b cause they take place at different levels of the syntactic tree (see, e.g Clahsen, 1989; Clahsen & Dalalakis, 2000; Friedmann & Grodzinsky, 1997)

Two types of experimental probes were utilized in our agreement stud *storybooks*, which served to elicit productions in present tense (feminin singular, feminine plural, masculine plural) as well as certain forms in pa tense (third person feminine singular and third person plural forms), and *series of enactments* that were designed as a guessing/description game. T game was created for the elicitation of the remaining past tense forms (fi and second person singular and plural).

Each book contained drawings and everyday scripts such as a birthd party, a trip to the zoo, a walk outside, a visit to the water park, and a day the beach. The experimenter told the child that she and the child were ing to look together at the pictures and tell the story. She then began telling the story, and she paused at predetermined points while pointing to a certain picture to allow the child to complete the story. The sentence context and accompanying drawing obligated the child's use of a verb with a particular agreement inflection. For example, "Afterwards they returned to the pool and they wanted to jump in the water. Danny jumped (*kafats [third* person masculine singular]). And Shlomit also ____ (*kaftsa[third* person feminine singular])."

To elicit productions requiring first person singular and plural inflections, the child and two experimenters participated in an enactment task. One experimenter left the room and the remaining experimenter and child performed predetermined actions with the props. For example, in one scenario, the child ate some chocolate and the remaining experimenter built a small tower with blocks. When the first experimenter returned, the other experimenter told the child, "Tell (experimenter's name) who ate, and who built with blocks." ("Who" questions employ the basic third person masculine singular form in Hebrew.) Consequently, a response such as "I ate (*axalti* [past, *first* person singular]), and she built (*banta* [past, third person feminine]) with blocks" was expected from the child. Several variations of this activity were employed to create obligatory contexts for first person plural, as well as second person masculine and feminine singular and second person plural inflections in the past.

The results for agreement marking by the HSLI children in the different verb patterns of Hebrew indicated abilities that were somewhat weaker than earlier findings had suggested. Within present tense, the HSLI children were less accurate than the ND-MPU controls in their use of agreement inflections for one of the four verb patterns, B5. This verb pattern has a complex phonological template and often conveys notions such as reflexivity, reciprocity, and inchoativeness. Within past tense, the differences between the HSLI children and the ND-MPU controls did not center on particular patterns but on particular agreement inflections. Those inflections producing the greatest difficulty for the HSLI children relative to the control children were precisely those that involved a distinction according to person as well as number and gender.

These included the second person masculine singular, the second person feminine singular, and the third person feminine singular. Forms involving distinctions of number and gender only, such as first person plural and third person plural, presented much less difficulty (Dromi et al., 1999).

These served as evidence that HSLI children do not always use grammatical morphology as accurately as would be expected by their language level. It seems that the relative complexity of the targeted form as measured by the number of underlying abstract distinctions that are marked by a single morpheme, as well as the methodology used for assessing morphological skills, might determine the level of mastery for a given inflection. In other words, data showed that even in Hebrew, if the morphological paradigms are too complex, then grammatical morphology itself might require greater processing capacity than HSLI children possess. Dromi et al. concluded that the verb agreement paradigm of past tense in Hebrew represents a case where the processing requirements approach the limits of HSLI children's available resources, leading to the noted differences between them and ND-MPU controls.

Leonard, Dromi, Adam, and Zadunaisky-Erlich (2000) investigated how HSLI children manipulate tense when there was no requirement to simultaneously change agreement. This study explored HSLI children's use of the basic verb forms of Hebrew (masculine singular in present tense, third person masculine singular in past tense) as well as infinitive forms. The motivation to examine the manipulation of tense was related to the finding that agreement inflections within past tense were more difficult for HSLI children than agreement inflections within present tense. It was not clear if past tense itself contributed to the difficulty. Infinitives were included because they are structurally more complex in Hebrew than basic forms (see Table 11.1). This raised the question of whether, when infinitives are required in obligatory contexts, they might be replaced by morphologically simpler forms such as the basic present or basic past tense forms.

The same five storybooks that were used in the agreement study were utilized in the tense study for the elicitation of target forms in obligatory contexts. In the study of tense, the experimenter paused at those points in the story that formed obligatory contexts for infinitives and present or past basic forms. The verb forms produced by the experimenter in the preceding sentence differed from the target in tense or finiteness, to ensure that the child's selection of the appropriate verb form could not involve imitation of the tense or finiteness feature just heard. For example, one excerpt from a story is: . . . *Yoav* went to the pool because he wanted to swim (*lisxot* [infinitive]). He entered the pool and ___ (*saxa* [past, third person singular]).

Results indicated that across all target types and patterns, mean percentages for the HSLI children (82%) and ND-MPU children (86%) were quite high. For three of the four patterns (B1, B4, and B5), the HSLI and ND-MPU controls did not differ significantly in the use of basic present tense, basic past tense, and infinitive forms. However, the HSLI had more difficulty than the younger ND children in the production of all target forms in the remaining pattern, B3. This pattern most typically (although not always) conveys the notion of causality. For this pattern, the HSLI children's overall performance was significantly lower than their overall performance for B1. Interestingly, many children's responses to B3 targets were productions of the corresponding form in B1. For many verbs, B1 expresses simple transitive events (e.g., *wear*), whereas B3 expresses causality (e.g., *dress [someone else]*).

To sum up, the results from the study on agreement inflections suggest that morphological problems of HSLI children become evident as paradigms become more complex. The difficulties uncovered reinforce previously raised suspicions on the relation between prosody and morphology in Hebrew. In elicited tasks, HSLI children often produce reduced renditions of a target form by omitting a segment or syllable, or they change to a verb pattern with a simpler syllable structure (e.g., they use B1 instead of B3). Although errors are seen, they seem to be a function of the number of distinctions (e.g., person as well as number and gender) rather than the result of a problem with any specific features. Similarly, the results for tense distinctions suggested problems with a particular pattern, but not with tense. Thus, tense and finiteness probably do not form the core of the problem faced by Hebrew-speaking children with SLI. Of course, these studies involved probes requiring specific verbs in specific patterns, with a particular tense and with particular agreement features. It was not known how the HSLI children's limitations were reflected in their everyday speech. For this reason, a study of the spontaneous speech of HSLI children and their ND-MPU controls was conducted.

THE USE OF VERB FORMS BY HSLI CHILDREN IN SPONTANEOUS LANGUAGE SAMPLES

The goal of this study was to examine the use of verb morphology by HSLI children in spontaneous speech. One previous study (Rom & Leonard, 1990) reported spontaneous use of inflections by HSLI. The language samples in that study were very short and the analysis collapsed morphological categories and verb patterns. In the study reported below, speech samples of more than 200 different utterances were collected from each participant, obligatory contexts for each morpheme were defined, and the analysis was focused on the distribution of the various finite and nonfinite verb forms in the different verb patterns of Hebrew. Furthermore, the participants in the present study were the same participants assessed through probes. This methodological decision facilitated comparisons between the spontaneous use and the elicited use of the same morphological forms by the same children (a detailed description of subjects as well as procedures of transcription and analysis appear in Blass, 2000).

It was hypothesized that during spontaneous conversations, HSLI children would produce less diverse verb forms than ND-MPU controls. It was presumed that HSLI children would utter more basic verb forms than forms marked for agreement.

Fifteen HSLI children who were previously diagnosed as children with SLI and therefore were already enrolled in intensive language preschool programs in Tel Aviv participated in the study. Their ages ranged from 4;2 to 6;1. All scored more than 1.25 standard deviations below the mean for their chronological age and socioeconomic status (SES) on a language screening test (Guralnik, 1995). Their Performance IQs (Wechsler, 1989) were within the normal range. Their MLUs in words ranged from 2.25 to 3.90 ($M = 3.02$, $SD = .56$) and MPUs in morphemes ranged from 2.87 to 5.42 ($M = 4.03$, $SD = .87$).

The ND-MPU group consisted of 15 children who ranged in age from 2;8 to 3;11. Their MLU scores in words were from 2.0 to 4.0 ($M = 3.06$, $SD = .58$), and their MPUs in morphemes very closely approximated those of the children with SLI, showing a range from 2.80 to 5.41 ($M = 4.0$, $SD = .81$). The ND-MPU children were pair matched with the HSLI children on the basis of MLU, MPU, sex, and SES (see Dromi et al., 1999; Leonard et al., 2000).

The spontaneous language samples were recorded from participants while they were engaged in playing or in a conversation with an experienced experimenter in a quiet room in the preschool. In all cases, the language sample was recorded prior to the elicitation of the probed data. Books, toys, and several sets of pictures were used to scaffold the speech of all children as minimally as possible, and yet to support a flow of connected speech. Detailed contextual notes were taken during the recording. Language samples were phonetically transcribed as shortly as possible following the recording while incorporating the contextual notes, which were then used for the identification of obligatory contexts for using each grammatical morpheme. A total of 200 to 300 spontaneous, nonrepetitive utterances were recorded from each child and resulted in an overall sample of 3,683 utterances from the HSLI and 3,269 utterances from the matched ND-MPU participants.

As a first step in the analysis, all constituents containing lexical verbs were identified. The two groups did not differ significantly in the number of constituents containing verbs that they used. As a second step, each verb form identified in the sample went through an identical descriptive procedure of its form. The following characteristics were noted for each verb: root, tense, pattern, number, gender, person, and the context for its use. The grammatical context for each verb was determined on the basis of the linguistic frame in which it appeared, the preceding question or comment provided by the experimenter, or an event or action that was performed when the verb was uttered. A total of 2,141 different verb productions from the HSLI children and 2,168 verb productions from the ND-MPU children were included in the computerized database. Analysis of variance was performed on the number of verb forms produced, using subject group as a between factor and verb pattern as a within factor. A main effect for pattern $F(4,112) = 1232.22$, $p < .01$, along with a significant subject group by pattern

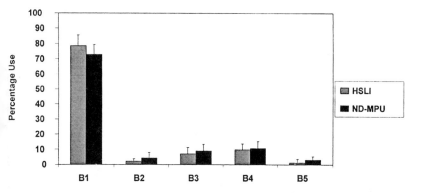

FIG. 11.1. The relative distribution of the different verb patterns in HSLI and ND-MPU groups.

teraction, $F(4,1120) = 3.83$, $p < .01$, was found. As shown in Fig. 11.1, 78.6% of verbs produced by the HSLI and 72.7% of all verbs produced by the ND-PU children belonged to pattern B1. This pattern is considered the simest in structure and most frequently used by Hebrew-speaking children as ell as adults (Berman, 1997). Post hoc comparisons revealed that the HSLI rticipants produced B1 verbs significantly more than the ND-MPU partici-nts. No significant differences were found between the two groups with spect to the use of other verb patterns. No other patterns were used with gh frequency by either of the two groups of children. The relative distri-tion of the different verb patterns by the HSLI and ND-MPU groups is pre-nted in Fig. 11.1.

A closer look at the B1 forms produced by the two groups further indi-ed that all subjects produced finite forms of B1 verbs much more often in nonfinite forms (69% finite and 6% nonfinite). This difference was sig-cant, $F(1,28) = 2758.12$, $p < .001$. Figure 11.2 presents the distribution of the erent finite verb forms in B1 that appeared in the sample collapsed for two subject groups. The dominance of finite verb forms was true for h groups of children.

Figure 11.3 presents the distribution of pattern 1 finite verb forms col-sed for the two groups. Out of the 24 different verb inflection categories t are possible in Hebrew, only 12 were produced by our HSLI and ND-U participants. As was hypothesized, verbs in present tense were re-ded much more frequently than past or future verb forms. The most fre-ntly used verb form in present was the basic form (masculine, singular). ast tense, the only category that exceeded 5% was again the basic form rd person, masculine, singular). Please note that neither group ever d a second person past tense form. Recall that these target forms are ong the most complex past tense forms in Hebrew as they simulta-usly encode tense, person, number, and gender.

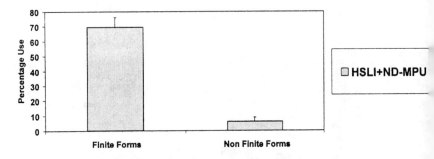

FIG. 11.2. The distribution of the different finite verb forms in B1 that appeared in the sample collapsed for the two subject groups.

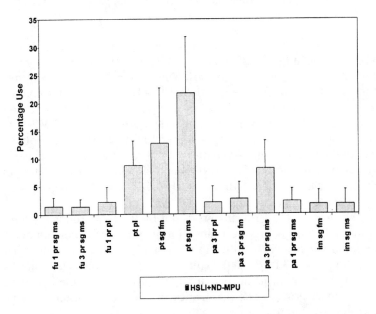

FIG. 11.3. The distribution of pattern 1 finite verb forms collapsed for the two groups.

As already noted, inspection of the nonfinite verb forms in the samp revealed that the HSLI and ND-MPU participants did not differ significan in their relative use of infinitives in B1. Only about 6% of infinitive v forms were identified in this most commonly used pattern. In other v patterns, however, the ND-MPU participants used infinitives nearly twice frequently as the HSLI children (4.4%–2.75%), a difference that was sigr cant ($p < .05$).

An interesting significant difference between the two groups was ide fied with respect to the occurrence of *stripped verb forms*. Stripped v forms are immature verb forms that lack overt morphological marking that can assist in identifying their precise grammatical function. For example, if a child says *saper*, it is impossible to determine whether he tried to say *lesaper* 'to tell' (infinitive), *mesaper* 'he tells' (present masculine singular), or *mesaperet* 'she tells' (present feminine singular), because so much morphological information is missing. Yet, it is clear that the stripped verb form was constructed from the consonantal root /s/./p/./r/. embedded in the target verb pattern B4. Stripped forms are often recorded in very young Hebrew-speaking children and they almost disappear in ND children when their lexicons exceed 20 different verbs (Armon-Lotem, 1996; Dromi et al., 1999). Although stripped forms were not frequent in the data, the HSLI participants produced such forms almost three times more frequently than our much younger ND-MPU participants (i.e., 22 occurrences in HSLI; 8 occurrences in ND-MPU). This difference was statistically significant, $t(28) = 2.00$, $p < .05$.

A COMPARISON BETWEEN SPONTANEOUS AND ELICITED VERB FORMS IN HEBREW

The HSLI and ND-MPU controls were similar in their spontaneous use of verb forms. The two groups used a limited set of morphological categories, with the greatest use concentrating on the simplest verb forms of Hebrew. The use of the B1 pattern by all children overrode their use of other verb patterns. These other patterns can be regarded as more complex than B1 both in terms of phonology and semantics. HSLI children, however, uttered verbs belonging to B1 even more often than the younger ND participants.

A range of finite forms were used by the two groups. It should be noted that present tense forms that are regarded the simplest in the paradigm (masculine singular) were produced in many more contexts than other finite forms. Basic forms in past tense (third person masculine singular) were the most frequent forms, with a complete absence of second person productions. Infinitives were used more often in B1 than in other patterns by children in the two groups. Infinitives in verb patterns other than B1 were used much more often by the ND-MPU children than by the HSLI children. Finally, immature stripped forms that are ungrammatical and usually disappear by age 2 in ND children were more frequent in the HSLI group.

On one hand, the results obtained from the analysis of spontaneous speech data supported previous findings that were based on the elicited data, and on the other hand, these new data differed from it. To what extent do these results corroborate with what has been found by utilizing probes?

- In the spontaneous data, as well as in the probed data, agreement in present tense did not represent a special difficulty for HSLI children. At the same time, agreement in past was problematic in the probes and was rarely recorded in the speech samples.

- The preference observed for the use of B1 in the spontaneous data corresponds with the finding that in the probes HSLI children did not differ in the use of agreement in three out of four patterns, including B1. Indeed, the HSLI children were most accurate on B1. However, the HSLI children often failed to provide correct agreement in B5, which has a complex phonological template and often conveys complex meanings. Verbs in B5 were not observed in the naturalistic data.

- The predominance of simple agreement categories (agreement in number and gender in present tense) and the absence of complex agreement categories in the spontaneous data (agreement in person, number, and gender in past and future tense) supports the claim that the more problematic categories in the probes—for which significant differences were recorded between the HSLI and ND-MPU children—were indeed the most difficult categories.

- Infinitives were used correctly but in low frequencies by the HSLI children as well as by ND-MPU controls. In both groups, 70% of the verbs appeared in their finite form. The claim that in Hebrew infinitives do not constitute a default form is supported by the naturalistic data.

- The very high prevalence of basic verb forms in present and in past tense is in accordance with the probe findings that these tensed forms were easier for HSLI children. These forms therefore, might have a special status as default forms in Hebrew. In the probe data, basic forms were common substitutes for more complex target forms.

- The higher rate of stripped forms in the spontaneous speech of the HSLI children relative to that observed in the ND-MPU controls highlights a related finding that was marginally significant in the agreement study. In the analysis of errors of agreement (see Dromi et al., 1999), stripped forms were sometimes recorded; although they appeared at a low rate in the HSLI data (occurring 17 times), they were nearly nonexistent in the ND-MPU control children's data (occurring only twice).

To what extent then do the spontaneous data differ from the probe data?

- The spontaneous data did not allow for the analysis of agreement within each verb pattern. There were very few instances in the samples of agreement forms in other than B1 and in other than present tense.

- The spontaneous data did not allow for the identification of specific difficulties that HSLI children might have had because such forms seemed to be avoided altogether by these children. Good examples are: the complete avoidance in the spontaneous samples of the phonological complex present tense B4 verb forms, or the avoidance of B5 verb forms that are regarded semantically complex as they encode notions such as reflexivity.

In sum, the method of collecting morphological data has a significant impact on pattern of results obtained. Whereas in the probe studies children are directed to produce specific target forms and often fail to do so because of the task heavy requirements (see Levy, Tennenbaum, & Ornoy, 2000), in naturalistic conversational contexts children may simply avoid some verb forms that pose difficulty. Within this paradigm of research, the relative use of a given linguistic form in obligatory contexts has become a standard measure for productivity. A methodological concern, however, is that the nonconstraining method of elicitation of spontaneous speech is not always successful in evoking linguistic forms that are of special interest to the researcher.

The combined evidence from naturalistic and probed data strongly support the conclusion that any special difficulty that HSLI children have with verb morphology is selective rather than sweeping. In many cases, these children produce verb forms as successfully as their utterance length or morphemes per utterance lead researchers to expect. This is especially so when the children are relatively free to select the forms to be produced, as in spontaneous speech. However, for those forms requiring simultaneous distinctions of person, number, gender, and tense, or for those forms involving challenging phonological templates and/or semantic notions, HSLI children have extraordinary difficulties. Their tendency to rely heavily on simple morphological forms in spontaneous speech may be a symptom of this weakness.

ACKNOWLEDGMENTS

The studies reported in this chapter were supported by a research grant 5R01 DC 00-458) from the National Institutes of Deafness and Other Communication Disorders, National Institutes of Health. The authors' thanks are extended to Galit Adam and Sara Zadunaiski-Ehrlich for their deep ongoing involvement in subject identification, data collection, transcription, and analysis. Their able assistance throughout the years is greatly appreciated. Thanks also go to Noga Meir and Zohar Chalamish, who participated in data collection, and to Ricardo Tarrasch and Carol Miller for their valuable help with statistical analysis.

REFERENCES

Armon-Lotem, S. (1996). *The minimalist child: Parameters and functional heads in the acquisition of Hebrew.* Unpublished doctoral dissertation, Tel-Aviv University.

Beni-Noked, S. (1985). *Some underlying characteristics of conversations between mothers and their language impaired children.* Unpublished master's thesis, Tel Aviv University.

Berman, R. (1978). *Modern Hebrew structure.* Tel Aviv: Universities Publishing.

Berman, R. (1985). The acquisition of Hebrew. In D. Slobin (Ed.), *The crosslinguistic study of language acquisition* (Vol. 1, pp. 255–371). Hillsdale, NJ: Lawrence Erlbaum Associates.

Berman, R. (1997). The investigation of Hebrew acquisition as a first language: Early emergence of syntax and discourse structures. In J. Shimron (Ed.), *Psycholinguistic studies in Israel: Language acquisition, reading, and writing* (pp. 57–100). Jerusalem: Magnes.

Berman, R. A., & Armon-Lotem, S. (1996). How grammatical are early verbs? *Les Annales de university de Besancon.*

Blass, A. (2000). *Verb inflection in Hebrew-speaking children with specific language impairment.* Unpublished master's thesis, Tel Aviv University.

Brown, R. (1973). *A first language.* Cambridge, MA: Harvard University Press.

Cazden, C. B. (1968). The acquisition of noun and verb inflections. *Child Development, 39,* 433–448.

Clahsen, H. (1989). The grammatical characterization of developmental dysphasia. *Linguistics, 27,* 897–920.

Clahsen, H., & Dalalakis, J. (2000). Tense and agreement in Greek SLI: A case study. *Essex Research Reported in Linguistics, 28,* 1–25.

Cleave, P., & Rice, M. (1997). An examination of the morpheme BE in children with specific language impairment: The role of contractibility and grammatical form class. *Journal of Speech, Language and Hearing Research, 40,* 480–492.

Dromi, E., & Berman, R. (1982). A morphemic measure of early language development: Data from Israeli Hebrew. *Journal of Child Language, 9,* 169–191.

Dromi, E., Leonard, L. B., Adam, G., & Zadunaisky-Ehrlich, S. (1999). Verb agreement morphology in Hebrew speaking children with specific language impairment. *Journal of Speech and Hearing Research, 42,* 1414–1431.

Dromi, E., Leonard, L. B., & Shteiman, M. (1993). The grammatical morphology of Hebrew speaking children with specific language impairment: Some competing hypothesis. *Journal of Speech and Hearing Research, 36,* 760–771.

Friedman, N., & Grodzinsky, Y. (1997). Tens and agreement in agrammatic production: Pruning the syntactic tree. *Brain & Language, 56,* 397–425.

Guralnik, E. (1995). *A screening test for Hebrew speaking preschoolers.* Tel Aviv: Matan Publisher.

Leonard, B. L. (1998). *Children with specific language impairment.* Cambridge, MA: MIT Press.

Leonard, L. B., Dromi, E., Adam, G., & Zadunaisky-Ehrlich, S. (2000). Tense and finiteness in the speech of children with specific language impairment acquiring Hebrew. *International Journal of Language and Communications Disorders, 27,* 1–25.

Levy, Y., Tennenbaum, B., & Ornoy, A. (2000). Spontaneous language of children with specific neurological syndromes. *Journal of Speech Hearing and Language Research, 43,* 351–365.

Loeb, D., & Leonard, L. (1991). Subject case marking and verb morphology in normally developing and specifically language-impaired children. *Journal of Speech Hearing and Language Research, 34,* 340–346.

Oetting, J., & Horohov, J. (1997). Past tense marking by children with and without specific language impairment. *Journal of Speech Hearing and Language Research, 40,* 62–74.

Rice, M., Wexler, K., & Cleave, P. (1995). Specific language impairment as a period of external optional infinitive. *Journal of Speech and Hearing Research, 38,* 850–863.

Rom, A., & Bliss, L. (1981). Comparison of nonverbal and verbal communicative skills of language impaired and normal speaking children. *Journal of Communication Disorders, 14,* 133–140.

Rom, A., & Bliss, L. (1983). The use of nonverbal pragmatic behaviors by language-impaired and normal-speaking children. *Journal of Communication Disorders, 14,* 251–256.

Rom, A., & Leonard, L. B. (1990). Interpreting deficits in grammatical morphology in specifically language impaired children: Preliminary evidence from Hebrew. *Clinical Linguistics & Phonetics, 4*(2), 93–105.

Wechsler, D. (1989). *Wechsler Preschool and Primary Scale of Intelligence–Revised.* New York: Psychological Corporation.

III

LANGUAGE COMPETENCE IN POPULATIONS OTHER THAN SPECIFIC LANGUAGE IMPAIRMENT

AN INTRODUCTION

Yonata Levy

The Hebrew University, Jerusalem

Different populations of children are associated with variability in language competence. Most cases are considered disorders of language—such as the language of children with a variety of neurodevelopmental disorders or children with SLI. Yet, in other cases, the linguistic competence of the child indeed varies from what is most commonly observed yet it is not disordered. Ethnic dialects (e.g., African Americans; see de Villiers, chap. 17 in this volume) are such cases. Interestingly, if Sandler's view (chap. 15 in this volume) of sign languages is accepted, then sign languages also are an example of nondisordered natural variability in linguistic competence.

What is common to the study of these variants in linguistic competence is that together with normative spoken language they set the limits of what might be functionally possible for the human brain under a variety of structural-functional conditions. Furthermore, the question of the specificity of the linguistic profile of children with SLI, a main theme herein, can only be raised in the context of language in children with other syndromes and is not in fact different from the question of the uniqueness of the linguistic profiles of children with other disorders.

It is quite possible, as has been the case in other areas, that the variability seen in the behavioral measure (i.e., language) will not be enough to single out each syndrome with its own unique linguistic profile. If this turns out to be the case, then the expectation is that there may not be a specific linguistic profile that is *only* seen in children with a certain syndrome, but that various syndromes will share similar behavioral manifestations of perhaps differing genetic origin. Furthermore, the effects of environment cannot be ruled out and those may work in different directions. It may bring closer profiles that characterize different syndromes because each needs to achieve functional efficiency, or it may serve to produce effects that make similar profiles appear distant, again, so as to achieve maximal efficiency under difficult conditions. In other words, similarity across symptoms or across profiles is a first step toward the search for a common biological origin, but it is certainly not nearly enough to argue for such common basis.

Sandler's chapter (15) examines the language competence of a special yet nondisordered population: deaf people who use sign language. Her investigations lead her to offer a new way of thinking about human linguistic competence. The traditional approach to sign languages views manual signing as an alternative modality that the brain is forced to use for linguistic communication when the oral channel is unavailable. On this view, the manual modality is conceived of as secondary and although it imposes certain constraints that introduce particular changes in the grammatical system, in essence the manual language that emerges shares its core properties with spoken languages.

Sandler offers to view the spoken and the manual systems as similar in certain ways and different in others and thus complimentary. On this view, spoken and manual languages together constitute the complete human communication system. Sandler presents fascinating analyses of prosody, tonality, intonation, and verb agreement in both oral and sign languages, stressing both unique and complimentary properties of each of these systems. She then argues that gesture is required as augmentation to both systems. Whereas in spoken languages people gesture manually, in sign languages people gesture with their mouth. Both modalities are natural, each leaves its traces in the other and together they comprise the whole human language faculty.

From the perspective of language disorders, this way of viewing the linguistic system opens up the possibility of an enriched conceptualization of language disorders. For example, given this view, what is the prediction with respect to language in children with severe motor deficits? Clinical observations consistently note the comorbidity of developmental motor problems and SLI. Such comorbidity can be accounted for on the basis of connectedness between brain areas that subserve those two functions. Sandler's chapter, however, provides a model that offers a cognitive explanation. If indeed the human communication system is vocal as well as manual, that is, it has an auditory as well as a motor component, then a case can be made for such comorbidity.

Clahsen and Temple's (chap. 13) investigations of children with Williams syndrome highlight the central debate in the field of language acquisition, normal as well as pathological. It is the debate surrounding generative approaches to acquisition versus alternative approaches: connectionist models that assume general learning principles, and other functional-cognitive models that do not presuppose an abstract computational component that underlies children's grammatical knowledge and directs development (e.g., construction grammar; see Conti-Ramsden's intro to sec. II). This debate is often set in the context of a modular view of cognition and language versus a view of cognition that does not advocate domain specific processes and categories.

Children with Williams syndrome (WS) are a good population with which to investigate issues pertaining to the debate concerning the modularity of language. For a number of years, children with this syndrome were described as having intact linguistic abilities in the face of low IQ and very deficient visuomotor skills. For awhile it was believed that the field of developmental language disorders has succeeded in providing the much-sought-after case of double dissociation: Children with SLI were said to have intact cognition but deficient language, and children with WS had impaired cognitive abilities but intact language.

However, intensive research into the details of linguistic competence of children with Williams syndrome in recent years has revealed deficits in language that reopened the debate. Is it indeed the case that the uneven cognitive profile of children with Williams syndrome can best be explained in reference to the modularity of language, or can their relatively good linguistic skills be accounted for in reference to general cognitive mechanisms that are seen to affect their performance in other domains as well?

Clahsen and Temple report data that argue for the relative preservation of the computational component of grammar in children with Williams syndrome, supporting a modular view of language competence. The authors explicitly reject recent attempts to account for language in children with Williams syndrome in reference to connectionist models of learning. Clahsen and Temple position themselves very clearly within the generative camp and as such their data is rather convincing.

Clahsen and Temple's findings are also relevant to another central debate in the field of developmental language disorders. Decades of neuropsychological work with adult patients have taken as axiomatic the assumption that when a deficit is incurred, the brain does not reorganize in a completely new way. Rather, to the extent that there is functional reorganization, it mirrors normal cognition. This assumption is a precondition for learning from the normal about the disordered and vice versa. Such a premise, however, is not as intuitive when pathology is considered within a developmental context. In the case of a congenitally disordered system, whether the disorder is due to a genetic cause or to a very early injury or has a metabolic origin, the hypothesis that development may follow a different course than the normally observed one is not implausible. Given that the initial state of the child differs from the normal, one may predict that the ultimate knowledge structure, even if not the ultimate functional achievements, may differ from the normal. This is an empirical question, but it also commits a researcher to a theoretical framework.

Karmiloff-Smith (1998) has argued for the plausibility of the hypothesis that congenital disorders might affect the route to learning. Her empirical work relates to children with Williams syndrome. Clahsen and Temple's chapter is relevant to these questions because the hypotheses being tested in this work derive from the premise that a similar grammar underlies linguistic knowledge of children with Williams syndrome and normal children. Interestingly, the authors point out that what they see as characteristic of children with Williams syndrome is very different from that which has been attributed to children with SLI. In the latter, grammatical deficits seem to be a necessary part of the definition of the syndrome.

Although the children in Clahsen and Temple's study, as well as the children in most studies of SLI, are well beyond the early phases of language acquisition, it is still instructive to tie this work with the statement made in Levy's chapter. Levy (chap. 14) presents data arguing for the similarity of linguistic profiles of children with different neurological syndromes and typically developing children of the same MLU. This comparison is said to hold for early language phases when MLU does not exceed 3. Levy offers to account for this feat in reference to brain plasticity.

Brain plasticity is the capacity of the brain to compensate for damage through the recruitment of alternative brain areas. Levy suggests that this mechanism, hitherto reserved for the discussion of the effects of localized brain damage on the relevant performance, is responsible for the uniform developmental course and achievements that are observed across populations with neurodevelopmental disorders early on.

Notice that a crucial piece of evidence that will either support or reject this hypothesis is still missing. A detailed study of this type with children with SLI has not been done as yet. The logic behind the claim that there is plasticity in these cases predicts that children with SLI will likewise follow normal developmental course until MLU 3. Clearly, this does not preclude the possibility that there will be specific biological conditions that will prevent plasticity from operating in a given syndrome.

Tager-Flusberg (chap. 12) outlines the similarities between the language profile of autistic children and the typical profile of children with SLI. She focuses specifically on two characteristic features seen in SLI—deficits in nonword repetition and problems with tense marking on verbs, and reports of similar deficits in her autistic group. Although, to date, there are no diagnostic neurological signs that characterize SLI, Tager-Flusberg presents findings from genetic studies that point to possible connections between loci of deficient genes, as well as from brain research comparing and contrasting anatomical malformations seen in autism and in SLI.

Note, however, that difficulties with tense marking (the much discussed optional infinitives, OI; see Wexler, chap. 1) and its prolonged period in children with SLI (the extended optional infinitive stage, EOI) is seen in second language learners, reported in Crago and Pradis' chapter 3, and in African Americans, reported in de Villiers chapter 17, as well as in autism. In other words, so far there are three different populations—autistic kids, normally developing second language learners, and African Americans—in addition to children with SLI, who show an EOI stage. Clearly, this raises a question concerning the specificity of this trait to SLI. It calls for a discussion of the usefulness of singling out SLI from the rest of the population of children with disorders of language when issues such as the meaning and scope of language competence are brought to the fore.

In sum, new work on different populations of children suggests that an understanding of the relation between brain and language requires a comprehensive study of language competence across different populations of children. Similarities that begin to emerge between linguistic profiles in a variety of syndromes along with the familiar unique properties that continue to receive empirical support as studies accumulate, suggest that more complex theoretical models are required.

REFERENCE

Karmiloff-Smith, A. (1998). Is atypical development necessarily a window on the normal mind/brain? The case of Williams syndrome. *Developmental Science, 1*(2), 273–277.

12

Language Impairment in Children with Complex Neurodevelopmental Disorders: The Case of Autism

Helen Tager-Flusberg
Boston University

Delays and deficits in the acquisition of language are often reported for children with a wide range of neurodevelopmental disorders such as Down syndrome, fragile X syndrome, Prader-Willi syndrome, and autism (Tager-Flusberg, 1999a). A key issue in the field of language disorders is whether there are common or unique developmental profiles of language deficit among children with different kinds of disorders. More specifically, do children with certain neurodevelopmental disorders show patterns of language deficit similar to those that have been described for children with specific language impairment (SLI)? This chapter explores this question by focusing on children with autism. It first reviews the interesting parallels and potential overlaps between autism and SLI. It then presents evidence from an ongoing study supporting the view that there is a subgroup of children with autism that have deficits in language identical to those found in children with SLI. Consideration is then given to the implications of this overlap between autism and SLI in relation to common genetic and neurobiological mechanisms. The final section compares language impairments in both these complex disorders, autism and SLI, to other genetically based neurodevelopmental disorders, and addresses the question regarding the specificity of the profile of impairments found in SLI.

OVERVIEW OF RESEARCH ON LANGUAGE IN AUTISM

Defining Autism

Autism was first recognized as a distinct syndrome by Kanner (1943), a child psychiatrist who identified the core symptoms of social isolation and a behavioral pattern of narrowed interests and resistance to change in a group of 11 children. Kanner (1946) noted many unusual features in the children's language, including echolalic repetition of speech, pronoun reversal errors, and the use of words and phrases in an apparently meaningless but idiosyncratic way (called "metaphorical language"). However, he did not consider impairments in language or communication to be at the core of the disorder. Over time, this view changed, and today autism is diagnosed, both in *Diagnostic and Statistical Manual of Mental Disorders* (4th ed.; *DSM–IV*) and the *International Statistical Classification of Diseases and Related Health Problems, tenth revision (ICD–10)*, on the basis of impairments in three domains: social interaction, language and communication, and restricted repertoire of activity and interests.

Is Autism on a Continuum with SLI?

In the late 1960s, the first systematic studies of autism were conducted, and one hypothesis that received attention purported that autism represented an extreme form of SLI, or "developmental dysphasia" as it was then called (Churchill, 1972; Rutter, 1965). On this view, autism was part of a continuum of disorders along with other forms of developmental language impairment. Bartak and his colleagues conducted the most systematic comparison of children with autism and children with severe developmental language disorder using a series of standardized language tests and measures taken from a natural language sample (Bartak, Rutter, & Cox, 1975, 1977). The children in both groups, all boys, were selected on the basis of having severe problems in language comprehension and were matched on age (5–10 year old) and nonverbal IQ (over 70). There were both similarities and differences between the groups. Both groups had major deficits in structural aspects of language, including comprehension and production of syntax, morphology, and semantics, as well as limited lexical knowledge. However, the autistic children showed unique qualitative differences in their use of language, similar to the characteristics described by Kanner (1946). These features (pronoun reversals, echolalia, stereotyped utterances, inappropriate remarks, absence of gesture, and conversational deficits) clearly distinguished between the autism and SLI groups, suggesting that autism could not simply be the result of primary problems in language (Bartak et al.

7). Instead, the kinds of pragmatic deficits that distinguished between
: autistic and SLI children were taken as strong evidence that autism and
are fundamentally separate disorders.

:ntifying Language Deficits That Are Universal
Autism

lowing Bartak et al.'s seminal studies, the focus in autism language re-
.rch shifted toward identifying features of language impairment that were
que and universal among children with autism. Psycholinguistic re-
rch investigated aspects of phonological, grammatical, semantic, and
ical aspects of development, typically by comparing autistic children to
ups of mentally retarded and younger normal children (e.g., Bartolucci
Albers, 1974; Bartolucci & Pierce, 1977; Bartolucci, Pierce, Streiner, &
)el, 1976; Pierce & Bartolucci, 1977; Tager-Flusberg, 1985). Deficits in
se domains, when they were found, were shown not to be specific to au-
n, but were related to the retardation found in many children with au-
n. In contrast, later research found that pragmatic and discourse impair-
nts clearly distinguished between autistic and nonautistic children (e.g.,
ps, Kehres, & Sigman, 1998; Loveland, Landry, Hughes, Hall, & McEvoy,
8; Loveland & Tunali, 1993; Tager-Flusberg & Anderson, 1991; Tager-
sberg & Sullivan, 1995; Wetherby, 1986), leading to the consensus that
s domain of language represents a core area of dysfunction in autism.
r recent reviews, see Lord & Paul, 1997; Tager-Flusberg, 1999b; Wilkin-
i, 1998.)

MPARISON BETWEEN AUTISM AND SLI

uble Dissociation Between Autism and SLI

the 1990s, autism was seen as a disorder that could be used as strong ev-
nce for the dissociation between form and function in language. Autism
s characterized as a syndrome in which grammatical and lexical aspects
anguage developed normally, while pragmatics was seriously impaired
;., Tager-Flusberg, 1994). This perspective was used to support the view
t computational and communicative aspects of language depend on dis-
:t cognitive and neural mechanisms. During this same period, as studies
SLI began to accumulate, this language disorder was described in ex-
ly the opposite way: impaired grammatical and lexical development, but
ict pragmatic and communicative abilities (e.g., Miller, 1991; Schaeffer,
.p. 5 in this volume). It was argued that autism and SLI demonstrated a
ible dissociation in structural and functional aspects of language.

The claims regarding language dissociations in both autism and SLI are not as extreme as has been portrayed here. The majority of children with autism show significant delays in acquiring language, and about half remain essentially nonverbal (Bailey, Phillips, & Rutter, 1996). Many children who do acquire spontaneous use of language continue to lag behind their peers in vocabulary and the acquisition of complex syntax and morphology (c Bartak et al., 1975). Thus, in autism, there are often problems in both structural and functional aspects of language; however, the former are more variable, not unique to autism, and not necessarily correlated with the degree of functional deficits. Similarly, for SLI, there are studies that have shown deficits in some children in pragmatics and related aspects of social functioning (e.g., Hadley & Rice, 1991; but see Schaeffer, chap. 5 in this volume), however, they are generally considered to be secondary to the primary impairments in structural language. Thus, it is important to note that within each population there is considerable variability in both the characteristics and severity of language problems, which may impede the ability to identify specific and selective deficits associated with either autism or SLI.

Parallels Between Autism and SLI

Despite the different profiles of language impairment found among children with autism and SLI, there are some important parallels between these disorders. First, both are considered complex disorders that are diagnosed on the basis of behavioral characteristics. In this respect, autism and SLI show similarities to other complex disorders such as attention deficit hyperactivity disorder or dyslexia. There is considerable heterogeneity and variability in expression in both autism and SLI. For autism, diagnosis is based on the presence of the three core areas of impairment identified earlier, but many individuals also have other secondary symptoms such as mental retardation, sensory and motor problems, unusual savant skills, and atypical sleep, eating, and other behavior patterns. These secondary symptoms are recognized as being a part of the syndrome of autism, however, they are not counted among the diagnostic criteria. In SLI there is similar heterogeneity, for example, some children have phonological impairments, some have both receptive and expressive deficits, some have primarily expressive problems, and some have pragmatic deficits (e.g., Tomblin & Zhang, 199 However, SLI is not yet defined on the basis of core or primary symptoms that form the criteria for all children receiving this diagnosis. Another parallel between these disorders is that, in both autism and SLI, symptoms initially noticed in the toddler or early preschool years. Failure to acquire language is the most frequently presenting problem, and for both disorders, language delays and deficits are among the primary characteristics

Finally, there is strong evidence that both autism and SLI are inherited disorders. The main evidence for the genetic basis of autism came from early twin studies, which showed that there was a significantly higher concordance rate for autism among monozygotic (MZ) twins, who share 100% of their genes, than for dizygotic (DZ) twins, who share only 50% of their genes (Folstein & Rutter, 1974, 1977). This difference in the concordance rates for MZ and DZ twins provides evidence for the heritability of autism. A recent investigation, which combined twin data from three different samples, concluded that the heritability estimates for autism were over 90% (Bailey et al., 1995). According to the current view regarding the primary etiology of autism, there are probably a few genes (between 2 and 6) that interact with each other to cause the autism phenotype (Santangelo & Folstein, 1999). There have also been several twin studies on SLI. Across these studies, MZ twins show significantly higher concordance rates than DZ twins, suggesting strong heritability of this disorder (Bishop, North, & Donlan, 1995; Dale et al., 1998; Tomblin & Buckwalter, 1998), which is also thought to be caused by several interacting genes (Tomblin & Zhang, 1999).

Overlap Between Autism and SLI

Family studies of children with autism and SLI have found that although the majority of first-degree relatives do not share the same diagnosis, they may have some related features, referred to as the "broader phenotype" (Piven, 1999; Tomblin, Freese, & Records, 1992). For example, the father of a child with autism may be socially withdrawn, but not have other symptoms of autism; the mother of a child with SLI may not have been diagnosed with this disorder in childhood, but she might have had difficulties learning to read and received a diagnosis of dyslexia.

Among family members of children with autism, there are significantly elevated rates of documented histories of language delay and language-based learning deficits that go well beyond pragmatic difficulties (Bailey, Palferman, Heavey, & Le Couteur, 1998; Bolton et al., 1994; Fombonne, Bolton, Prior, Jordan, & Rutter, 1997; Piven et al., 1997). In the original autism twin sample, co-twins who were discordant for autism had high rates of language deficits that resemble the pattern described as SLI (Folstein & Rutter, 1977; see also Le Couteur et al., 1996). There are no good epidemiological studies, but these family and twin studies suggest that SLI may occur significantly more frequently in autism families than in the general population.

There is also evidence that in families identified on the basis of having a child with SLI, there is a significantly elevated risk of autism among the siblings. Hafeman and Tomblin (1999) recently reported that in a population-based sample of children diagnosed with SLI, 4% of the siblings met criteria for autism. This rate is much higher than would be expected based on the current prevalence estimates of about 1 in 500 (Fombonne, 1999). This rate of 4% is not significantly different from the 6% risk recurrence rates in autism families.

The findings from these family studies suggest that autism and SLI may represent partially overlapping populations. Another piece of evidence for potential overlap between autism and SLI comes from studies of children with so-called semantic-pragmatic disorder (cf. Bishop & Rosenbloom, 1987; Rapin & Allen, 1983). In the original studies by Bartak and his colleagues (Bartak et al., 1975, 1977), there was a small group of children (10% of the sample) who could not easily be categorized as either autistic or SLI; they seemed to fall between the two disorders. More recently, there have been more systematic studies showing that some children with SLI have discourse impairments similar to those found in autism (Bishop, Chan, Hartley, Adams, & Weir, 2000; Conti-Ramsden, Crutchley, & Botting, 1997). The diagnostic category of semantic-pragmatic disorder remains controversial because it seems to be so closely related to the autism spectrum (Boucher, 1998; Lister-Brook & Bowler, 1992). However, Bishop (2000) provided a persuasive argument that more research is needed on the potential overlap between language impairments in autism and SLI before eliminating it from classification schemes.

Existing data on these syndromes has a serious limitation in that most research on autism and SLI relies on completely different measures of language. Most investigations of language in autism have used pragmatic, conversational, narrative, or other discourse measures, whereas studies of SLI have included lexical, syntactic, or morphological measures. Studies on autism and SLI that rely on nonoverlapping measures cannot be expected to yield evidence of potential overlap in deficits in these disorders. The next section summarizes the findings from an ongoing study designed explicitly to explore the full range of language deficits in children with autism by including a variety of language measures that are typically used in studies of SLI.

AN INVESTIGATION OF LANGUAGE IMPAIRMENTS IN AUTISM

Background

Over the past two decades, almost no studies have investigated the wide variability in language patterns in autism. Understanding the nature of structural language deficits in children with autism has been seriously neglected, even though it is well known that language ability is the single most significant predictor of long-term outcome in this population (Rutter, 1970; Ventner, Lord, & Schopler, 1992). Using a set of standardized tests of vocabulary and grammatical ability, Jarrold, Boucher, and Russell (1997) claimed to show no variability in the profiles of the autistic children and adolescents. There are, however, methodological problems with this study, and its conclusions contradict the clinical reality of widely varying language abilities in autism.

As part of a wider interdisciplinary research program on autism, a large cohort of children with autism and a comparison group of children with a history of language impairment are being followed. This longitudinal project is designed to measure the heterogeneity in autism in language, cognitive, and neuropsychological functioning using both standardized and experimental measures with the goal of linking this heterogeneity in symptom expression to underlying genes and individual differences in brain structure and function. This chapter presents data from the autistic children on a subset of the language measures; comparisons between the autism and language impaired comparison group are still in progress.

The Sample

A total of 89 children with autism were initially included in the language study (see Kjelgaard & Tager-Flusberg, 2001). They were selected on the basis of having at least some language, defined as the ability to use some two-word utterances. The children were between the ages of 4 and 14 ($M = 7;4$), and all met *DSM–IV* criteria for autistic disorder. The diagnosis was made on the basis of the Autism Diagnostic Interview–Revised (ADI–R; Lord, Rutter, & LeCouteur, 1994) and the Autism Diagnostic Observation Schedule (ADOS; Lord et al., 2000). The ADI–R is a lengthy interview that was completed with one or both parents. Diagnosis is made on the basis of a subset of questions that ask about the child's social, communication, and behavior patterns between ages 4 and 5. The ADOS is a semi-structured interactive observation that assesses current social and communicative behaviors relevant to a diagnosis of autism. There were 80 boys and 9 girls in the sample, which is not surprising given that autism is significantly more prevalent in males. The IQ of each child was assessed using either the preschool or school-age version of the Differential Ability Scales (mean IQ = 68; range = 25–141).

Language Measures

A standard battery of tests was administered individually to the children, measuring their phonological, lexical, and higher order semantic and grammatical language abilities. Testing generally took place over two sessions, with each session including several breaks for the children. This chapter presents data from the following tests:

- *Goldman–Fristoe Test of Articulation* (Goldman & Fristoe, 1986). The Goldman–Fristoe measures the accuracy of productive phonology for the consonant sounds of English. The test presents the child with a series of pictures to name, such that across the set of pictures, all the consonant sounds of English are tested in the word initial, medial, and final position.
- *Peabody Picture Vocabulary Test–III* (PPVT; Dunn & Dunn, 1997). The PPVT–III tests lexical comprehension by presenting an auditory word and asking the child to pick the correct picture from an array of four pictures.
- *Expressive Vocabulary Test* (EVT; Williams, 1997). The EVT measures expressive vocabulary by asking the child to name pictures. As the test advances to more difficult items, children are asked to produce synonyms for words represented in pictures.
- *Clinical Evaluation of Language Fundamentals* (CELF: Preschool or III; Semel, Wiig, & Secord, 1995; Wiig, Secord, & Semel, 1992). The CELF is an omnibus test designed to measure morphology, syntax, semantics, and working memory for language. It is comprised of six subtests that are used to calculate measures of receptive (three subtests) and expressive (three subtests) language skills.
- *Repetition of Nonsense Words* (NWRT). The subtest from the NEPSY was used, which is a comprehensive developmental neuropsychological assessment battery (Korkman, Kirk, & Kemp, 1998). This measure assesses the ability to analyze and reproduce phonological knowledge by asking the child to repeat nonsense words that are presented on an audiotape.

Relations Between Language Testing, Age, and IQ

Because of the wide variability in the language skills of the children, in many cases all the tests were not completed. Data was obtained on the Goldman–Fristoe, the PPVT, and EVT for almost all the children in the sample, but only about one half could be scored on the CELF and the NWRT. There were no differences in the ages of the children who were able to complete the more complex language tests and those who could not (with the exception that the NWRT was not administered to children under age 5), thus age itself was not the limiting factor. On the other hand, IQ was a good indicator of who could complete the CELF and NWRT. In general, those children with higher IQ scores were more likely to complete these higher level tests, which have considerable attentional, working memory, and other nonlinguistic test-related factors associated with them.

Language Profiles and Subgroups in Autism

For each test, the child's standard score was computed, based on a mean of 100 and a standard deviation of 15 points. Although the tests are not all equivalent in that they have different floor and ceiling scores, using the standard scores allowed for a comparison of the children's profiles across the different measures. Overall, there was no profile of scores that captured the entire sample of children. For example, looking at the two vocabulary measures, the majority of children (80%) showed no discrepancy (defined as more than 1 standard deviation score difference) between the PPVT and EVT. However, 16% of the children had significantly higher PPVT scores (suggesting better receptive knowledge), and 4% had significantly higher EVT scores (suggesting better expressive knowledge). Similarly, among the children who completed the CELF, no uniform pattern characterized the children in this study. Instead, there was considerable variability in performance across the different receptive and expressive subtests. Table 12.1 presents the average standard scores obtained on each language measure, and the large standard deviations illustrate this variability.

To explore this variability further, the children were divided into subgroups, based on their scores on one of the language tests. The first subgroup analysis used the PPVT to divide the sample, because almost all the children were scored on this test. The following three subgroups were created:

- *Normal language*—A standard score on the PPVT of 85 or higher. Twenty-five percent of the children in this study were in this group.
- *Borderline language*—a PPVT standard score between 70 and 84, between 1 and 2 standard deviations below the mean. Twelve percent of the children were in this group.
- *Impaired language*—a PPVT standard score below 70, more than 2 standard deviations below the mean. Sixty percent of the children were in this group.

TABLE 12.1
Performance on the Language Tests

Test	M	SD
Goldman–Fristoe	90.17	17.03
Peabody Picture Vocabulary Test–III	70.37	22.68
Expressive Vocabulary Test	68.99	23.62
Clinical Evaluation of Language Fundamentals	72.32	17.71
Repetition of Nonsense Words	81.88	13.89

The study then looked at the children's profile of language skills for each of these subgroups across the other language measures that most children completed: the EVT and the Goldman–Fristoe. For the normal language group, scores on all the language tests were within the normal range, yielding a flat test profile. For the other two groups, the EVT and PPVT, scores were similar to one another, significantly below the mean. However, scores on the Goldman–Fristoe were in the normal range (for the borderline group, $M = 104$; for the impaired group, $M = 85$). This pattern indicates that articulation skills at the one-word level is spared in autism overall, although there were a few children, generally those below age 6, who did have deficits on the Goldman–Fristoe. Across the sample, scores on the vocabulary measures and IQ were significantly correlated (for PPVT: $r(77) = .83$, $p < .001$; for EVT: $r(77) = .77$, $p < .001$). Nevertheless, IQ itself did not determine language subgroup. Over 25% of the children in the impaired language subgroup had IQ scores above 70, and 40% of the children in the normal language subgroup had IQ scores in the borderline or mentally retarded range (i.e., IQ scores below 85).

This first subgroup analysis captured most of the sample because it focused on the language tests that most children could do. However, it yielded only limited information about profiles within each subgroup because it omitted the broader range of language measures administered. A second subgroup analysis was conducted focusing on the children who were able to complete the CELF. Most of the 44 children in this analysis had nonverbal IQ scores in the normal range. These children were divided into normal, borderline, and impaired language groups based on total CELF standard scores using similar definitions as before. Thus, the normal language subgroup had CELF scores above 85 and just under 25% of the sample were included in this group. The borderline subgroup had CELF scores between 70 and 84, representing 30% of the sample. The impaired subgroup, whose CELF scores were below 70 (more than two standard deviations below the mean), represented almost half this sample of relatively high IQ children.

The language profiles for each subgroup are shown in Fig. 12.1. For this graph, the scores on the PPVT and EVT, which were normed on the same population, were combined to yield an overall vocabulary standard score. For the normal language subgroup, the scores on all the language measures were well within the normal range, representing a relatively flat profile. These children had normal phonological, lexical, and morphosyntactic abilities, as measured by the standardized tests used in this study. In contrast, the children in the other subgroups had deficits in higher order syntax and semantics (as measured by the CELF), vocabulary, and the ability to represent and reproduce novel phonological sequences, as measured by the NWRT. The children in the borderline and impaired subgroups did not,

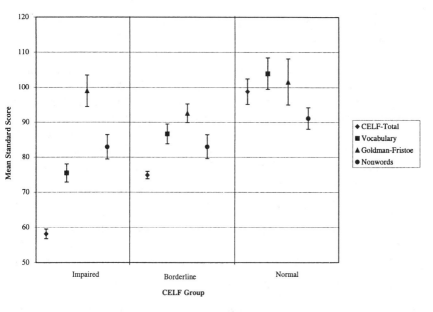

FIG. 12.1. Language profiles for each subgroup.

however, have deficits in basic articulation skills, replicating the pattern found for the larger sample in the previous subgroup analysis. The language test profiles for the borderline and language impaired subgroups are particularly revealing about the nature of language impairments in autism. They provide good evidence for the hypothesis that there is overlap between a subgroup of autism and SLI. First, deficits in simple articulation skills are not part of the description of language disorder in autism, confirming earlier studies (Bartolucci et al., 1976; Boucher, 1976). Second, the patterns of performance across the different language tests shown in Fig. 12.1 matches the profile found across these same kinds of tests in children with SLI (Tomblin & Zhang, 1999; see Rice, chap. 2 in this volume). For example, scores on the vocabulary measures were somewhat higher than the CELF scores, suggesting that lexical knowledge is generally less impaired than higher order language abilities. Nevertheless, vocabulary was below the mean for both the borderline (*M* = 87) and impaired (*M* = 75) subgroups.

Perhaps the most interesting finding was the poor performance by the language impaired subgroups on the NWRT. Given that children with autism are known for their excellent echolalic skills (defined as the ability to repeat words and phrases out of context and in the apparent absence of comprehension) and good articulation, it might have been predicted that across the board, the children in this study would have done well on the NWRT. Surprisingly, this was clearly not the case. Performance on the

NWRT distinguished well between children with normal language (M = 91) and children with borderline (M = 83) or impaired (M = 83) language.

What is the significance of finding that a subgroup of children with autism has great difficulty repeating nonsense words? The NWRT was included in the language battery because it is a standardized language test on which children with SLI demonstrate significant deficits (e.g., Bishop, North, & Donlan, 1996; Dollaghan & Campbell, 1998; Gathercole & Baddeley, 1990; Weismer et al., 2000). Indeed, poor performance on nonword repetition tests is now considered one of the primary clinical markers of SLI (Tager-Flusberg & Cooper, 1999). Data suggest that children with autism who have impaired language as measured on standard tests, such as the PPVT or CELF, also show difficulties in overall performance on nonsense word repetition.

A recent follow-up conducted a detailed analysis of the kinds of errors that autistic children make on a nonsense word repetition test to explore whether their error patterns were similar or different to those found in SLI (Condouris, Smith, Tager-Flusberg, & Arin, 2001). Using the nonsense word repetition test taken from the Comprehensive Test of Phonological Processing, 30 children with autism were audiotaped as they repeated the stimuli presented. The tapes were carefully transcribed phonetically, and then coded. The autistic children were able to maintain the overall syllabic structure of the stimuli, but made primarily substitution and deletion errors. Their errors confirm that the performance of language impaired children with autism on nonsense word repetition tasks is both quantitatively and qualitatively similar to children with SLI.

FOLLOW-UP STUDY ON LANGUAGE IMPAIRMENT IN AUTISM

Tense Marking in SLI

Current research on SLI has identified another important clinical marker of this disorder, at least for English speakers. This second marker involves measures of children's knowledge and processing of finite verb morphology. Thus, a number of studies have found that children with SLI tend to omit several finite verb-related morphemes in obligatory contexts, including the third person present tense *-s* (e.g., *John leave-s*) or the past tense regular (e.g., *John walk-ed*) or irregular (e.g., *John left*) forms (for a summary of the research and the theoretical model, see Wexler, chap. 1 in this volume; see also Bedore & Leonard, 1998; Rice & Wexler, 1996; Rice, Wexler, & Cleave, 1995; Rice, Haney, & Wexler, 1998). These findings of potential overlap between autism and SLI were followed by the exploration of whether the children with autism in the initial study who fell into the impaired language group would also show problems in marking tense (Roberts, Rice, & Tager-Flusberg, 2000). It is important to note, however, that the use of other morphological markers in these autistic children was not probed, leaving open the possibility that they had deficits in grammatical morphology that were not restricted to marking tense. Nevertheless, earlier studies on the use of grammatical morphemes in the spontaneous speech of children with autism identified selective deficits in marking the past tense (Bartolucci, Pierce, & Streiner, 1980; Howlin, 1984; Tager-Flusberg, 1989).

Methods

One year after completing the first study, the majority of the children returned for longitudinal follow-up studies. Data were collected from 62 (54 boys, 8 girls) of the children in the original sample of 89. Children were administered the following standardized language tests: PPVT, EVT, and NWRT. They were also given two experimental tasks, drawn from Rice and Wexler's groundbreaking work on tense in SLI (Rice et al., 1995). One task used linguistic probes to elicit the past tense, the other used probes to elicit the third person singular present tense marker.

On the past tense task, children were shown pictures of people engaged in activities and asked questions such as "*What happened?*" or "*What did he do with the rake?*" There were 11 trials designed to elicit regular past tense forms on lexical verbs (e.g., wash, color) and 8 intermixed trials to elicit irregular forms (e.g., catch, fall). On each trial, the experimenter first modeled the verb and then asked the probe questions. For the third person task, 12 pictures depicting people in various occupations (e.g., doctor, painter) were presented to the children. They were asked questions, such as "*Tell me what a doctor does.*" and "*What does a painter do?*" Children were probed until they produced a verb (any verb) in the third person (e.g., *He help/s people*).

Performance on Experimental Tense Tasks

Using the same definitions as in the previous study, PPVT standard scores were used to divide the 62 children into three language subgroups (normal, borderline, impaired). Most children were classified into the same subgroups as they were placed the year before, however their current PPVT standard scores were used to create the groups for this data analysis. Figure 12.2 shows the performance of the children on the tense marking tasks for the normal (25 children) and impaired subgroups (20 children). The normal language group gave almost twice as many correct responses as the impaired group, whose performance was between 30% and 40% correct on

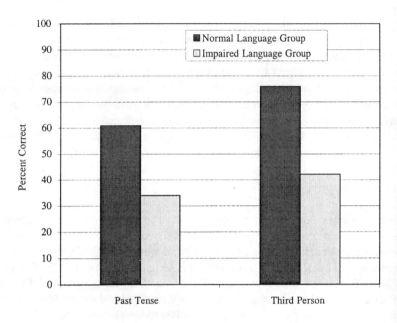

FIG. 12.2. Performance of the children on the tense marking tasks.

both tasks. The most common error pattern was to omit any morphologic‹ marking on the verb stem, the error most frequently reported for childre with SLI. On the past tense task the children were equally likely to produc these bare stem errors on the regular and irregular verbs, and made fe‹ overregularization errors (e.g., *falled*). Again, studies on children with S report similar findings (Marchman, Wulfeck, & Weismer, 1999; Rice, 1999‑

The older children in the sample performed somewhat better than tł younger children. The correlations between age and percent correct r sponses were $r(60) = .28$, $p = .05$ on the third person singular task and $r(60)$ .31, $p = .05$ on the past tense task. These findings suggest some improv ment over time in the morphological abilities of children with autism. Sir lar developmental change has been found in longitudinal studies of cł dren with SLI (See Rice, chap. 2 in this volume; Rice, Wexler, & Hershberg‹ 1998). In contrast, there were no significant relations between IQ and p‹ formance on the experimental tasks.

The final analysis explored the relation between the two clinical marke for SLI used in this study: the ability to mark grammatical tense and n‹ sense word repetition. For the third person singular task, the correlati with NWRT was $r(60) = .42$, $p < .01$, and for the past tense task the corre tion was $r(60) = .51$, $p < .01$. Similar findings have been found for childr with SLI (Conti-Ramsden, Botting, & Faragher, 2001). There are a number different explanations about why these measures of phonological repres‹

tation and grammatical morphology might be related in SLI (e.g., Chiat, 2001), however, the data do not address this more theoretical issue.

This follow-up study demonstrated that autistic children in the impaired language subgroup closely resembled children with SLI on a second clinical marker, namely, difficulties marking tense in finite clauses. These findings confirm that there are important parallels between the language profile of a subgroup of children with autism, and what is known about the language characteristics of children with SLI. Taken together, the studies reported provide strong evidence that there is a subgroup of children with autism whose language deficits essentially meet all known criteria for SLI.

IMPLICATIONS OF CURRENT RESEARCH

Autism and SLI as Overlapping Populations

How might these close links between autism and SLI be interpreted? As noted earlier, Churchill (1972) proposed that autism was simply an extreme form of SLI, but this theory was rejected on the basis of detailed comparative studies by Bartak et al. (1975, 1977). The view presented here is closer to Rutter's (1965) perspective, in that it is hypothesized that autism and SLI are *overlapping populations* (cf. Bishop, 2000). More specifically, there is a subgroup of children with autism who also have SLI. On this view, language impairment or SLI is a co-occurring disorder in some, but not all, children with autism. Thus, SLI is not a defining feature of autism because there are clearly children with autism but without any linguistic deficits (as in the normal language group), but it does occur in a significantly large subgroup of the population.

Genetic Links Between Autism and SLI

Evidence for overlap of autism and SLI from family studies was presented earlier. In addition to this behavioral evidence, recent genetic linkage and association studies offer further clues to some shared genetic basis for these disorders. The first genetic study of SLI was conducted on a unique family living in England, known as the KE family. Half the members of this large three-generation family are affected by a severe speech and language disorder that is transmitted as an autosomal dominant single gene trait. The gene was localized to the long arm of chromosome 7 (in the region of 7q31), and dubbed SPCH1 (Fisher, Vargha-Khadem, Watkins, Monaco, & Pembrey, 1998; Lai et al., 2000). Tomblin and his colleagues followed up this important finding in an association study, using their population-based sample of children with SLI (Tomblin, Nishimura, Zhang, & Murray, 1998).

They found a significant association between SLI and an allele of the CFTR gene, which is in the 7q31 region where SPCH1 is located. Thus, there is strong evidence that there is a gene (or genes) located on the long arm of chromosome 7 that contributes to SLI.

In autism, there are no pedigrees as rich as the KE family in the literature. Instead, the primary strategy for finding genes associated with this disorder thus far has been to study multiplex families in which more than one family member, usually siblings, received a diagnosis of autism. Genome-wide scans of such families suggest linkage between autism and the long arm of chromosome 7, in the neighborhood of the SPCH1 gene (e.g., Barrett et al., 1999; IMGSAC, 1998, 2001). There have also been several recent studies of small pedigrees with known chromosomal abnormalities in this region, associated with either language disorder or autism (e.g., Ashley-Koch et al., 1999).

At this point, the cumulative evidence for some shared gene in autism and SLI is becoming quite strong both from family and genetic linkage studies. The current working hypothesis is that this putative gene on chromosome 7q.31 codes for at least some aspects of the language disorder found in a subgroup of individuals with autism, and for aspects of the phenotype of SLI (cf. Folstein & Mankoski, 2000). Further research is needed to pinpoint the specific gene or genes on 7q.31 associated with these disorders, and epidemiological studies should be conducted that will identify the proportion of the autistic population that shares the SLI language profile.

Neurobiological Links Between Autism and SLI

Genetic factors lead to phenotypes, or the cognitive and behavioral impairments associated with a neurodevelopmental disorder, by influencing the development and organization of the brain from the earliest embryological stages. If subgroups within autism and SLI have common underlying genetic abnormalities, then it would be hypothesized that they would show similar atypical patterns of brain structure and function. Thus far there have been several studies of brain structure in SLI, but almost no published work or functional neuroimaging methods, using language-related tasks in either autism or SLI.

The most consistent finding in studies of children and adults with SLI is that they show different patterns of brain asymmetry when compared to non-SLI controls. In normal individuals, left cortical regions, especially in key language areas (perisylvian region, planum temporale and Heschel's gyrus), are enlarged relative to the size of those regions in the right hemisphere. In contrast, individuals with SLI or with language-based learning disorders show reduced or reversed asymmetries in these areas (Clark & Plante, 1998; Galaburda, 1989; Jernigan, Hesselink, Sowell, & Tallal, 1991; Leonard et al., 1996; Plante, Swisher, Vance, & Rapcsak, 1991).

There have been no comparative studies of autistic and SLI children, and there are no published studies investigating cortical asymmetry in autism. A magnetic resonance imaging (MRI) study was completed comparing 16 boys with autism (all with normal nonverbal IQ scores) to 15 age, sex, and handedness matched normal controls (Herbert et al., 2002). The main findings were that the autistic boys had significant *reversal* of asymmetry in the inferior lateral frontal cortex, which was 27% larger in the right hemisphere as compared to 17% larger in the left hemisphere for the controls. These findings parallel the MRI findings from boys with SLI, and further confirm similarities between these two groups.

COMPARING SLI TO OTHER NEURODEVELOPMENTAL DISORDERS

This chapter has argued that the primary characteristics of language impairment that define SLI may also be found in a subgroup of children with a different complex disorder, namely, autism. These parallels between autism and SLI open up the question of whether there are other neurodevelopmental disorders in which similar language impairments may be found (see also Crago & Paradis, chap. 3, and de Villiers, chap. 17, in this volume). The next section explores the language deficits found in Down syndrome.

Language Impairment in Down Syndrome

Down syndrome (DS) is the most common genetically based (chromosomal) neurodevelopmental disorder, identified by the presence of an extra copy of chromosome 21. Generally, IQ scores range between 45 and 55, although, as in all neurodevelopmental disorders, there is wide variability (cf. Tager-Flusberg, 1999c). Recent investigations of the phenotype of DS suggest that language is relatively more impaired than other cognitive functions, although the sources and nature of this deficit have not yet been resolved (Chapman, 1995; Fowler, 1990; Miller, 1988, 1992). Because DS is identified at birth, studies of language impairment in this population have the advantage of allowing prospective developmental studies beginning before the onset of language.

During the first stages of development, language and related communicative abilities show significant delays, which are most evident in delayed babbling and phonological deficits that persist into later childhood (e.g., Lynch, Oller, Eilers, & Basinger, 1990; Stoel-Gammon, 1980). These delays are beyond those expected given the cognitive mental age levels of the children with DS in these studies.

The most significant deficits in language during later stages are in expressive language, particularly in the acquisition of syntax and grammatical morphology (e.g., Chapman, 1997). Although most studies on DS language have been descriptive, rather than driven by linguistic theory, these primary deficits in grammar parallel those found in SLI. Morphological deficits in DS are quite striking (Bol & Kuiken, 1990), but are generally more severe compared to SLI. Finally, it is interesting to note that, as in SLI, nonword repetition is significantly impaired in DS (Laws, 1998). Taken together, these findings indicate that language impairment in DS shares the same primary clinical markers identified for SLI, and in studies of language impaired children with autism. Although fewer studies have explored language deficits in other neurodevelopmental disorders, there are some signs that similar features may be found, for example, in fragile X syndrome or in Prader-Willi syndrome (see Tager-Flusberg, 1999a, for a review, and see Levy, chap. 14 in this volume).

Similarities of Language Impairment Across a Range of Populations

What is the significance of these shared patterns of language impairment across a number of different populations? Do they challenge the hypothesis presented earlier, which states that the similarity between autism and SLI suggests common underlying genes influencing the language impairments in these populations? These are difficult questions, but they address the heart of the issue regarding the uniqueness and significance of SLI as a distinct developmental language disorder (see Crago & Paradis, chap. 3, and deVilliers, chap. 17, in this volume for discussion of these issues). It is also impossible to provide definitive answers because there are no good comparative and detailed studies that may begin to dissect the language phenotypes associated with any of these neurodevelopmental disorders.

One possibility is that although these disorders seem to be related to one another, the similarities noted here are quite superficial; in fact, they might be fundamentally different, with little in common between DS and SLI. On this view, the distinct genetic etiology of DS on the one hand, and shared genetic etiology of autism and SLI on the other, lead to different patterns of language impairment that are only parallel to one another at a descriptive level. Another possibility is that the pattern of language impairment found in SLI, autism, and these other disorders represent a final common pathway. Different genes may influence language acquisition in the same way, leading to the same language phenotype by exerting a similar influence on how the brain becomes organized for language from the earliest embryological stages. There is, at this point, insufficient evidence that would allow choosing between these and other possible interpretations of the apparent similarities between SLI and other neurodevelopmental disorders. Nevertheless, future research should be directed toward identifying the genetic, neurobiological, and cognitive mechanisms that underlie language impairments across a broad range of neurodevelopmental disorders in order to answer some questions about parallel patterns of language deficit.

CONCLUSIONS

For over 30 years, researchers have considered the relation between autism and developmental language disorders, especially SLI (cf. Bishop, 2000). The research summarized in this chapter presents new evidence that there is overlap between the populations. Specifically, there is now strong evidence that a subgroup of children with autism share the same phenotypic features of language impairment that characterize SLI; genetic studies point to linkage to the same region of SLI; and the same pattern of atypical brain asymmetry has been found in studies using MRI.

The language impaired subgroup in autism suggests that SLI can occur within autism, but it is not part of the diagnostic criteria for autism. Given the evidence for biological overlap, it seems appropriate to consider SLI as a comorbid disorder in autism. In a similar way, other psychiatric disorders, such as affective disorder or obsessive-compulsive disorder, can also be present in autism and count as co-morbidities (e.g., Kerbeshian & Burd, 1996; Lainhart & Folstein, 1994; McDougle et al., 1995). Interestingly, current classification schemes (e.g., APA, 1994) rule out the diagnosis of SLI in the presence of autism. It may, however, prove useful and appropriate to allow SLI as a secondary diagnosis when a person meets all the other inclusionary diagnostic criteria for the disorder. The most important reason for giving a child a diagnosis is to provide guidelines for the kinds of therapeutic interventions that may be offered. Perhaps, therefore, the greatest significance of the research program discussed in this chapter is that it may offer new perspectives on developing interventions for language impairment in children with autism, SLI, and perhaps other neurodevelopmental disorders.

ACKNOWLEDGMENTS

Preparation of this chapter was supported by grants from the National Institute on Deafness and Other Communication Disorders (PO1 DC 03610) and the National Institute on Neurological Diseases and Stroke (RO1 NS 38668).

REFERENCES

APA (1994). *DSM–IV: Diagnostic and statistic manual of mental disorders* (4th ed.). Washington, DC: American Psychiatric Association.

Ashley-Koch, A., Wolpert, C. M., Menold, M. M., Zaeem, L., Basu, S., Donnelly, S. L., Ravan, S. A., Powell, C. M., Qumsiyeh, M. B., Aylsworth, A. S., Vance, J. M., Gilbert, J. R., Wright, H. H., Abramson, R. K., DeLong, G. R., Cuccaro, M. L., & Pericak-Vance, M. A. (1999). Genetic studies of autistic disorder and chromosome 7. *Genomics, 61*, 227–236.

Bailey, A., Le Couteur, A., Gottesman, I., Bolton, P., Simonoff, E., Yuzda, E., & Rutter, M. (1995). Autism as a strongly genetic disorder: Evidence from a British twin study. *Psychological Medicine, 25*, 63–77.

Bailey, A., Palferman, S., Heavey, L., & Le Couteur, A. (1998). Autism: The phenotype in relatives. *Journal of Autism and Developmental Disorders, 28*, 369–392.

Bailey, A., Phillips, W., & Rutter, M. (1996). Autism: Towards an integration of clinical, genetic, neuropsychological, and neurobiological perspectives. *Journal of Child Psychology and Psychiatry, 37*, 89–126.

Barrett, S., Beck, J. C., Bernier, R., Bisson, E., Braun, T. A., Casavant, T. L., Childress, D., Folstein, S., Garcia, M., Gardiner, M., Gilman, S., Haines, J. L., Hopkins, K., Landa, R., Meyer, N., Mullane, J., Nishimura, D., Palmer, P., Piven, J., Purdy, J., Santangelo, S., Searby, C., Sheffield, V., Singleton, J., & Slager, S. (1999). An autosomal genomic screen for autism. Collaborative linkage study of autism. *American Journal of Medical Genetics, 88*, 609–615.

Bartak, L., Rutter, M., & Cox, A. (1975). A comparative study of infantile autism and specific developmental receptive language disorder: I. The children. *British Journal of Psychiatry, 126*, 127–145.

Bartak, L., Rutter, M., & Cox, A. (1977). A comparative study of infantile autism and specific developmental receptive language disorders: II. Discriminant function analysis. *Journal of Autism and Childhood Schizophrenia, 7*, 383–396.

Bartolucci, G., & Albers, R. J. (1974). Deictic categories in the language of autistic children. *Journal of Autism and Childhood Schizophrenia, 4*, 131–141.

Bartolucci, G., & Pierce, S. (1977). A preliminary comparison of phonological development in autistic, normal, and mentally retarded subjects. *British Journal of Disorders of Communication, 12*, 137–147.

Bartolucci, G., Pierce, S., & Streiner, D. (1980). Cross-sectional studies of grammatical morphemes in autistic and mentally retarded children. *Journal of Autism and Developmental Disorders, 10*, 39–50.

Bartolucci, G., Pierce, S., Streiner, D., & Eppel, P. (1976). Phonological investigation of verbal autistic and mentally retarded subjects. *Journal of Autism and Childhood Schizophrenia, 6*, 303–315.

Bedore, L. M., & Leonard, L. B. (1998). Specific language impairment and grammatical morphology: A discriminant function analysis. *Journal of Speech Language and Hearing Research, 41*, 1185–1192.

Bishop, D. (2000). Pragmatic language impairment. In D. V. M. Bishop & L. B. Leonard (Eds.), *Speech and language impairments in children: Causes, characteristics, intervention and outcom* (pp. 99–113). East Sussex: Psychology Press Ltd.

Bishop, D., Chan, J., Hartley, J., Adams, C., & Weir, F. (2000). Conversational responsiveness in specific language impairment: Evidence of disproportionate pragmatic difficulties in a subset of children. *Development and Psychopathology, 12*, 177–199.

Bishop, D., North, T., & Donlan, C. (1995). Genetic basis of specific language impairment: Evidence from a twin study. *Developmental Medicine and Child Neurology, 37*, 56–71.

Bishop, D., North, T., & Donlan, C. (1996). Nonword repetition as a behavioural marker for inherited language impairment: Evidence from a twin study. *Journal of Child Psychology and Psychiatry, 36*, 1–13.

Bishop, D., & Rosenbloom, L. (1987). Classification of childhood language disorders. In W. Yule & M. Rutter (Eds.), *Language development and disorders: Clinics in developmental medicine* (pp. 16–41). London: MacKeith Press.

Bol, G., & Kuiken, F. (1990). Grammatical analysis of developmental language disorders: A study of the morphosyntax of children with specific language disorders, with hearing impairment and with Down's syndrome. *Clinical Linguistics and Phonetics, 4,* 77–86.

Bolton, P., Macdonald, H., Pickles, A., Rios, P., Goode, S., Crowson, M., Bailey, A., & Rutter, M. (1994). A case-control family history study of autism. *Journal of Child Psychology and Psychiatry, 35,* 877–900.

Boucher, J. (1976). Articulation in early childhood autism. *Journal of Autism and Childhood Schizophrenia, 6,* 297–302.

Boucher, J. (1998). SPD as a distinct diagnostic entity: Logical considerations and directions for future research. *International Journal of Language and Communication Disorders, 33,* 71–81.

Capps, L., Kehres, J., & Sigman, M. (1998). Conversational abilities among children with autism and children with developmental delays. *Autism, 2,* 325–344.

Chapman, R. (1995). Language development in children and adolescents with Down syndrome. In P. Fletcher & B. MacWhinney (Eds.), *The handbook of child language* (pp. 641–663). Oxford, England: Blackwell.

Chapman, R. S. (1997). Language development in children and adolescents with Down syndrome. *Mental Retardation and Developmental Disabilities Research Reviews, 3,* 307–312.

Chiat, S. (2001). Mapping theories of developmental language impairment: Premises, predictions and evidence. *Language and Cognitive Processes, 16,* 113–142.

Churchill, D. W. (1972). The relation of infantile autism and early childhood schizophrenia to developmental language disorders of childhood. *Journal of Autism and Childhood Schizophrenia, 2,* 182–197.

Clark, M. M., & Plante, E. (1998). Morphology of the inferior frontal gyrus in developmentally language-disordered adults. *Brain & Language, 61,* 288–303.

Condouris, K., Smith, J. L., Tager-Flusberg, H., & Arin, D. (2001, November). *Children with autism's performance on a nonword repetition task: Evidence of an SLI subgroup.* Paper presented at the meeting of the American Speech and Hearing Association, New Orleans, LA.

Conti-Ramsden, G., Botting, N., & Faragher, B. (2001). Psycholinguistic markers for specific language impairment. *Journal of Child Psychology and Psychiatry, 42,* 741–748.

Conti-Ramsden, G., Crutchley, A., & Botting, N. (1997). The extent to which psychometric tests differentiate subgroups of children with SLI. *Journal of Speech, Language, and Hearing Research, 40,* 765–777.

Dale, P., Simonoff, E., Bishop, D. V. M., Eley, T. C., Oliver, B., Price, T. S., Purcell, S., Stevenson, J., & Plomin, R. (1998). Genetic influence on language delay in two-year-old children. *Nature Neuroscience, 1,* 324–328.

Dollaghan, C., & Campbell, T. (1998). Nonword repetition and child language impairment. *Journal of Speech, Language, and Hearing Research, 41,* 1136–1146.

Dunn, L. M., & Dunn, L. M. (1997). *Peabody Picture Vocabulary Test* (3rd ed.). Circle Pines, MN: American Guidance Service.

Fisher, S. E., Vargha-Khadem, F., Watkins, K. E., Monaco, A. P., & Pembrey, M. E. (1998). Localisation of a gene implicated in a severe speech and language. *Nature Genetics, 18,* 168–170.

Folstein, S., & Rutter, M. (1974). Genetic influences and infantile autism. *Nature, 265,* 726–728.

Folstein, S., & Rutter, M. (1977). Infantile autism: A genetic study of 21 twin pairs. *Journal of Child Psychology and Psychiatry, 18,* 297–321.

Folstein, S. E., & Mankoski, R. E. (2000). Chromosome 7q: Where autism meets language disorder? *American Journal of Human Genetics, 67,* 278–281.

Fombonne, E. (1999). The epidemiology of autism: A review. *Psychological Medicine, 29,* 769–786.

Fombonne, E., Bolton, P., Prior, J., Jordan, H., & Rutter, M. (1997). A family study of autism: Cognitive patterns and levels in parents and siblings. *Journal of Child Psychology and Psychiatry, 38*, 667–684.

Fowler, A. (1990). Language abilities in children with Down syndrome: Evidence for a specific syntactic delay. In D. Cicchetti & M. Beeghly (Eds.), *Children with Down syndrome: A developmental perspective* (pp. 302–328). New York: Cambridge University Press.

Galaburda, A. (1989). Ordinary and extraordinary brain development: Anatomical variation in developmental dyslexia. *Annals of Dyslexia, 39*, 67–79.

Gathercole, S., & Baddeley, A. (1990). Phonological memory deficits in language disordered children: Is there a causal connection? *Journal of Memory and Language, 29*, 336–360.

Goldman, R., & Fristoe, M. (1986). *Goldman–Fristoe Test of Articulation.* Circle Pines, MN: American Guidance Service.

Hadley, P., & Rice, M. (1991). Conversational responsiveness of speech and language impaired preschoolers. *Journal of Speech and Hearing Research, 34*, 1308–1317.

Hafeman, L., & Tomblin, J. B. (1999). Autism behaviors in the siblings of children with specific language impairment. *Molecular Psychiatry, 4* (Suppl. 1), S14.

Herbert, M., Adrie, K., Makris, N., Kennedy, D., Lange, N., Bakardjiev, A., Hodgson, J., Takeoka, M., Tager-Flusberg, H., & Caviness, V. (2002). *Abnormal asymmetry in language association cortex in autism.* Unpublished manuscript.

Howlin, P. (1984). The acquisition of grammatical morphemes in autistic children: A critique and replication of the findings of Bartolucci, Pierce, and Streiner, 1980. *Journal of Autism and Developmental Disorders, 14*, 127–136.

International Molecular Genetic Study of Autism Consortium. (1998). A full genome screen for autism with evidence for linkage to a region on chromosome 7q. *Human Molecular Genetics, 7*, 571–578.

International Molecular Genetic Study of Autism Consortium (IMGSAC). (2001). Further characterization of the autism susceptibility locus AUTS1 on chromosomal 7q. *Human Molecular Genetics, 10*, 973–982.

Jarrold, C., Boucher, J., & Russell, J. (1997). Language profiles in children with autism: Theoretical and methodological implications. *Autism, 1*, 57–76.

Jernigan, T., Hesselink, J., Sowell, E., & Tallal, P. A. (1991). Cerebral structure on magnetic resonance imaging in language- and learning-impaired children. *Archives of Neurology, 48*, 539–545.

Kanner, L. (1943). Autistic disturbances of affective contact. *Nervous Child, 2*, 217–250.

Kanner, L. (1946). Irrelevant and metaphorical language. *American Journal of Psychiatry, 103*, 242–246.

Kerbeshian, J., & Burd, L. (1996). Comorbidity among Tourette's syndrome, autistic disorder and bipolar disorder. *Journal of the American Academy of Child & Adolescent Psychiatry, 35*, 681–685.

Kjelgaard, M., & Tager-Flusberg, H. (2001). An investigation of language impairment in autism: Implications for genetic subgroups. *Language and Cognitive Processes, 16*, 287–308.

Korkman, M., Kirk, U., & Kemp, S. (1998). *NEPSY: A developmental neuropsychological assessment.* San Antonio: The Psychological Corporation.

Lai, C. S., Fisher, S. E., Hurst, J. A., Levy, E. R., Hodgson, S., Fox, M., Jeremiah, S., Povey, S., Jamison, D. C., Green, E. D., Vargha-Khadem, F., & Monaco, A. P. (2000). The speech region of human 7q.31: Genomic characterization of the critical interval and localization of translocations associated with speech and language disorder. *American Journal of Human Genetics, 67*, 357–368.

Lainhart, J. E., & Folstein, S. E. (1994). Affective disorders in people with autism: A review of published cases. *Journal of Autism & Developmental Disorders, 24*, 587–601.

Laws, G. (1998). The use of nonword repetition as a test of phonological memory in children with Down syndrome. *Journal of Child Psychology and Psychiatry, 39*, 1119–1130.

Le Couteur, A., Bailey, A., Goode, S., Pickles, A., Robertson, S., Gottesman, I., & Rutter, M. (1996). A broader phenotype of autism: The clinical spectrum in twins. *Journal of Child Psychology and Psychiatry, 37,* 785–801.

Leonard, C., Lombardino, L. J., Mercado, L. R., Browd, S., Breier, J., & Agee, O. (1996). Cerebral asymmetry and cognitive development in children: A magnetic resonance imaging study. *Psychological Science, 7,* 79–85.

Lister-Brook, S., & Bowler, D. (1992). Autism by another name? Semantic and pragmatic impairments in children. *Journal of Autism and Developmental Disorders, 22,* 61–82.

Lord, C., & Paul, R. (1997). Language and communication in autism. In D. J. Cohen & F. R. Volkmar (Eds.), *Handbook of autism and pervasive development disorders* (2nd ed., pp. 195–225). New York: Wiley.

Lord, C., Risi, S., Lambrecht, L., Cook, E. H., Leventhal, B. L., DiLavore, P. C., Pickles, A., & Rutter, M. (2000). The autism diagnostic observation schedule-generic: A standard measure of social and communication deficits associated with the spectrum of autism. *Journal of Autism and Developmental Disorders, 30,* 205–223.

Lord, C., Rutter, M., & Le Couteur, A. (1994). Autism Diagnostic Interview–Revised: A revised version of a diagnostic interview for caregivers of individuals with possible pervasive developmental disorders. *Journal of Autism and Developmental Disorders, 24,* 659–685.

Loveland, K., & Tunali, B. (1993). Narrative language in autism and the theory of mind hypothesis: A wider perspective. In S. Baron-Cohen, H. Tager-Flusberg, & D. J. Cohen (Eds.), *Understanding other minds: Perspectives from autism* (pp. 247–266). Oxford, England: Oxford University Press.

Loveland, K., Landry, S., Hughes, S., Hall, S., & McEvoy, R. (1988). Speech acts and the pragmatic deficits of autism. *Journal of Speech and Hearing Research, 31,* 593–604.

Lynch, M., Oller, K., Eilers, R., & Basinger, D. (1990, June). *Vocal development of infants with Down's syndrome.* Paper presented at the symposium for Research on Child Language Disorders, Madison, WI.

Marchman, V. A., Wulfeck, B., & Weismer, S. E. (1999). Morphological productivity in children with normal language and SLI: A study of the English past tense. *Journal of Speech Language and Hearing Research, 42,* 206–219.

McDougle, C. J., Kresch, L. E., Goodman, W. K., Naylor, S. T., Volkmar, F. R., Cohen, D. J., & Price, L. H. (1995). A case-controlled study of repetitive thoughts and behavior in adults with autistic disorder and obsessive-compulsive disorder. *American Journal of Psychiatry, 152,* 772–777.

Miller, J. (1988). The developmental asynchrony of language development in children with Down syndrome. In L. Nadel (Ed.), *The psychobiology of Down syndrome* (pp. 167–198). Cambridge, MA: MIT Press.

Miller, J. (1992). Development of speech and language in children with Down syndrome. In I. T. Lott & E. E. McCoy (Eds.), *Down syndrome: Advances in medical care* (pp. 39–50). New York: Wiley-Liss.

Miller, J. (1991). Research on language disorders in children: A progress report. In J. Miller (Ed.), *Research on child language disorders* (pp. 3–22). Austin, TX: Pro-Ed.

Pierce, S., & Bartolucci, G. (1977). A syntactic investigation of verbal autistic, mentally retarded and normal children. *Journal of Autism and Childhood Schizophrenia, 7,* 121–134.

Piven, J. (1999). Genetic liability for autism: The behavioral expression in relatives. *International Review of Psychiatry, 11,* 299–308.

Piven, J., Palmer, P., Landa, R., Santangelo, S., Jacobi, D., & Childress, D. (1997). Personality and language characteristics in parents from multiple-incidence autism families. *American Journal of Medical Genetics, 74,* 398–411.

Plante, E., Swisher, L., Vance R., & Rapcsak S. (1991). MRI findings in boys with specific language impairment. *Brain & Language, 41,* 52–66.

Rapin, I., & Allen, D. (1983). Developmental language disorders: Nosologic considerations. In U. Kirk (Ed.), *Neuropsychology of language, reading, and spelling* (pp. 155–184). New York: Academic Press.

Rice, M. L. (1999). Specific grammatical limitations in children with specific language impairment. In H. Tager-Flusberg (Ed.), *Neurodevelopmental disorders* (pp. 331–359). Cambridge, MA: MIT Press.

Rice, M. L., Haney, K. R., & Wexler, K. (1998). Family histories of children with SLI who show extended optional infinitives. *Journal of Speech Language and Hearing Research, 41*, 419–432.

Rice, M. L., & Wexler, K. (1996). Toward tense as a clinical marker of specific language impairment in English-speaking children. *Journal of Speech and Hearing Research, 39*, 1239–1257.

Rice, M. L., Wexler, K., & Cleave, P. L. (1995). Specific language impairment as a period of extended optional infinitive. *Journal of Speech & Hearing Research, 38*, 850–863.

Rice, M. L., Wexler, K., & Hershberger, S. (1998). Tense over time: The longitudinal course of tense acquisition in children with specific language impairment. *Journal of Speech Language & Hearing Research, 41*, 1412–1431.

Roberts, J., Rice, M., & Tager-Flusberg, H. (2000, June). *Tense marking in children with autism: Further evidence for overlap between autism and SLI.* Paper presented at the symposium on Research in Child Language Disorders, Madison, WI.

Rutter, M. (1965). The influence of organic and emotional factors on the origins, nature, and outcome of childhood psychosis. *Developmental Medicine and Child Neurology, 7*, 518–528.

Rutter, M. (1970). Autistic children: Infancy to adulthood. *Seminars in Psychiatry, 2*, 435–450.

Santangelo, S. L., & Folstein, S. E. (1999). Autism: A genetic perspective. In H. Tager-Flusberg (Ed.), *Neurodevelopmental disorders* (pp. 431–447). Cambridge, MA: MIT Press.

Semel, E., Wiig, E. H., & Secord, W. A. (1995). *Clinical Evaluation of Language Fundamentals* (3rd ed.). San Antonio: The Psychological Corporation.

Stoel-Gammon, C. (1980). Phonological analysis of four Down's syndrome children. *Applied Psycholinguistics, 1*, 31–48.

Tager-Flusberg, H. (1985). Constraints on the representation of word meaning: Evidence from autistic and mentally retarded children. In S. A. Kuczaj & M. Barrett (Eds.), *The development of word meaning* (pp. 139–166). New York: Springer-Verlag.

Tager-Flusberg, H. (1989). A psycholinguistic perspective on language development in the autistic child. In G. Dawson (Ed.), *Autism: New directions in diagnosis, nature and treatment* (pp. 92–115). New York: Guilford.

Tager-Flusberg, H. (1994). Dissociations in form and function in the acquisition of language by autistic children. In H. Tager-Flusberg (Ed.), *Constraints on language acquisition: Studies of atypical children* (pp. 175–194). Hillsdale, NJ: Lawrence Erlbaum Associates.

Tager-Flusberg, H. (1999a). Language development in atypical children. In M. Barrett (Ed.), *The development of language* (pp. 311–348). Hove, Sussex: Psychology Press.

Tager-Flusberg, H. (1999b). A psychological approach to understanding the social and language impairments in autism. *International Review of Psychiatry, 11*, 325–334.

Tager-Flusberg, H. (1999c). Introduction to research on neurodevelopmental disorders from a cognitive neuroscience perspective. In H. Tager-Flusberg (Ed.), *Neurodevelopmental disorders* (pp. 3–24). Cambridge, MA: MIT Press.

Tager-Flusberg, H., & Anderson, M. (1991). The development of contingent discourse ability in autistic children. *Journal of Child Psychology and Psychiatry, 32*, 1123–1134.

Tager-Flusberg, H., & Cooper, J. (1999). Present and future possibilities for defining a phenotype for specific language impairment. *Journal of Speech, Language, and Hearing Research, 42*, 1001–1004.

Tager-Flusberg, H., & Sullivan, K. (1995). Attributing mental states to story characters: A comparison of narratives produced by autistic and mentally retarded individuals. *Applied Psycholinguistics, 16*, 241–256.

Tomblin, J. B., & Buckwalter, P. (1998). Heritability of poor language achievement among twins. *Journal of Speech, Language, and Hearing Research, 41*, 188–199.

Tomblin, J. B., Freese, P. R., & Records, N. L. (1992). Diagnosing specific language impairment in adults for the purpose of pedigree analysis. *Journal of Speech and Hearing Research, 35*, 832–843.

Tomblin, J. B., Nishimura, C., Zhang, X., & Murray, J. (1998). Association of Developmental Language Impairment with Loci at 7q31. *American Journal of Human Genetics* (Suppl. 63), A312.

Tomblin, J. B., & Zhang, X. (1999). Language patterns and etiology in children with specific language impairment. In H. Tager-Flusberg (Ed.), *Neurodevelopmental disorders* (pp. 361–382). Cambridge, MA: MIT Press.

Ventner, A., Lord, C., & Schopler, E. (1992). A follow-up study of high-functioning autistic children. *Journal of Child Psychology and Psychiatry, 33*, 489–507.

Weismer, S. E., Tomblin, J. B., Zhang, X., Buckwalter, P., Chynoweth, J. G., & Jones, M. (2000). Nonword repetition performance in school-age children with and without language impairment. *Journal of Speech, Language, and Hearing Research, 43*, 865–878.

Wetherby, A. (1986). Ontogeny of communication functions in autism. *Journal of Autism and Developmental Disorders, 16*, 295–316.

Wiig, E. H., Secord, W., & Semel, E. (1992). *Clinical Evaluation of Language Fundamentals—Preschool*. San Antonio: The Psychological Corporation.

Wilkinson, K. (1998). Profiles of language and communication skills in autism. *Mental Retardation and Developmental Disabilities Research Reviews, 4*, 73–79.

Williams, K. T. (1997). *Expressive Vocabulary Test*. Circle Pines, MN: American Guidance Service.

13

Words and Rules in Children with Williams Syndrome

Harald Clahsen
Christine Temple
University of Essex

Williams syndrome (WS) is a genetic disorder, with an incidence of 1 in 25,000, associated with learning difficulties (Greenberg, 1990). It is caused by a microdeletion on the long arm of chromosome 7 at 7q11.23, which affects one allele of the elastin gene and other contiguous genes (Ewart et al., 1993; Frangiskakis et al., 1996; Tassabehji et al., 1996). Within cognitive skills, there is a spatial disorder, for example, in drawing and relative strength in language. The development of language is also uneven, but there is dispute about the actual performance on language tasks and the best theoretical interpretation of this performance.

Investigating morphosyntactic skills in subjects with WS, Clahsen and Almazan (1998, 2001) found that the subjects with WS do not show any syntactic impairment, and they perform excellently on regular past tense and regular plural inflection. On the other hand, their scores on irregular past tense and irregular plural forms were found to be lower than those of unimpaired mental age controls, and the subjects with WS were seen to use regular rules of inflection excessively, even in circumstances in which unimpaired children (and adults) would not use them. Another finding from these studies was that the grammatical profile of WS does not extend to children with specific language impairment (SLI). A comparison of the results from the WS subjects to those of SLI studies using the same experimental tasks revealed differences, with the SLI children showing weaknesses on syntactic tasks and regular inflection paired with relatively well-preserved lexical skills.

Clahsen and Almazan (1998, 2001) proposed an account of the unusual pattern of morphosyntactic skills in WS, in terms of a modular view of the language faculty in which the knowledge of language is assumed to consist of two separate components, a lexicon of stored entries and a computational system of combinatorial operations to form larger linguistic expressions (e.g., Chomsky 1995; Pinker, 1999). They argued that these two core modules of language are dissociated in WS such that the computational (rule-based) system for language is selectively spared, whereas lexical representations and/or their access procedures are impaired. They also argued that this pattern of skill dissociation does not hold for SLI.

This chapter provides new evidence from three sources for a modular account of the linguistic skills of subjects with WS. Results are presented on the use of comparative adjectives, receptive and productive vocabularies, and reading skills in WS. It is argued that the new findings provide further support for a modular account and for the hypothesis of a selective lexical deficit in WS. In addition, a critique is presented of the nonmodular connectionist model that Thomas and Karmiloff-Smith (1999) and Thomas et al. (2001) proposed to explain the past tense performance of subjects with WS.

COMPARATIVE ADJECTIVES IN WS

Previous studies of morphological skills in subjects with WS have focused on two phenomena, the past tense and noun plurals (Bromberg, Ullman, Marcus, Kelly, & Coppola, 1994; Clahsen & Almazan, 1998, 2001; Thomas et al., 2001; Zukowski, 2001). To determine whether the findings from these studies generalize to other morphological phenomena, this chapter examines how subjects with WS form comparative adjectives. Moreover, in order to assess to what extent the WS data are similar or different to the way SLI subjects form comparative adjectives, results from an SLI study on comparative adjective formation are reported in which the same experimental task was used that was employed for the WS subjects.

Gradable adjectives in English can form comparatives by -er suffixation (*big–bigger*) and/or by a periphrastic form with *more* (*unusual–more unusual*). In addition, a small number of highly frequent adjectives have suppletive comparative forms (*good–better, bad–worse*). For most adjectives, the suffixed and the periphrastic comparative are in complementary distribution, but for some adjectives, both options exist (see Aronoff, 1976; Barber, 1964; Frank, 1972). The use of -er suffixation is to a certain extent constrained by syllable structure, in addition to other factors: monosyllabic adjectives typically form -er comparatives, likewise disyllabic adjectives ending in -y (e.g., *happy*), but the comparative of most other adjectives with more than one syllable is formed periphrastically (e.g., *more modern*). This distribution, however, is not without exceptions. Aronoff (1976) cited **apter* versus *stupider* as exceptions. Note also that monosyllabic adjectives can readily be used with *more*, when a speaker wants to emphasize the idea of comparison, for example, by adding a *than* clause (*John is more mad than Bob*) and in the so-called correlative construction (*The more old he is, the more wise he becomes*). Moreover, borrowed gradable adjectives, even monosyllabic ones, resist *-er* suffixation (*chic–*chicer, macho–*machoer*). Even though most disyllabic adjectives take periphrastic comparatives, there are many that require the suffixed comparative, for example, adjectives ending in *-ple, -ble, -tle,* and *-dle* (*simpler, nobler, subtler, idler*). Finally, disyllabic adjectives ending in *-ly, -ow, -some,* and *-er* (e.g., *lovely, narrow, handsome, clever*), as well as those with initial or final syllable stress (e.g., *pleasant, profound*) have both comparative options available, according to Frank (1972).

The linguistic analysis of periphrastic and suppletive comparative forms is fairly straightforward and uncontroversial. Suppletive comparatives such as *worse, better,* and *further* are probably lexically listed, and the periphrastic construction involves the insertion/merger of *more* for adjectives that do not have a morphologically formed comparative. Graziano-King (1999) presented an analysis of the *more* + Adj construction in terms of Chomsky (1995), in which the periphrastic construction is formed in the syntax as a last resort to check an abstract degree feature when a bare adjective form is unable to do so; in other words, *more* insertion is blocked by the presence of a suppletive or suffixed comparative form. By contrast, the linguistic representation of *-er* comparatives is controversial. Several linguists have posited an *-er* suffixation rule that is said to be morphophonologically conditioned such that it only applies to monosyllabic adjectives and disyllabic ones with certain endings (see, e.g., Aronoff, 1976; Di Sciullo & Williams, 1987). The difficulty, however, has been to capture all the exceptions that resist *-er* suffixation. Consider, for example, **apter* versus *stupider* mentioned earlier, or *handsomer* versus **irksomer*. Moreover, Graziano-King (1999) observed that all of the exceptions to *-er* suffixation are low frequency adjectives. On these grounds, she suggested that there is no *-er* suffixation rule for English comparatives and the existing *-er* comparatives are lexically listed. Support for these claims comes from an acceptability judgment task performed with 70 adult native speakers, 36 4-year-olds and 36 7-year-olds in which an *-er* comparative preference was found for high frequency monosyllabic adjectives, but not for low frequency ones.

Unimpaired children have been reported to produce both *-er* and *more* comparatives early on. Graziano-King (1999) analyzed corpora from the CHILDES database (MacWhinney, 1995) of two children (age range: 0;7–8;0) and found 220 instances of *-er* comparatives and 22 *more* forms. There were also 13 cases of double markings, such as *more lighter, more specialer, more* *cleaner.* Similar results were obtained from elicited production experiments. Children of all age groups studied produced *-er* and *more* comparatives, even though they were more successful at correctly marking adjectives requiring *-er* forms. Gathercole (1985, p. 96), for example, found that even the youngest children in her sample (i.e., those from 2;5 to 3;0) produced the suffixed and the periphrastic comparatives, with correctness scores of 28% and 15%, respectively.

The following section reports the results of an elicited production experiment that was administered to 4 subjects with WS and to two control groups of 10 unimpaired children each with chronological ages similar to the mental ages of the WS children.[1]

Participants

The four subjects with WS are the same as those examined in previous studies from the group (see Clahsen & Almazan, 1998, 2001; Temple et al., 2001). Details of their cases histories are given in the Appendix. The subjects' chronological ages are as follows: Jane 11;2, Florence 12;7, Emily 13;1, and Martin 15;4. All subjects live with their parents and attend a special school where they interact with other mentally handicapped children. Their mental ages were derived from scores on the Wechsler Intelligence Scale for Children–III (Wechsler, 1992). By this method, Emily and Jane had mental ages of 5;4 and 5;7, whereas Florence and Martin had mental ages of 7;5 and 7;7, respectively.

The data from the WS subjects is compared to two control groups of monolingual English-speaking children who live in native homes and were randomly selected by date of birth from state schools in Essex and Suffolk, England. The first control group consists of 10 children with a mean chronological age of 5;4 years (range: 5;1–5;10), and the second group is made up of 10 children with a mean chronological age of 7;1 years (range: 7;1–7;11). Subjects who had any known neurological abnormality, learning difficulties, or a history of special needs were excluded.

The responses of the WS subjects are also compared to the results of Dalalakis (1994), who studied comparative formations in SLI subjects using the same elicited production task employed in the present study. Dalalakis examined comparatives in the KE family, a large family spanning three gen-

---

[1]The experiment was administered to the WS children by Mayella Almazan and to the unimpaired children by Melanie Ring. Normal mental age controls were used rather than other children with learning difficulties of similar mental age. This avoided spurious apparent discrepancies based on comparisons to another atypical group. For example, as discussed by Temple et al. (2001), comparisons of children with WS in a linguistic study to children with DS for whom impoverished language development in relation to mental age has been long documented is like investigating precocious reading by utilizing a dyslexic control sample.

erations of which seven members have been argued to suffer from SLI (see Gopnik & Goad, 1997; Ullman & Gopnik, 1999; Vargha-Khadem, Watkins, Fletcher, & Passingham, 1995).

Method

The materials and procedures were adopted from Dalalakis' (1994) elicited production task; see also Layton and Stick (1979) and Gathercole (1985) for similar tasks. Twenty pairs of pictures were used in which two items were depicted that differed in terms of a gradable attribute (e.g., size). The pictures were accompanied by two sentences, which were read aloud to the children. For example: *This circle is big. This is even* ___? The children were prompted to complete the sentence with a comparative form. Five kinds of target adjectives were used, as shown in Example 1:

(1) *ER adjectives*	*MORE adject.*	*EITHER*	*IRREGULARS*	*NONCE*
big	dangerous	round	good	weff
funny	expensive	straight	bad	kell
sad	modern	tasty		bimmy
young	unusual	bitter		toshal
little	open			

According to Dalalakis (1994), the adjectives in the first column require -*er* comparative forms in adult English, those in the second column have periphrastic comparatives, and those in the third column may take either form. The adjectives *good* and *bad* have irregular (suppletive) comparatives. The first three nonce adjectives were expected to elicit -*er* comparatives, *weff* and *kell* because they are monosyllabic, and *bimmy* because of the -*y* ending, whereas *toshal* should be more likely to yield a periphrastic comparative.

The stimulus materials were presented to each child individually. One of the unimpaired control children failed to complete the experiment, and her responses were not included in the analysis. All other unimpaired and WS children did not show any difficulty understanding the task. The children's responses were written down and tape-recorded for verification.

Results

The results for the five kinds of adjectives tested are shown in Table 13.1 for the four groups of participants. The analysis included responses that incorporated the target stem (i.e., either one of the comparative forms or a bare stem form of the target adjectives). The mean scores and standard devia-

TABLE 13.1
Elicited Production of Comparative Adjectives

	5-year-old controls		WS-5	7-year-old controls		WS-7
	M in %	SD	M in %	M in %	SD	M in %
ER Adjectives						
-er	96.7	(10.44)	100	88.3	(25)	100
More	0	(0)	0	11.7	(25)	0
Bare stem	3.3	(3.3)	0	0	(0)	0
MORE Adjectives						
-er	30.5	(35.3)	89	52.7	(36.8)	90
More	9.3	(15.7)	0	31.2	(43)	10
Bare stem	60.2	(33.6)	11	16.1	(25)	0
EITHER Adjectives						
-er	67.5	(28.9)	88	76	(33)	88
More	2.5	(7.9)	0	19	(34.5)	0
Bare stem	30	(28.4)	12	5	(10.5)	12
IRREGULAR Adjectives						
Correct	10	(21.1)	0	20	(25.8)	0
-er	85	(24.2)	100	60	(39.4)	100
More	0	(0)	0	20	(42.1)	0
Bare stem	5	(15)	0	0	(0)	0
NONCE Adjectives						
-er	65.1	(26.0)	50	73.9	(37.2)	100
More	5.8	(12.4)	0	23.6	(38.1)	0
Bare stem	19.1	(17.9)	50	2.5	(7.9)	0

tions present a breakdown of the relative percentages of these responses. Responses in which the children produced (unintelligible) mispronunciations or in which they substituted the target adjective with some other lexeme were not included in the analysis; such responses made up 15.5% of the total responses of the 5-year-old controls, 10.5% for the 7-year-old controls, and just 1% of the total responses in the WS data.

Consider first the data from the unimpaired children. Table 13.1 shows that the 5-year-olds and the 7-year-olds produced *-er* comparatives as well as periphrastic forms with *more*, even though in both groups of children the suffixed forms were used more frequently than the periphrastic construction. Moreover, Table 13.1 shows that the comparatives of ER adjectives are most often correctly formed by both groups of children, whereas for MORE adjectives they are less successful. There were also 10 cases of double markings—9 from the 7-year-olds, 1 from the 5-year-olds—in which the children produced both *more* and a suffixed form (e.g., *more straighter*). These results from the control children replicate those of the previous studies of unimpaired children's comparative formations mentioned earlier.

The data from the WS children differ in several ways from those of the control children. Table 13.1 shows that the WS children achieve similar correctness scores to the normals for adjectives for which -er forms are grammatical, but they perform worse on adjectives that require MORE comparatives and on adjectives that require suppletive forms; the latter are all incorrect in the WS data, and only one of the MORE adjectives is correctly formed by the WS children. With respect to error types, Table 13.1 shows that the WS subjects produce many -er comparative forms for MORE adjectives and for IRREGULARS. A by-item paired *t* test for the adjectives that require periphrastic or suppletive comparative forms reveals that the WS children (taken as a group) had significantly more -er errors than the unimpaired children, $t(6) = 5.91$, $p < .01$. For MORE adjectives and for IRREGULARS, each WS subject produced significantly more -er errors than the unimpaired controls (mean percentage for controls: 54.07, $SD = 19.12$). Emily and Martin produced -er forms in all such cases, $z = 2.40$, $p < .01$, and Jane and Florence had -er forms in all but one instance, $z = 1.65$, $p < .05$. This difference also holds for individual items; for each item that requires a periphrastic or suppletive comparative form in English, the WS children (taken as a group) produced more -er errors than the mean for the unimpaired children. These results indicate that, with respect to -er errors, each WS child behaves differently from the groups of unimpaired children tested. Examining the individual subject data of the two control groups, there was one child among the 5-year-olds and three among the 7-year-olds who used -er for MORE adjectives and for IRREGULARS as frequently as the WS children. The remaining 15 control children overapplied -er less often than any of the 4 WS children. The WS children, relative to unimpaired controls, on the other hand, underuse the periphrastic construction. The WS children do not produce any comparatives with *more* for ER adjectives, for nonce forms, or for adjectives that allow both -er and *more*. There are also no cases of double markings (*more bigger*) in the WS data. Another difference between the WS children and the unimpaired controls concerns the use of stem forms (i.e., cases in which the adjective was simply repeated without any comparative marking). For MORE adjectives, the 5-year-olds frequently produced bare stems indicating they were unwilling to apply -er or *more* comparative formation in these cases, and the WS children produced just one bare stem form in this condition, yielding a marginally significant difference ($z = 1.46$, p < .07) for the 5-year-olds. Instead, the WS children most often applied -er suffixation.

Summarizing, the data from the WS children show that they have just one way of forming comparatives, and this is -er affixation, which they apply freely to any adjective. This holds for both groups of WS children studied here. In contrast, the unimpaired children produce not only -er comparatives, but also periphrastic comparative constructions, suppletive comparatives, and double markings (*more straighter*). The data also show that the use of *-er* is more constrained in the unimpaired children than in the subjects with WS.

Discussion

The WS data from the present experiment show that these children excessively overapply *-er* comparative adjective formation, and that the lexical exceptions and constraints on *-er* comparatives in English do not influence their comparative formations. These observations indicate that they have developed an *-er* suffixation rule that can freely generalize to any adjective. Subjects with SLI, on the other hand, have been shown to perform differently on the same task. Dalalakis (1994) found that the most frequent error produced by the impaired members of the KE family were omissions of comparative markings (i.e., they either repeated the unmarked bare stem form of the adjective or an unmarked form of a different lexeme). Dalalakis took this finding to mean that the SLI subjects are impaired in making use of grammatical rules for comparative formation. Whatever the precise nature of this impairment, the present set of findings shows that it does not hold for WS.

As already mentioned, the linguistic representation of *-er* comparatives in the grammar of English is controversial, and it is not the purpose of the present study to decide between these accounts. One suggestion has been that *-er* comparatives are derived from a (morphophonogically conditioned) rule. Under this account, the WS children would have a *generalized* suffixation rule, where the adult grammar has a *lexically restricted* one. The alternative view is that *-er* comparatives are stored in the lexicon and there is no comparative suffixation rule in English. If this is correct, then adjectives that allow *-er* comparatives would have subentries for these forms; the adjective *hot*, for example, would have subentries for *hotter* and (probably also for) *hottest*. Under this account, the WS children would have developed an *-er* suffixation rule where the adult grammar has structured lexical entries, and it might be speculated that the transparency of *-er* comparative forms (which makes them easily decomposable into stems and affixes) promotes the development of such a rule. Irrespective of the proper treatment of *-er* comparatives in English, the WS data suggest that these children either fail to store or activate comparative forms in the lexicon and that such forms are generated by a general *-er* suffixation that can apply to any adjective. The observation that the WS children underuse periphrastic comparatives is also compatible with this interpretation. In the adult language, *more* comparatives apply when there is no *-er* or suppletive comparative form available. For WS children, however, there are no such cases because their general *-er* rule can apply to any adjective.

The comparatives data fit in with that found on WS children's performance in the past tense and their use of noun plurals (Clahsen & Almazan, 1998, 2001). WS children have difficulty retrieving or accessing irregular past tense and plural forms, which are lexically stored as subnodes of complex lexical entries. The lexeme *drive*, for example, comprises a base form (*drive*) and two subentries (*driven, drove*). The children with WS can access the base form when required, but their performance on the lexical exceptions (i.e., the subentries) seems to be impaired. Rules of affixation, on the other hand, are used excessively in the WS children, hence their high correctness scores on the regular past tense and plural formation and their frequent -*ed* and -*s* plural overregularization errors. The comparatives data confirm the dissociation found for past tense and plural formation in WS. The WS children generate comparatives by a general -*er* rule, which appears to be insensitive to the constraints and lexical exceptions of -*er* comparative formation in English.

LEXICAL SKILLS IN WS

Several studies have reported superior performance on receptive vocabulary using the Peabody Picture Vocabulary Test (PPVT) or British Picture Vocabulary Scale (BPVS). Subjects with WS performed significantly better than normal mental age matched controls (Bellugi, Bihrle, Jernigan, Trauner, & Doherty, 1990) and above the level of the subjects' mental ages derived from other measures (Tyler et al., 1997). Superior performance has also been reported on tasks of oral fluency, in which words have to be selected from the lexicon to conform to specified phonological (e.g., beginning with the letter *f*) or semantic (names of animals) constraints (Bellugi, Bihrle, Neville, Jernigan, & Doherty, 1992; Volterra, Capirci, Pezzini, Sabbadini, & Vicar, 1996), even though not every study reports this quantitative advantage (Rossen, Klima, Bellugi, Bihrle, & Jones, 1996). Issues have also been raised about atypical language use in WS. It has been described as having many of the qualities of cocktail party speech (Bradley & Udwin, 1989; Udwin, Yule, & Martin, 1987) with frequent use of social phrases and idioms. Individual word use has also been reported as unusual. Bellugi et al. (1992) provided the example "I'll have to evacuate the glass" meaning "empty the glass." Unusual selections within oral fluency responses for the children with WS are also reported with increased numbers of low frequency responses (e.g., terandon, unicorn, in animal fluency) and significantly more items of low frequency among later items in lists, even where overall performance levels numerically are similar (Rossen et al., 1996).

These issues of possible lexical talent and impairment and atypical use of vocabulary have been explored in a study of the four children with WS

TABLE 13.2
Psychometric Test Scores on Lexicosemantic Tasks

	Emily	Jane	Florence	Martin
Chronological age	13;1	11;2	12;7	15;4
Mental age	5;4	5;7	7;5	7;7
Receptive vocab. age	9;6	6;8	10;2	7;9
Semantic concept age	6;10	9;2	9;2	12;2
Naming age	6;3–6;5	4;3–4;8	6;3–6;5	4;3–4;8

(Temple et al., 2001). Consider, first, the results of various psychometric measures to assess the children's lexicosemantic skill in relation to their mental age. Receptive vocabulary age was determined from scores on the BPVS (Dunn, Dunn, Whetton, & Pintilie, 1982) and naming age was determined from the naming subtest of the British Ability Scales (Elliot, Murray, & Pearson, 1983). Age equivalent scores for knowledge of semantic concepts were determined from the similarities subtest of the WISC–III (Wechsler, 1992). This requires the child to judge how two words are the same, an easy item being *wheel* and *ball* and a difficult item being *liberty* and *justice*. The child is told that there is a similarity, the items are the same in some way, and they must identify the similarity. The scores on these psychometric measures are summarized in Table 13.2. This indicates that all the children with WS have receptive vocabulary scores above the level of their mental ages. They also have semantic concept ages above the level of their mental age. Yet, all the children have naming ages below the receptive vocabulary levels and are therefore all anomic in relation to these measures of lexicosemantic representation.

Receptive vocabulary was further examined by using multiple examples of items from the same semantic field. Children heard a spoken word and had to select a picture matching that word. This format was the same as for the BPVS. However, in the BPVS, the requirement is to select a picture, which matches the word, from an array containing three distracters, some of which resemble the target but are not semantically linked. In contrast, here the child had to select the target from an array containing 23 semantic distracters, all of which were from the same semantic field. The items employed were names for animals (including birds and sea creatures), indoor objects, foods and clothes, with stimuli selected from Snodgrass and Van derwart (1980). When the children had to select in this way from multiple distracters in the same semantic field, their receptive vocabulary levels were significantly weaker than those of normal mental age controls. For example Martin is correct on 75% of items compared to a mental age control score of 94%: $SD = 2.92$, $z = 6.50$, $p < .001$. Thus, when detailed semantic specification is required, the system that has developed for the child with WS is less effective than normal. It is possible that the system improves with age, but it is also possible that the elevated levels of receptive vocabulary reported in adults with WS (e.g., Bellugi et al., 1990; Tyler et al., 1997) are only superficially correct, because they are also based on results from the BPVS or the similar PPVT (Dunn & Dunn, 1981).

Testing of older cases of WS with the multiple semantic distracters employed by Temple et al. (2001) would resolve this issue. In the design of this study, the distracters were more numerous than in the BPVS, raising the issue of an alternative explanation in terms of attentional or visuoperceptual difficulties. A current study addresses these alternative hypotheses (Temple & Sherwood, in preparation), but variation here in task performance renders this explanation unlikely. For example, naming performance (Temple et al. (2001) (discussed later) where items are presented individually is much poorer than ability to point to a picture from a spoken name where there are 23 distracters. Moreover, performance with 23 distracters remains well above chance and there are accuracy levels of 69% or above for all cases of WS. So general attentional and perceptual factors are unproblematic two thirds of the time. Further, the two older children, Florence and Martin, show category-specific effects, with weaker performance on clothes and foods, respectively, but good performance on animals, the category that has been suggested as containing exemplars that are the most perceptually similar. Finally, the semantic errors generated in reading discussed later, where there are no pictorial stimuli or multiple distracters, argue against perceptual or attentional explanations. These cross task differences argue against generalized attentional or visuoperceptual difficulties being relevant to the pattern of results.

The pervasive naming impairment reported in the psychometric measures was found in the more detailed analysis to be most marked in the children with older mental ages. Overt error analysis was possible in comparison to control performance but also in comparison to recently published error data on the children's naming of the Snodgrass and Vanderwart stimuli (1980) by Cycowicz, Friedman, and Rothstein (1997). This analysis indicated that for every child with WS, error responses included a significantly larger proportion of responses that were atypical, than those made by mental age controls. Examples of atypical responses made by the children with WS are *caterpillar* → 'antelope' (Emily), *lobster* → 'ostrich' (Martin), *broom* → 'saucepan', *spanner* → 'corkscrew'. Despite these naming difficulties, Temple et al. (2001) found that oral fluency scores were significantly above mental age level for three of the four children with WS. Yet, responses also had atypical characteristics with all the children showing a significantly elevated proportion of responses of low frequency.

Finally, reaction times were measured to naming pictures, colors, and some other sets of stimuli. This study was conducted only with Florence

TABLE 13.3
Mean Reaction Times for Correct Naming Responses

	Pictures (msecs to name)	Colors (msecs to name)
Florence (MA 7 yrs)	786	938
Martin (MA 7 yrs)	586	694
7-year-old controls	1218(171)	1063(140)
10-year-old controls	982(133)	933(153)

and Martin, who were found to have the most marked anomia in the detailed analysis. The stimuli were selected to be as easy as possible in terms of being of high frequency, high familiarity, and with early age of acquisition. Accuracy was high, above 89% in all categories for both controls and the children with WS. The mean response times for naming pictures and colors accurately are given in Table 13.3. These results indicated that both Martin and Florence's reaction times were significantly faster than mental age controls at naming pictures. Martin is also significantly faster at naming colors. Data from normal 10-year-old controls are also given in Table 13.3. Martin is also significantly faster in naming pictures than these children who are 3 years above his mental age level. Florence is 1.5 *SD*s above the speed of naming pictures for these children.

There is a pattern of high skill in receptive vocabulary when the distracters are neither too numerous nor too similar in semantic specification; high skill in identifying similarities between pairs of words when told that there is such a similarity and it should be identified, with no time constraint; and high skill in finding words according to a single general semantic or phonological cue in oral fluency when selections have to be as fast and numerous as possible. Also, when naming is accurate, it is significantly faster than normal.

In contrast, there is weak skill in receptive vocabulary when fine grain semantic knowledge is required. There are naming difficulties and naming errors are atypical and more loosely related in meaning to targets than for controls. Responses in oral fluency also include higher proportions of num bers of atypical low frequency responses.

Discussion

Temple et al. (2001) proposed that lexical access in WS is constrained differ ently from normal, with looser criteria for target identification but a mor rapid arrival at selected targets. This leads to fast-sloppy access and, i some cases, only partial activation of the full semantic specification for lex cal targets. They proposed that this enhanced speed contributes to the lar guage advantage seen on some tasks but with incomplete activation increasing the error rate and affecting the pattern of errors on others. The rapid incomplete activation may be sufficient to generate good performance in receptive vocabulary when broad semantic knowledge is required, but is insufficiently detailed for good performance in the face of multiple semantically similar competing distracters in the more detailed task. The fast but inadequate activation leads to naming errors and high rates of atypical errors. It enables high rates of selection in oral fluency when the word can be any one in a broad semantic field, without the requirement for fine grain semantic specification. It also enables good performance on the similarities subtest when the children are told there is a relation between pairs of items and they must keep looking for it with no time constraints, which may reduce the "sloppy activation."

Temple et al. (2001) proposed a modular explanation for these effects in WS, integrating them with a modular model of lexical access. The good receptive vocabulary scores on the BPVS and good similarities performance would argue for good development of the semantic system itself. Poor picture naming would then occur at a word selection/search stage intermediate between the semantic system and the speech output lexicon. However, the poor performance on the receptive vocabulary task where there are multiple semantic distracters suggests that specification of entries within the semantic system is poor or that less constrained selection occurs earlier than at the level of the speech output lexicon, because it affects a pointing response. The impairment affects the representation in the semantic system or their activation via fast-sloppy access.

Enhanced performance on pointing from spoken names over naming suggests that at least part of the problem relates to activation or the use of existent lexical/semantic entries. The impaired performance on receptive vocabulary in comparison to controls could be argued to indicate that there may also be a representational deficit in which some entries are specified poorly. However, if the deficits were representational, it is not clear why semantic fluency is so good, why performance on verbal concepts is good, why accurate naming is fast, and why semantic errors in reading are generated to specific items known to have intact representations.

The account in terms of fast-sloppy access fits in with the proposed interpretation of the results on inflectional morphology in children with WS. If to access the irregular past form a blocking operation inhibiting the regularly inflected form is required (Pinker, 1999), then the children with WS may have a lexical system where access is too fast with insufficient editing of responses. The regular past form may then be processed effectively but also elicited where an irregular past form would be more appropriate. A similar mechanism could operate on the comparatives data presented earlier.

Some of the results concerning lexical skills are not incompatible with a connectionist network within which there is less weight than normal on semantic representations. Such an explanation could account for naming difficulties and possibly for atypical errors and selections in oral fluency. Increased weight on phonological representations might even be able to account for elevated initial letter performance on oral fluency. However, it is not clear why reduced weight on semantic representations would also lead to elevated performance on semantic fluency, or why performance with verbal concepts (*similarities*) is so good, or why naming when accurate would be faster than normal. Modular theories have greater flexibility in providing explanations for such a range of effects.

READING IN WS

If lexical retrieval is characterized by fast-sloppy selection and semantic specification may be impoverished or atypical, then there should be difficulties in the development of the lexicosemantic reading route. If phonological reading skills were nevertheless good, then the reading of regular words might be good but with frequent regularization to irregular words. If phonological reading skills are impaired or inaccessible and reliance was on the lexicosemantic reading route, then high rates of paralexias would be predicted, including semantic paralexias.

Delayed reading development in WS in terms of reading age has been reported in group studies of children and adults (Howlin, Davies, & Udwin 1998; Udwin et al., 1987). However, there have not yet been any of the detailed psycholinguistic analyses of individual cases of reading in relation to models of normal function that have characterized many contemporary analysis of developmental dyslexia (e.g., Castles & Coltheart, 1993; Temple, 1997a, 1997b). There has also been no detailed discussion in case studies or group analyses of the initial patterns of reading development in WS as reading begins to emerge. Temple (in press) provided a psycholinguistic case description of early reading development in one of the cases of WS discussed earlier, which includes an error analysis of paralexic responses. Initial investigations of a second case indicate that the pattern discussed is not unique in children with WS as they just start to read, but further descriptions are needed to determine whether it characterizes all cases at the very start of reading.

On a standard test, the Schonell, Emily has a reading age of 5;1. In total, across word lists, 361 words were presented for reading aloud, of which 25 were read correctly and 320 induced paralexic errors. The words read aloud correctly were high in frequency and the nouns and adjectives read aloud correctly were highly imageable. Of the overt paralexic errors, 51 (16%) were semantic paralexias (e.g., *queen* → 'people', *blue* → 'red', *chimney* → 'house', *five* → 'seven', *garden* → 'beach'); 19 (6%) were visuosemantic (sharing semantic features and 50% of letters, e.g., *ball* → 'lead', *stupid* → 'silly', *bird* → 'bee', *mother* → 'mum', *sock* → 'mask'), and 17 (5%) were visual + semantic (i.e., a visual error followed by a semantic error; e.g., *shampoo* → 'light' [via lamp], *floor* → 'stupid' [via fool], *glass* → 'everyone' [via class], *shampoo* → 'light' [via lamp], *cloud* → 'naughty' [via loud]).

Thus, in total, 27% of errors had a semantic component. Both the error rates for semantic paralexias and for paralexias with a semantic component were significantly higher than the equivalent rates generated by random pairings of stimuli and responses, where only 5% of errors were semantic paralexias and 7.5% in total had a semantic component. They were also significantly higher than the rates reported by Seymour and Elder (1986) for normal beginning readers learning in a scheme emphasizing whole words, where "phonics" were not explicitly taught. Even the Seymour and Elder children (1986) had a rate of semantic paralexias of only 2% versus Emily's rate of 16%.

The reading disorder for which semantic errors are the key characteristic is deep dyslexia (Marshall & Newcombe, 1966). There have been few case descriptions of this disorder in children (Johnston, 1983; Siegel, 1985; Stuart & Howard, 1995; Temple, 1988). The number of distinct semantic errors (n = 50) made by Emily is the highest reported in any of these cases of developmental deep dyslexia. Emily also displays the other characteristics of deep dyslexia. No nonwords can be read aloud correctly and the majority of errors in attempting to read nonwords are lexicalizations. Spelling is also impaired. This pattern of reading development would normally be interpreted as reflecting failure to develop a sublexical phonological reading route or a direct route from print-to-sound with dependence on a partially established lexicosemantic route, within which a word's pronunciation is activated only after its meaning is first derived (Coltheart, Patterson, & Marshall, 1980) and this explanation would also apply to Emily.

Emily was able to name correctly and recognize the spoken names for the majority of items that she read incorrectly. For a subset of items (n = 33), data was available from reading, naming, and pointing to a picture from a spoken name, enabling cross-task comparison for the same items. Each of the 33 items generated errors in reading, of which 13 items generated errors with a semantic component. For 28 of the 33 items, Emily was able to name the item correctly and for 26 she could recognize the spoken name by selecting the matching picture from 23 semantically related distracters. Of the 13 items that generated errors with a semantic component in reading, 10 were named correctly from pictures. The semantic errors cannot therefore be attributed to absence of semantic specification for the item or to any generalized difficulty with lexical production of the item name. Activation of only partial semantic features may have occurred so that incorrect lexical entries were activated, an interpretation consistent with fast-sloppy access in reading as well as in naming. However, despite the anomia discussed earlier, sloppy access to lexical entries appears to arise in reading to an even greater degree than in naming, because semantic paralexias are generated even to those items that can be read or understood correctly. The pattern of lexical access appears to differ in degree dependent on the modality of input (written words vs. pictures). However, the qualitative pattern of the impairment is very similar and the differential performance across tasks confirms that it is access or activation that is problematic rather than the representation itself.

It is of interest in relation to the issues already discussed that Emily is able to do successfully a number of both implicit and explicit phonological processing tasks and there is no evidence of impairment here in relation to mental age. Emily can also sound 16 of 26 letters of the alphabet. Yet, she seems unable to use this skill and her other explicit phonological skills to stop the production of semantic errors. Thus, for example, Emily can sound out all the component letters of the word *friend*, except for the letter *e*. Yet, when asked to read the word *friend* aloud, she says "boy." This pattern of performance strengthens the argument for modular impairments and the independence during development of the lexicosemantic reading route and the phonological reading route, within which the grapheme-phoneme skills, reflected by the ability to sound out letters, are processed. Basic initial phonological skills have been mastered, but they cannot be used in the lexicosemantic domain. There is certainly no evidence that they impinge on or constrain the lexicosemantic skills in any way.

The form of some semantic errors—for example, a tendency to say "people" for living things, whether animals or actual people—supports the view that there may be difficulty in activating lower nodes in a hierarchical structure. In similar fashion, problems with irregularly inflected word forms may reflect restricted activation or representation of lower nodes within morphological structures.

It will be of interest to study whether Emily's pattern of initial reading is characteristic of all children with WS as they first develop reading. It will also be of interest to study Emily further as reading develops, because it is clear that not all older children and adults with WS have deep dyslexia. For Emily, initial reading is abnormal. Follow-up studies will indicate whether subsequent reading development emerges with the emphasis on an expanding lexicosemantic reading route as in phonological dyslexia or emphasis on an expanding phonological reading route as in surface dyslexia.

A CRITIQUE OF THE NONMODULAR CONSTRUCTIVIST ACCOUNT OF WS

A nonmodular "constructivist" model has been proposed by Karmiloff-Smith and her collaborators (Thomas & Karmiloff-Smith, 1999; Thomas et al., 2001) to explain the past tense performance of subjects with WS. According to this account, the linguistic performance of a subject with WS is argued to reflect shifted constraints in the representation and development of language, whereby there is greater reliance on phonology and a reduced contribution of semantic information. More specifically, it is claimed that in WS "phonological representations may be too specific to support robust generalisation" (Thomas et al., 2001, p. 170), which prevent subjects with WS from learning the past tense properly and from generalizing inflectional patterns to novel items. Moreover, it is claimed that the apparent deficit in irregular past tense formation in WS is simply delayed language development and is not different from the normal developmental progression.

The following section first criticizes the design and statistical analysis of Thomas et al. (2001) and offers a reanalysis of their data. It then discusses their theoretical conclusions focusing on the hypotheses of delayed language development and a phonological deficit in WS.

Reanalyzing Thomas et al.'s (2001) Data

As Thomas et al. (2001, p. 148) pointed out, "It is not enough to demonstrate that irregular past tense formation is poorer than regular past tense formation. Rather, it must be shown that their level of past tense formation is poorer than we would expect *given their level of language development*." Yet, their study failed to make this direct comparison to address the issue. Instead, they discussed average performance collapsed across 18 cases of WS, with ages ranging from 11 to 53 years and mental ages ranging from 5 to 16 years. There is no explicit matching of groups of children with mental ages at particular levels to normal controls of the same age level. Performance across the 10-year linguistic band is collapsed into one set of averaged figures in the error analysis, which is the key issue for comparison. In the only statistical endeavor to take account of the wide range of mental ages, Thomas et al. (2001) engaged in a variety of data manipulations that seem questionable. They collapse normal children from 5 to 10 years and treat them as if they are a single group, collapse results across two disparate paradigms of spontaneous or phonologically cued past tense production, compare normals (age 5–10) with cases of WS subjects (mental age = 5;7–16;5), note that the data for their linear regression is not in any way linear and attempt to address this by using inverse squares of chronological and mental age, conduct regression analyses using these age factors, show main effects of group and of verb type, but argue their case on the basis of failure to find a significant interactional effect of verb type and group after all these manipulations. This is their case for absence of a selective deficit for irregulars in WS.

Yet, if their data on WS is averaged, a more direct and straightforward comparison can be made, which, in contrast to their interpretation, confirms the deficit in irregular past tense formation. Table 2 of Thomas et al. (2001) provided the verbal mental ages for the cases of WS. It gave a mean verbal mental age of 7;11, but Thomas et al. (2001) noted that three subjects were unable to do their task, and if they are removed, then the verbal mental age for the group is 8;4. If the error data for this group of cases of WS with mental age of 8;4 is then compared with the normal subject group who have a mean mental age of 8;1 years, then for irregular past tense forms, correct irregulars are produced in 69% of cases for the normal group but only 52% for the WS group. In contrast, incorrect regularizations or stems are produced in 32% of cases for the normal 8-year-olds but in 45% of cases for the subjects with WS. This is a significant difference in proportions; $\chi^2 = 3.93$, $p < .05$. Similarly, for Task 2, with cued responses, for irregular past tense forms, correct irregulars are produced in 77% of cases for the normal group but in only 54% of the WS group. In contrast, incorrect regularizations or stems are produced in 20% of cases for the normal 8-year-olds but in 32% of cases for the subjects with WS. This is also a significant difference in proportions between the groups, $\chi^2 = 5.45$, $p < .05$. Thus, even in the Thomas et al. (2001) data, the level of irregular past tense formation in WS is significantly poorer than would be expected from their level of language development. Moreover, an analysis of variance performed on Thomas et al.'s data (which was presented in an earlier version of their study) revealed that the WS group produced significantly fewer irregularizations than both of their control groups, the chronological age controls, $F(1, 61) = 49.91$, $p < .001$, and their mental age controls, $F(1, 61) = 11.63$, $p = .001$. Thus, Thomas et al.'s data indeed showed that children with WS perform worse on irregular than unimpaired children and produce significantly fewer overapplication of irregular inflection than mental age controls.

Also note that a selective deficit in irregular inflection is not only evident from Thomas et al.'s data, but also from the WS data presented in Clahsen and Almazan (1998) for the past tense, from Clahsen and Almazan's (2001) study of noun plurals, and from Bromberg et al.'s (1994) study with 6 WS participants (speaking American English), which reported spared production of regular past tense formation, but impaired production of irregulars with overregularizations largely produced instead. Moreover, in a study of noun plural formation with 12 children with WS and 12 control children, Zukowski (2001) found that the WS children apply the regular plural affix t existing nouns and to nonce nouns at near-ceiling rates (86%–95%) just like control children, but they performed worse than the unimpaired children on irregulars (29% correct irregulars for WS vs. 41% for controls). These results suggest that selective difficulties with irregular inflection seem to be a rather robust characteristic of children with WS, in contrast to the claims made by Thomas et al. (2001).

Delayed Language Development in WS?

Thomas and Karmiloff-Smith (1999; Thomas et al., 2001) made two broad arguments with respect to this question. On the one hand, they presented data that they argued suggest that language development is delayed in WS and follows the normal developmental progression (although the previous analysis differs). Yet, on the other hand, they simultaneously argued that "WS does not merely represent a case of delayed language development, but a case of language development following an atypical developmental trajectory" (Thomas et al., 2001, p. 169), and when they modeled the overspecified phonological representations that they argued create this trajectory, they showed that a deficit in irregular verb formation results. Thus, on the one hand, they argued that a documented deficit in WS is not a specific deficit, and on the other hand, they proposed a model that they claimed predicts just this deficit.

An empirical difficulty for the hypothesized delay of language development results from the fact that, in some important respects, the subjects with WS studied by Thomas et al. (2001) perform worse when they get older. This is evident from their Figs. 4 and 5, which show that both in terms of chronological and verbal mental age, the older subjects with WS produce more -ed overregularizations to nonce words that rhyme with existing irregular verbs than the younger ones. A different pattern is found for the unimpaired controls: Initially they produce more -ed regularizations with age, then performance levels off and then the older they get, the less often they add -ed to rhyming irregulars. This difference is hard to reconcile with the view that the linguistic profile of subjects with WS simply represents a delay of normal language development.

Another challenge for the delay hypothesis comes from the results of a recent study of plural formation and compounding (Clahsen & Almazan, 2001). Results from three experiments showed that the subjects with WS excessively overapplied the regular plural -s, even in circumstances in which typically developing children hardly ever use -s plurals, namely, as nonhead elements inside compounds. In contrast to unimpaired controls, the subjects with WS maintained regular -s plurals inside compounds, producing ungrammatical derived compounds such as *rats-eater, as well as many ungrammatical root compounds with regular -s plurals as nonhead elements (e.g., *foots cake, *gooses fax*, etc.). In an additional comprehension experiment, the children with WS were found frequently to misinterpret compounds like *red rats eater* as the eater being red rather than the victims. This indicated that, in contrast to unimpaired children, the presence of a regular plural did not have any effect on the interpretation of the compound by children with WS. The results from these three experiments show that in subjects with WS, regular plurals can occur freely inside compounds. This is different from adult English and from early child language. Gordon (1985) and Alegre and Gordon (1995) found that even the youngest children in their samples (i.e., the 3-year-olds) were sensitive to the difference between regular and irregular plurals inside compounds. Clahsen, Rothweiler, Woest, and Marcus (1992) and Clahsen, Marcus, Bartke, and Wiese (1996) replicated Gordon's results for German child language. All age groups of unimpaired children in the Clahsen et al. studies produced irregular plurals inside compounds and avoided regular plurals. Hence, the pattern of plurals inside compounds observed in WS does not correspond to any developmental stage found in unimpaired children. These results cast doubt on Thomas and Karmiloff-Smith's delay hypothesis.

The comparatives data presented earlier do not confirm the delay hypothesis either. It was found that the children with WS relied almost exclusively on *-er* comparative affixation and heavily overapplied it without any obvious restriction. The two control groups of unimpaired children tested here, as well as groups of younger unimpaired children, behaved differently. Recall, for example, the findings from Gathercole (1985), which are based on a similar kind of elicitation task. She observed that even the youngest children in her sample (i.e., those 2;5 to 3;0) produced not only *-er* comparatives but also periphrastic (*more*) comparatives, and not only *-er* was used in overapplication errors, but *more* was also overapplied to ER adjectives. Thus, it seems as if the WS comparative behavior does not simply represent delayed language development.

Impaired Phonological Representations in WS?

Thomas and Karmiloff-Smith argued that subjects with WS differ from unimpaired children and adults in their phonological representation system. The idea is that the language of subjects with WS develops under a different set of constraints from normal child language development and subjects with WS have "greater reliance on phonology and relatively weaker semantics" (Thomas et al., 2001, p. 170) This idea of greater reliance on phonology has been implemented in a connectionist network for past tense formation in which the phonological input representations are overspecified in a way such that the network is unable to detect similarities between different phonological representations. In other words, phonological representations in subjects with WS are said to be "overly-detailed" (Thomas et al., 2001, p. 171) and more specific than those of unimpaired children. Thomas et al. (2001) argued that this difference explains why WS children perform worse on irregular past tense formation than unimpaired controls; this is presumably because the stem and past tense forms of irregular verbs tend to be phonologically more different from each other than those of regular verbs (compare *teach–taught* vs. *walk–walked*). Overly detailed phonological representations are also said to explain why the WS group produces fewer irregularizations (i.e., overapplications of irregular past tense forms) than typically developing children (Thomas et al., 2001, p. 164); in their account, this could be due to the fact that overspecified phonological representations of existing past tense forms in WS may prevent associative generalizations to new items.

A difficulty for this account concerns observed differences between overapplication of regular and irregular patterns in the WS data. Such differences have been found in different samples of WS subjects, as well as for different morphological phenomena. Bromberg et al. (1994) found that the six WS participants they studied were impaired in producing irregulars and that instead they most often produced overregularizations. This is parallel to what Clahsen and Almazan (1998, 2001) found for a different group of subjects with WS. With respect to the past tense, these WS subjects (incorrectly) supplied the -*ed* affix to 38% of the existing irregular verbs tested (as opposed to 13% for the unimpaired controls), and to 65% of the nonce verbs that rhymed only with existing irregular verbs (compared to 19% for the unimpaired children), whereas irregularizations occurred in less than 10%. Similar results were obtained for noun plurals by Clahsen and Almazan (2001). The subjects with WS heavily overapplied the regular plural affix, with rates twice as high as those of unimpaired control children, whereas irregular patterns were not overapplied. Moreover, in Thomas et al.'s data, the WS group produced significantly fewer irregularizations than typically developing children (as shown by the analysis of variance reported earlier), and a reanalysis of their data revealed that the WS children studied by Thomas et al. produced significantly more -*ed* overregularizations than unimpaired controls. The contrast between overregularizations and irregularizations is also confirmed by the results of a recent study with German-speaking subjects with WS (Krause & Penke, 2000). It was found that the subjects with WS overregularized the regular -*t* participle, even to high frequency irregular verbs, an error that did not occur in the control data. It was also found that, in contrast to the unimpaired controls, overapplications of irregular plural patterns were almost nonexistent in the WS data. These findings replicate those on English indicating that inflectional rules may be excessively used in subjects with WS. From Thomas and Karmiloff-Smith's phonological deficit account, it would be expected that subjects with WS would be impaired in generalizing all kinds of inflectional patterns because their phonological representations are overly detailed. The finding, however, that subjects with WS seem to be more willing to overextend regular inflectional patterns than irregular ones is left unexplained.

It is also difficult to see how the phonological deficit hypothesis might account for the incorrect compound formations with regular plurals as nonhead elements (e.g., *rats-eater) made by subjects with WS. These kinds of errors do not result from any difficulty with irregular inflection or an impairment in generalizing to nonce words. The two competing forms (e.g., rat and rats) are both existing word forms, and even if subjects with WS had "overly detailed phonological representations," this would not explain why children with WS frequently use the plural form inside compounds, whereas typically developing children almost always use the singular form. From a morphological perspective, however, the behavior of the subjects with WS in compounding fits in with their frequent overapplications of the regular past tense -ed and the regular plural -s. What is common to these processes is that an otherwise productive morphological operation (e.g. -ed affixation, -s affixation, lexical compounding) is constrained or has exceptions in adult language, and it is these exceptions and constraints that cause difficulty for the subjects with WS.

A final problem with the theory of phonological deficit in which subjects with WS place "more weight on phonological information and less weight on semantic information" is the difficulty for this formulation in accounting for differences in ability in WS, between skills on different forms of lexicosemantic tasks. Several studies, including those discussed earlier, have described areas of lexicosemantic advantage in the performance of subjects with WS, with enhanced receptive vocabulary and oral fluency (Bellugi et al., 1990; Temple et al., 2001; Tyler et al., 1997; Volterra et al., 1996). These areas of lexicosemantic advantage contrast with areas in which lexicosemantic impairment is indicated, such as impoverished ability in defining words (Bellugi et al., 1990) and naming (Bromberg et al., 1994; Temple et al. 2001). These task-specific effects pose problems for generalized theories such as Thomas and Karmiloff-Smith's. Even if one accepted that there were "relatively weaker semantics," the theory does not account for these task specific manifestations. The theory could account for impaired naming where a word has to be retrieved in response to a picture. However, i could not simultaneously account for enhanced receptive vocabular where a picture is selected from a spoken word and enhanced semantic flu ency where a word is retrieved in response to a semantic cue. Wherea task-specific effects are often problematic for generalized theories, they ar less problematic for modular theories.

Initial investigations of early reading skills in WS have produced simila contrasts (Temple, Almazan, & Sherwood, 2001). The pattern of reading de scribed is characterized by semantic errors and complete inability to read nonwords and parallels that of deep dyslexia (Coltheart et al., 1980; Marshall & Newcombe, 1966). Phonological processes in the reading in WS have developed to the extent that some individual letters can be sounded correctly. However, this fails to block semantic errors, which indicates modularity between phonological and semantic processes in reading rather than 'a different balance between semantic and phonological information, specifically a greater reliance on phonology and relatively weaker semantics" (p. 170). The severe impairment of phonological skills in reading occurs despite some competent oral phonological abilities, which also argues for modularity within phonological processes themselves (Temple, 2001).

Overall, the results discussed indicate that the proposal of delay in normal language development in WS resulting from overly detailed phonological representations is unable to account for the pattern of linguistic performance observed in WS.

CONCLUSIONS

The results of this study show that that the profile of morphosyntactic skills in WS is different from that of SLI. Subjects with SLI have been found to show difficulty and delays in core aspects of syntax, such as feature checking (Clahsen et al., 1997; Wexler, Schütze, & Rice, 1998), A-chains, and binding principles (van der Lely, 1998), whereas subjects with WS appear to be unimpaired in these domains. Moreover, subjects with SLI do not excessively overapply regular rules of inflection (Dalalakis, 1994; Ullman & Gopnik, 1999). By contrast, children with WS were found to excessively overapply the past tense -ed, the plural -s, and the comparative -er, and they perform worse than controls on lexically constrained inflection, such as irregular past tense and plural forms and on exceptions to -er comparative formation. This was interpreted as a selective lexical deficit in which children with WS have difficulty retrieving or accessing inflected word forms that are stored in memory (as subnodes of complex lexical entries). Combinatorial operations, on the other hand, are unaffected, enabling high scores for accuracy on regular inflection and frequent use of overgeneralizations. It is clear that WS and SLI have different grammatical profiles. The further question, however, of whether any of these profiles is unique to each of the two syndromes or whether it may also be found in other kinds of developmental language impairments, requires further comparative studies.

In processing base lexical items, it was found that comprehension of spoken words involving the activation of semantic representations is effective in subjects with WS where general information is required and there are few similar competing responses in forced choice arrays. However, when fine grain semantic knowledge is required to distinguish the item for multiple others from the same semantic class, performance is significantly poorer than controls. Thus, error rates in naming are high and errors have fewer semantic features in common with targets than normal. Performance is significantly enhanced on oral fluency where access to the general semantic field of the entry is all that is required. Access in naming highly familiar items is also faster than normal. The results were interpreted as indicating fast-sloppy access with enhanced skills where only partial activation of semantic specification is required but impaired skill where a more detailed representation must have been established and must be available.

The pattern of early reading development in one case of WS was that of deep dyslexia. The form of some semantic errors—for example, a tendency to say "people" for living things, whether animals or actual people (e.g., *fish* → 'people', *dog* → 'people', *queen* → 'people', *daddy* → 'people')—supports the view that there may be difficulty in activating lower nodes in a hierarchical structure. Nonwords could not be read, although some letters could be sounded. The impairment was interpreted as reflecting absence of a direct reading route, and dependency on an impoverished lexicosemantic route that appears disconnected from information about letter sounds within the phonological reading route.

A connectionist account of WS has been proposed by Thomas and Karmiloff-Smith (1999) and Thomas et al. (2001). However, this explanation is inadequate in accounting for the morphological results on past tense formation, compounding, and comparatives. It also appears unable to account for either the distinction in lexicosemantic skill dependent on the task demands outlined earlier or the disconnection of phonological information from lexicosemantic selection in reading.

In contrast, a modular account of these results with WS argues for difficulty in storing or activating subnodes and subentries of lexical representations for inflected word forms, and difficulty in activating or storing distant subnodes specifying fine grain semantic information within lexicosemantic entries, with intact combinatorial and rule-governed skills in forming morphologically complex words and enhanced speed and effectiveness of lexical access when only general semantic specification is required. In early reading development, the impaired lexicosemantic access, which triggers semantic paralexias, is combined only with letter sound knowledge in the phonological domain.

Also, children with WS display patterns of performance that normal children do not display at any age. For example, in WS children regular plurals can freely occur in compounds, whereas normal children produce irregular plurals in compounds but avoid regular ones. This avoidance is a characteristic of all ages and the production and response to regular plurals in WS is not a feature of any normal developmental stage. Similarly, the children with WS relied almost exclusively on -er comparative formation and heavily overapplied -er without any obvious restriction, a pattern of performance that differs from that of the two control groups of unimpaired children tested, as well as from reports of comparative formations in younger unimpaired children. The production of atypical responses in naming and oral fluency is also not a feature of any normal developmental stage. Indeed, although as children get older their knowledge of low frequency words increases, the proportion of these produced in fluency tasks actually reduces rather than increases (Temple et al., 2001) so that the elevated proportions of these responses in WS is also atypical in comparison to older children. Finally, the early reading skills in the case of WS included a semantic error rate to single words, which is significantly higher than any described in normal children of any age.

On the other hand, no data suggest that the structure of the underlying linguistic system is different from normal or there are any new modular components that are not seen in normal children or evidence of distinct patterns of interconnections between modules, which differ from normal. Instead, the linguistic performance of the WS subjects can be explained in terms of selective deficits of an otherwise normal modular system. Thus, in the construction of morphological forms, the children with WS are able to form -ed past tense forms, -s plurals, and -er comparative adjectives. In the adult language, these morphological operations are constrained or have exceptions, and it is these exceptions and constraints that cause difficulty for the subjects with WS. In literacy, letters could be sounded, but this phonological ability did not contribute to the recognition of words. Words were read via a lexicosemantic reading system within which a phonological output representation could only be triggered subsequent to the activation of meaning. Within modular theories, the linguistic performance of subjects with language impairments may reflect the architecture of the normal system but with selective components of this system under- or overdeveloped. It is this interpretation that seems most parsimonious in accounting for the data in WS.

ACKNOWLEDGMENTS

We are grateful to the children who participated in this study as well as their parents and teachers. We also thank Janine Graziano-King, Martina Penke, Andrew Radford, Andrea Zukowski, and the editors of the present book for helpful comments on an earlier version. The research on Williams syndrome is supported by grants from the Economic and Social Research Council (R000223511) and the Research-Promotion Fund (RPF) of the University of Essex.

REFERENCES

Alegre, M. A., & Gordon, P. (1995). Red rats eater exposes recursion in children's word formation. *Cognition, 60*, 65–82.

Aronoff, M. (1976). *Word formation in generative grammar.* Cambridge, MA: MIT Press.

Barber, C. (1964). *Linguistic change in present-day English.* University of Alabama Press.

Bayley, N. (1970). *Bayley Scales of Infant Development.* New York: Psychological Corporation.

Bellugi, U., Bihrle, A., Jernigan, T., Trauner, D., & Doherty, S. (1990). Neuropsychological, neurological and neuroanatomical profile of Williams Syndrome. *American Journal of Medical Genetics, 6*, 115–125.

Bellugi, U., Bihrle, A., Neville, H., Jernigan, T., & Doherty, S. (1992). Language, cognition and brain organisation in a neurodevelopmental disorder. In M. Gunnar & C. Nelson (Eds.), *Developmental behavioural neuroscience: The Minnesota symposium on child psychology* (Vol. 24, pp 201–232). Hillsdale, NJ: Lawrence Erlbaum Associates.

Bradley, E. A., & Udwin, O. (1989). Williams' syndrome in adulthood: A case study focusing on psychological and psychiatric aspects. *Journal of Mental Deficiency, 33*, 175–184.

Bromberg, H., Ullman, M., Marcus, G., Kelly, K., & Coppola, M. (1994, November). *A dissociation of memory and grammar: Evidence from Williams syndrome.* Paper presented at the 18th annual Boston University Conference on Language Development, Boston.

Castles, A., & Coltheart, M. (1993). Varieties of developmental dyslexia. *Cognition, 47*, 149–180.

Chomsky, N. (1995). *The minimalist program.* Cambridge, MA: MIT Press.

Clahsen, H., & Almazan, M. (1998). Syntax and morphology in children with Williams syndrome *Cognition, 68*, 167–198.

Clahsen, H., & Almazan, M. (2001). Compounding and inflection in language impairment: Evidence from Williams Syndrome (and SLI). *Lingua, 111*, 729–757.

Clahsen, H., Bartke, S., & Goellner, S. (1997). Formal features in impaired grammars: A comparison of English and German SLI children. *Journal of Neurolinguistics, 10*, 151–171.

Clahsen, H., Marcus, G., Bartke, S., & Wiese, R. (1996). Compounding and inflection in German child language. *Yearbook of Morphology 1995*, 115–142.

Clahsen, H., Rothweiler, M., Woest, A., & Marcus G. (1992). Regular and irregular inflection in the acquisition of German noun plurals. *Cognition, 45*, 225–255.

Coltheart, M., Patterson, K. E., & Marshall, J. C. (Eds.). *Deep dyslexia.* London: Routledge & Kegan Paul.

Cycowicz, Y. M., Friedman, D., & Rothstein, M. (1997). Picture naming by young children: Norms for name agreement, familiarity and visual complexity. *Journal of Experimental Child Psychology, 65*, 171–237.

Dalalakis, J. (1994). English adjectival comparatives and familial language impairment. In Matthews (Ed.), *Linguistic aspects of familial language impairment* (pp. 50–66). Montreal McGill University.

Di Sciullo, A. M., & Williams, E. (1987). *On the definition of word.* Cambridge, MA: MIT Press

Dunn, L. M., & Dunn, L. M. (1981). *Peabody Picture Vocabulary Test–Revised manual.* Circle Pines, MN: American Guidance Service.

Dunn, L. M., Dunn, L. M., Whetton, C., & Pintilie, D. (1982). *The British Picture Vocabulary Scale* Windsor, Berks: NFER-Nelson.

Elliott, C. D., Murray, D. J., & Pearson, L. S. (1983). *The British Ability Scales. Manual 3.* Windsor Berks: NFER-Nelson.

Ewart, A. K., Morris, C. A., Atkinson, D., Weishan, J., Sternes, K., Spallone, P., Stock, A. D., Leppert, M., & Keating, M. T. (1993). Hemizygosity at the elastin gene locus in a developmental disorder, Williams syndrome. *Nature Genetics, 5*, 11–16.

Frangiskakis, J. M., Ewart, A. K., Morris, C. A., Mervis, C. B., Bertrand, J., Robinson, B. F., Klein B. P., Ensing, G. J., Everett, L. A., Green, E. D., Proschel, C., Gutowski, N. J., Noble, M., Atkins

D. L., Odelberg, S. J., & Keating, M. T. (1996). LIM-kinase 1 hemizygosity implicated in impaired visuospatial constructive cognition. *Cell, 86,* 59–69.

Frank, M. (1972). *Modern English: A practical reference guide.* Englewood Cliffs, NJ: Prentice-Hall.

Gathercole, V. V. (1985). More and more and more about more. *Journal of Experimental Child Psychology, 40,* 73–104.

Gopnik, M., & Goad, H. (1997). What underlies inflectional patterns in genetic dysphasia. *Journal of Neurolinguistics, 10,* 109–137.

Gordon, P. (1985). Level ordering in lexical development. *Cognition, 21,* 73–93.

Graziano-King, J. (1999). *Acquisition of comparative forms in English.* Unpublished doctoral dissertation, CUNY Graduate Center, New York.

Greenberg, F. (1990). Introduction. *American Journal of Medical Genetics* (Suppl. 6), 85–88.

Howlin, P., Davies, & Udwin, O. (1998). Cognitive functioning in adults with Williams syndrome. *Journal of Child Psychology & Psychiatry, 39,* 183–189.

Johnston, R. S. (1983). Developmental deep dyslexia? *Cortex, 19,* 133–139.

Krause, M., & Penke, M. (2000, October). *Inflectional morphology in German Williams Syndrome.* Paper presented at the second international conference on the Mental Lexicon, Montreal.

Layton, T., & Stick, S. (1979). Comprehension and production of comparatives and superlatives. *Journal of Child Language, 6,* 511–527.

MacWhinney, B. (1995). *The CHILDES project: Tools for analyzing talk.* Hillsdale, NJ: Lawrence Erlbaum Associates.

Marshall, J. C., & Newcombe, F. (1966). Syntactic and semantic errors in paralexia. *Neuropsychologia, 4,* 169–176.

Pinker, S. (1999). *Words and rules.* London: Weidenfeld & Nicolson.

Reynell, J., & Huntley, M. (1985). *The Reynell Developmental Language Scales* (2nd rev.). Windsor, Berks: NFER-Nelson.

Rossen, M., Klima, E. S., Bellugi, U., Bihrle, A., & Jones, W. (1996). Interaction between language and cognition: Evidence from Williams syndrome. In J. H. Beitchman, N. J. Cohen, M. M. Konstantareas, & R. Tannock (Eds.), *Language learning and behaviour* (pp. 367–392). New York: Cambridge University Press.

Seymour, P. H. K., & Elder, L. (1986). Beginning reading without phonology. *Cognitive Neuropsychology, 3,* 1–37.

Siegel, L. S. (1985). Deep dyslexia in childhood? *Brain & Language, 26,* 16–27.

Snodgrass, J. G., & Vanderwart, M. (1980). A standardised set of 260 pictures: Norms for name agreement, image agreement, familiarity and visual complexity. *Journal of Experimental Psychology: Human Learning & Memory, 6,* 174–215.

Stuart, M., & Howard, D. (1995). KJ: A developmental deep dyslexia. *Cognitive Neuropsychology, 12,* 793–824.

Tassabehji, M. K., Metcalfe, K., Fergusson, W. D., Carette, M. J. A., Dore, J. F., Donnai, D., Read, A. P., Prochel, C., Gutowski, N. J., Mao, X., & Sheer, D. (1996). LIM-Kinase 1 detected in Williams syndrome. *Nature Genetics, 13,* 272–273.

Temple, C. M. (1988). Red is read but eye is blue: A further comparison of developmental and acquired dyslexia. *Brain & Language, 34,* 13–37.

Temple, C. M. (1997a). Cognitive neuropsychology and its application to children. *Journal of Child Psychology and Psychiatry, 38,* 27–52.

Temple, C. M. (1997b). *Developmental cognitive neuropsychology.* Hillsdale, NJ: Lawrence Erlbaum Associates.

Temple, C. M. (in press). Deep dyslexia in Williams syndrome. *Journal of Neurolinguistics.*

Temple, C. M., Almazan, M., & Sherwood, S. (in press). Lexical skills in Williams syndrome: A cognitive neuropsychological analysis. *Journal of Neurolinguistics.*

Temple, C. M., & Sherwood, S. (in preparation). Vocabulary skills in Williams syndrome.

Thomas, M. S. C., & Karmiloff-Smith, A. (1999, September). *Connectionist modelling of past tense formation.* Paper presented at the Cognitive Psychology Section of the British Psychological Society, York, UK.

Thomas, M. S. C., Grant, J., Barham, Z., Gsödl, M., Laing, E., Lakusta, L. Tyler, L. K., Grice, S., Paterson, S., & Karmiloff-Smith, A. (2001). Past tense formation in Williams syndrome. *Language & Cognitive Processes, 16,* 143–176.

Thorndike, R. L., Hagen, E. P., & Sattler J. M. (1986). *Stanford–Binet Intelligence Scale.* Chicago: Riverside.

Tyler, L. K., Karmiloff-Smith, A., Voice, J. K., Stevens, T., Grant, J., Udwin, O., Davies, M., & Howlin, P. (1997). Do individuals with Williams syndrome have bizarre semantics? Evidence for lexical organisation using an on-line task. *Cortex, 33,* 515–527.

Udwin, O., Yule, W., & Martin, N. (1987). Cognitive abilities and behavioural characteristics of children with idiopathic infantile hypercalcaemia. *Journal of Child Psychology and Psychiatry, 28,* 297–309.

Ullman, M., & Gopnik, M. (1999). The production of inflectional morphology in hereditary specific language impairment. *Applied Psycholinguistics, 20,* 51–117.

van der Lely, H. (1998). SLI in children: Movement, economy and deficits in the computational-syntactic system. *Language Acquisition, 7,* 161–192.

Vargha-Khadem, F., Watkins, K., Fletcher, P., & Passingham, R. (1995). Praxic and nonverbal cognitive deficits in a large family with a genetically transmitted speech and language disorder. *Proceedings of National Academy of Science, USA. Psychology, 92,* 930–933.

Volterra, V., Capirci, O., Pezzini, G., Sabbadini, L., & Vicari, S. (1996). Linguistic abilities in Italian children with Williams syndrome. *Cortex, 32,* 663–677.

Wechsler, D. (1976). *Wechsler Intelligence Scale for Children–Revised.* New York: The Psychological Corporation.

Wechsler, D. (1992). *Wechsler Intelligence Scale for Children* (3rd ed.). Sidcup, Kent: The Psychological Corporation.

Wexler, K., Schütze, C., & Rice, M. (1998). Subject case in children with SLI and unaffected controls: Evidence for the Agr/Tns omission model. *Language Acquisition, 7,* 317–344.

Zukowski, A. (2001). *Uncovering grammatical competence in children with Williams syndrome.* Unpublished doctoral dissertation, Boston University.

APPENDIX

Emily

Emily is a 13-year-old girl. She was diagnosed with WS by a pediatrician at age 10 and the diagnosis was confirmed by chromosomal analysis. She was born at full term following a normal pregnancy. There were no complications during delivery or the neonatal period. Birth weight was 2,920 grams. Emily sat at 9 months and walked at 18 months. At age 3, mild developmental delay led to a referral to a child development clinic. Pure tone audiometry at this time indicated bilateral mild hearing loss at high frequencies. Sensitivity to loud noises was also noted. At age 7;6, speech was reported as clear although immature. At age 8;11, language development was reported as delayed, with a vocabulary level of 4;0 on an unspecified test. Verbal reasoning scores were reported as higher but no details are available. At th time of current assessment, mental age derived from scores on the WISC–III (Wechsler, 1992) was 5;4. Verbal IQ was 50, Performance IQ was 46, and Full Scale IQ was 44.

Jane

Jane is an 11-year-old girl. Diagnosis of WS, by a genetics team, was at age 3. Jane was born at full term plus 11 days following a normal pregnancy and delivery. Birth weight was 3,080 grams. At 3 months, Jane was referred to a local hospital with feeding difficulties, even though her weight was 4,750 grams. Investigations at that time revealed mild pulmonary and aortic stenosis. At 2;1, mental age was 1;4 on Bayley's Mental Scale of Infant Development (Bayley, 1970). Difficulties were noted with fine motor skills and concentration. At 2;10, mental age was 2;3 on the Stanford–Binet Intelligence Scales (SBIS; Thorndike, Hagen, & Sattler, 1986). At 4;2, word combinations were reported. At 4;6, mental age was 2;8 on the SBIS (Thorndike, Hagen, & Sattler, 1986) and comprehension was 2;9 on the Reynell Developmental Language Scales (RDLS; Reynell & Huntley, 1985). At 4;9, comprehension level was 3;0 on an unspecified test. At age 7, on McCarthy's Scale of Children's Abilities, the General Cognitive score was 53. At age 8, pure tone audiometry revealed a mild hearing loss in both ears. At the time of current assessment, mental age derived from scores on the WISC–III (Wechsler, 1992) was 5;7. Verbal IQ was 66, Performance IQ was 48, and Full Scale IQ was 54.

Florence

Florence is a 12-year-old girl. Diagnosis of WS was at 6 months. Florence was born at 38 weeks, by lower caesarean section, in view of late decelerations on an antenatal cardiotacograph, which was performed because the mother was small for dates. Birth weight was 2,620 grams. Florence was noted to have dysmorphic features and a systolic murmur at 6 days. She has a small pulmonary artery stenosis. At age 4, she was diagnosed with a right convergent squint, for which she requires spectacles. At 4;11, on the RDLS (Reynell & Huntley, 1985), she attained a comprehension age of 3;8. Her expressive language, in the view of the speech therapist, was at an appropriate level for age. At age 6, on McCarthy's Scale of Children Abilities, her general cognitive score was 63. At age 11, she was reported as having a mild hearing loss at low frequencies in both ears. At age 12, poor motor coordination was noted. At the time of current assessment, mental age derived from scores on the WISC–III (Wechsler, 1992) was 7;5. Verbal IQ was 69, Performance IQ was 57, and Full Scale IQ was 61.

Martin

Martin is a 15-year-old boy. Diagnosis of WS was made by a consultant pediatrician at age 3. Pregnancy and delivery were normal. Birth weight was 3,020 grams. There were no neonatal problems, except for an umbilical and inguinal hernia operation at 3 months. Developmental milestones were delayed. Martin had a bilateral squint and an operation for correction was performed at 9 months, followed by another at 3 years, although a left convergent squint continued to be reported at 8 years. At age 4, mental age on the SBIS (Thorndike, Hagen, & Sattler, 1986) was 3;3, with an IQ of 70. Tested on the RDLS (Reynell & Huntley, 1985) at the age of 5;5, comprehension age was 4;8–4;9 and expressive age was 7;0, although rate of articulation was slow. At 7;4, on the WISC–R (Wechsler, 1976), Verbal IQ was 80 and Performance IQ was 69, but with considerable scatter between subtests. Martin had bilateral hearing loss at mid and high frequencies. Assessed on the Manchester word list, a test for speech discrimination, at the age of 11;6, 92% of his responses were correct. Hearing was interpreted as being unproblematic in one-to-one situations but with possible loss of consonant discrimination if there is background noise. At the time of current assessment, mental age derived from scores on the WISC–III (Wechsler, 1992) was 7;7. Verbal IQ was 69, Performance IQ was 46, and Full Scale IQ was 55.

14

Basic Language Skills in Children with Neurodevelopmental Disorders and the Notion of Brain Plasticity

Yonata Levy
The Hebrew University, Jerusalem

This chapter focuses on the linguistic profiles of children with diagnosed neurodevelopmental disorders (ND) that have marked cognitive sequelae, with emphasis on grammatical features. There is general consensus that the hallmark of language impairment in children with ND is delay in the onset of language and a generally slowed down developmental pace. Delay is typically seen in children who are later diagnosed as having SLI as well. The notion of a linguistic profile, as used in this chapter, excludes considerations of delay. Rather, the studies reported here focus on course of acquisition, typical errors, and acquisitional milestones, assuming that delay as well as a slowed down acquisitional pace will most probably be present in all or almost all the children studied. To use a traditional phrase, this chapter investigates the existence of deviance, accepting delay as characteristic of these populations.

It is of particular interest in the context of the current volume to be able to compare children with specific language impairment (SLI) with children with ND. Several chapters in the current volume have directly addressed the question: Is specific language impairment specific when compared to other populations with language impairments (e.g., Crago & Paradis, chap. 3, and Tager-Flusberg, chap. 12, in this volume)? Although this chapter does not offer a direct comparison between grammatical profiles of children with SLI and children with ND, it provides a detailed description of the profiles observed in children with ND that might serve as background against which such a comparison might be possible.

Published research relating to early linguistic phases in children with ND is summarized. Few studies have focused on morphosyntactic abilities in children with ND during the early developmental period. Yet, even when morphosyntactic abilities have not been studied directly, it is possible to glean evidence concerning children's abilities from the data presented. Then work done with children with ND of this basic level of language is presented.

The conclusion from almost all of the published research, in which the question of the grammatical profile of children with ND was often a side issue, is that at the basic level, children's grammatical profiles are remarkably similar across syndromes. The within-group variability is often as great as or even greater than the variability seen among the genotypically different syndromes. Furthermore, the linguistic profiles, specifically the grammatical profiles, observed in children with neurodevelopmental disorders, do not differ from those observed in typically developing children. The concluding section offers a way of conceptualizing the notion of brain plasticity to account for these data.

LINGUISTIC PROFILES OF CHILDREN WITH CONGENITAL SYNDROMES THAT HAVE COGNITIVE SEQUELAE

Down syndrome (DS) is among the most prevalent genetic disorders, occurring until recently in 1 of 800 live births. In 95% of the cases, it is the result of a third chromosome 21. The remaining cases are individuals in whom only parts of chromosome 21 have triplicates, so trisomy 21 is not complete. Lenneberg (1967) was the first to note that individuals with DS typically manifest language problems that are more serious than expected based on general cognitive functioning (Cardoso, C. B. Mervis, & C. A. Mervis, 1985; Sabsay & Kernan, 1993). Findings to that effect were interpreted by Fowler (1990) as pointing to the same phenomenon that is seen in SLI, namely, the dissociation of language and cognition.

Clinical reports of language in children with DS maintain that expressive language, specifically morphological and syntactic abilities, are among the most affected areas in individuals with DS. Many individuals with DS never acquire productive language skills that are more advanced than those shown by normal preschool children even though their other cognitive abilities progress beyond this level (Fowler, 1990).

However, despite significant delays in the onset of language and poor linguistic skills later on, MLU in children with DS was found to correlate highly with age. In the 1–3.5 range, MLU predicts grammatical complexity just as it does in typical children (Rondal, Ghiotto, Bredart, & Bachelet, 1988, but cf.

Bol, chap. 10 in this volume). Furthermore, it was shown that the language of children with DS within this range of MLU does not differ from that of children with retardation of unknown etiologies, nor in fact does it differ from the language of typically developing children of equivalent MLU (Pruess, Vadasy, & Fewell, 1987; Owens & MacDonald, 1982; Rondal, 1993; Tager-Flusberg, Calkins, Nolin, & Baumberger, 1990). Again, the first person to notice this was Lenneberg (1967), who argued that for the duration of the critical period, children with DS acquire language in much the same way as normal children. More recently, Fowler (1990) expressed a similar view.

Note, however, that there have been cases in the literature of individuals with DS who had good language. Perhaps the most detailed case is described in Rondal (1995). The existence of such individuals suggests that the genetic makeup that is typical of DS does not prevent good language, although such cases are rather rare.

Fragile X (FX) is considered the most common inherited cause of mental retardation in males in the general population, with a calculated prevalence of 1 in 4,000. As the name indicates, FX is an X-linked syndrome. Whereas the clinical manifestations and the chromosomal deficit have been known since the late 1970s, the genetic basis for the mental retardation was not identified until 1991 (Rousseau et al., 1991; Verkerk et al., 1991).

A common finding in individuals with FX concerns the production of deviant, repetitive language, which is distinct from the language of persons with either DS or autism (Sudhalter, Cohen, Silverman, & Wolf-Schein, 1990). The language of FX males is often described as jocular, narrative and staccato with short bursts of three and four word phrases and repetitive (Hagerman, 1991).

The production of such deviant language did not correlate, however, with the Index of Productive Syntax, whereas correlations between MLU and the Index of Productive Syntax as derived from naturalistic conversations were similar to those observed in normal preschoolers (Sudhalter, Scarborough, & Cohen, 1991). In other words, in individuals with FX too, MLU predicts syntactic complexity in naturalistic productions. Note that Sudhalter et al. (1991) studied males with FX syndrome of different ages and mostly beyond the early phases of language acquisition. However, a consideration of their younger children with MLU levels of up to 3 suggests that language in the early phases is comparable to normal, language matched controls. Furthermore, similar to individuals with Down syndrome, the general cognitive level in individuals with FX does not predict language level (Walzer, 1985). Differences in strategies employed by individuals with FX syndrome during conversation did not correlate with any of the semantic-syntactic measures either (Ferrier, Bashir, Meryash, Johnson, & Wolff, 1991).

Autism is a disorder of neurological development probably occurring before birth. The most obvious anatomical abnormalities of the brain appear to be selective and confined to the limbic system and the olive (Bauman, 1999). Whereas genetics is most probably playing a significant role involving multiple gene abnormalities, its mechanism is not known at present.

Disturbances in language development almost invariably appear in autism. A significant majority of autistic children fail to develop communicative skills, or are significantly delayed in developing language. A certain proportion of autistic children, most notably high functioning autistic children, do develop good linguistic skills. It is often the case in autistic children who develop language that output is limited and the communication patterns are severely deficient. Studies that looked at the linguistic characterization of autistic children who developed language suggest that the children follow the same developmental course as do typically developing children (Tager-Flusberg et al., 1990; see Tager-Flusberg, chap. 12 in this volume). Similar to normal development, growth in MLU at the earlier phases reflects structural complexity. MLU ceases to be a predictor of structural complexity beyond MLU 3 (Scarborough, Rescorla, Tager-Flusberg, & Fowler, 1991).

Tager-Flusberg et al. (1990) compared sentence length and structural complexity in spontaneous and imitative utterances in autistic children. They found that spontaneous utterances were significantly longer and included more advanced grammatical constructions than imitative sentences. It is concluded that grammar in autism is not impaired at least in the early phases. This led the authors to state that the normal route is the only route to acquisition and there are no alternative ways to acquire language. Note that this should be understood as an empirical claim, for, in theory, it is possible to conceive of more than one way to develop language.

Williams syndrome (WS) is a rare autosomal disorder present in 1 of 20,000 live births. It is a contiguous gene disorder caused by deletion on chromosome 7Q11.23, which includes the elastin gene. The function of 16 or so additional genes that are involved in the WS phenotype is not yet understood. A marked feature of the WS phenotype is their good language. Children with WS easily engage in conversations, have good vocabularies, excellent phonology and remarkable narrative skills. Although researchers differ as to the nature of their grammatical competence, there is general consensus that language is an area of relative strength in WS (see Clahsen & Temple, chap. 13 in this volume). Whereas grammatical knowledge in school-age children and adolescents with WS has been relatively well researched, not much is known about the early phases of grammatical development in children with WS apart from the familiar delay which, despite their ultimately good linguistic achievements, characterizes this syndrome in much the same way as it does other neurodevelopmental disorders.

Capirci, Sabbadini, and Volterra (1996) presented a case study of an Italian girl with WS who was followed between ages 2;6 and 4;10. In many re spects, this Italian child followed a normal course of language acquisition, but she did not master certain aspects of formal grammar and her production varied depending on context. Thus, unlike findings in other syndromes, this study suggests that there was a qualitative difference between the type of errors that this child made and errors that are encountered in typically developing children.

Levy (in press) presents a longitudinal study of 2 Hebrew speaking children with WS. The children were studied from the beginning of two word combinations for a period of 18 months. As expected, there was a significant delay in the onset of complex language. The children were 2;10–3;6 when word combinations began. The developmental course did not present a clear cut picture—with respect to some of the grammatical features the children were showing a similar to the normal course of development while in other respects they were progressing relatively more rapidly than normally developing children of similar MLU.

LINGUISTIC PROFILES OF CHILDREN WITH ANATOMICAL INJURIES

A different group of children within the population with neurodevelopmental disorders are children with congenital anatomical brain malformations. This group includes children who have suffered brain injuries either pre- or perinatally that have affected their development in cognitive as well as in other domains. The findings in this group mirror those reported for children with congenital neurological syndrome. Although there is considerable delay in the onset of language, a similar to the normal course of development is seen in the early phases.

Bishop (1988a) reviewed a series of studies of children with anatomical injuries and concluded that they show a similar-to-the-normal course of acquisition in the early phases of language development. Recall that in all of these studies, as well as in the present work, delay along with a slow developmental pace are presumed to be characteristic of most children with neurodevelopmental disorders and do not enter into the description of the children's linguistic profiles beyond this very general statement.

Thal et al. (1991) is the only study that failed to find the expected delay. Thal et al. (1991) investigated 53 children, from 10 to 44 months old, with a single unilateral brain injury to the right or to the left hemisphere incurred before 6 months of age. The authors stated that the expectation that there will be delays in grammatical development in children with left anterior lesions, associated with a potential "developmental agrammatism," has not been supported by the data, i.e., timing as well as course of development of grammar were normal.

Feldman, Holland, and Keefe (1989) described the language abilities of two pairs of twins in whom one twin sustained a brain injury to the left hemisphere (LH) around the time of birth. Results show that the handicapped twins scored at or above the normal range on all formal tests, although they were somewhat lower on vocabulary and on the Expressive scale of the Sequenced Inventory of Communicative Development (Hendrick, Prather, & Tobin, 1975).

Levy, Amir, and Shalev (1992) presented a case study of a child with congenital LH infarct affecting the middle cerebral artery. A detailed comparison of the course of acquisition in this child suggests that although there was delay in onset, a normal course of development was evident. Large-scale studies of children with unilateral brain injuries to the left or to the right hemisphere point to the same conclusions (Bates, Vicari, & Trauner, 1999).

The next section presents two studies of children with neurodevelopmental disorders who were acquiring Hebrew as their first and only language. The first study considers the grammatical profiles of 8 children with congenital neurological deficits or with anatomical abnormalities whose MLU is at or around 3. These findings were reported originally in Levy, Tennebaum, and Ornoy (2000). The second study considers linguistic knowledge as it is reflected in children's ability to appropriately repair their utterances in response to the listener's requests for clarification. Both studies compared children's performance to the performance of typically developing children of equivalent MLU.

By way of introduction to both studies, a brief exposition of the structure and acquisition of Hebrew is presented with a focus on the linguistic elements that figure in the analysis of the data from the children.

A BRIEF DESCRIPTION OF THE STRUCTURE OF HEBREW AND RELATED ACQUISITIONAL FACTS

The Structure of Hebrew

Hebrew is a Semitic language. Hebrew words are composed of consonantal roots cast in vocalic word patterns. The roots are usually triconsonantal and the patterns are in the form of vocalic infixes, prefixes, and suffixes. All verbs are analyzable into root + pattern. With respect to nouns, however, this generalization is only partial because some nouns do not have a recognizable root. There are seven verb patterns and about three dozen noun patterns. It is generally the case in Hebrew that the roots convey core meanings, whereas the patterns are essentially derivational paradigms that in part introduce meaning modulations.

Although the formal paradigms of this derivational system are highly systematic, their semantics is only partially predictable from their forms. As for nouns, it is often the case that derivational paradigms are strictly formal and do not convey meanings at all.

Hebrew has a rich inflectional morphology. Verbs in the past and future are inflected for tense, number, person, and gender. Present tense verbs are not marked for person. The following are examples of verbs and nouns from the root *G-D-L* (Root-consonants are in capitals; verbs are in third person, masculine, singular, past tense; nouns are in singular form): *GaDaL* 'grew-intransitive (verb)'; *GiDeL* 'grew-transitive (verb)'; *GuDaL* 'was grown-passive (verb)'; *hiGDiL* 'made bigger-active causative (verb)'; *huGDaL* 'made bigger-passive causative (verb)'. *GDiLa* 'growing-up (noun)'; *GiDuL* 'tumor; growth (noun)'; *GaDLut* 'grandeur (noun)'; *haGDaLa* 'enlargement (noun)'; *miGDaL* 'tower (noun)'.

Hebrew nouns are classified for gender and this classification determines forms of agreement and of plural marking. Agreement is required with respect to gender, number, and person. Subject-complement constructions that are without verbs, traditionally called "nominal sentences," are well formed in Hebrew. A direct object marker *et* is obligatory for marking accusative objects.[1]

---

[1]Examples 1–4 illustrate agreement patterns in Hebrew, and Examples 5–7 show nominal constructions and use of the direct object *et*.

1. ha-yeled   nixnas   la-   kit<u>a</u>   ha-xadash<u>a</u>
   the-boy entered-sg/m to(def)-class/f the-new/f
   'The boy entered the new class'

2. ha-yald<u>a</u>   nixnes<u>a</u>   la-   kit-<u>ot</u>   ha- xadash-<u>ot</u>
   the-girl entered-sg/f to(def)-classes/f/pl the-new/f/pl
   'The girl entered the new classes'

3. ha-yelad<u>im</u> nixnesu   la-   xadar<u>im</u>   ha-xadash<u>im</u>
   the-boys   entered-pl to(def)-room/m/pl the-new/m/pl
   'The boys entered the new rooms'

4. ha-yelad<u>ot</u> nixnesu   la-   xadar<u>im</u> ha-xadash<u>im</u>
   the-girls   entered-pl to(def)-rooms/m the-new/pl/m
   'The girls entered the new rooms'

5. ha-yeled xaxam
   the-child clever
   'The child (is) clever'

6. ima   ba-   bayt
   mother in(def)-home
   'Mother (is) at home'

7. ima   ra'ata   et   ha-yeled
   mother saw-past/f/sg (acc.marker) the(def)-boy
   'Mother saw the boy'

Although being fully marked for person in the past and the future, Hebrew has a "mixed" pattern of subject omission. Omission of overt subject is typically grammatical in the first and second persons in the future and past tense but ungrammatical in the third person in those tenses. It is likewise ungrammatical to omit overt subjects in the present tense because present tense forms are not marked for person.[2]

Acquisition

The acquisition of Hebrew morphology has been studied extensively in recent years. Berman (1985, 1994) investigated the development of verb morphology. She argued that early verb use is rote learned and thus item based. Typically, the child has one verb form per root. Once the child begins to vary verb forms, there will be many more forms for each root, because roots will occur in different patterns and in different inflectional endings (Levy, 1997).

Hebrew-speaking children start out with *semantically* unanalyzed forms of verbs yet at the same period they can effectively control the necessary formal manipulations of the various root + pattern combinations. For quite some time, children continue to use a rich variety of verb forms in morphosyntactically appropriate contexts, not knowing that these formal manipulations may be systematically used to achieve modulations of meanings. It is only around age 4, a long time after they have been using most verb patterns productively, that children's errors indicate that they begin to appreciate the semantics of the system (Berman, 1985, 1994). Data show that 2-year-old Hebrew speakers, although unaware of the semantics of the derivations, differentiate between the consonantal roots of words and the vocalic word patterns. It seems that the componential nature of Hebrew words is appreciated by Hebrew speakers at a very early stage in their linguistic development (Levy, 1988a).

Previous studies of the acquisition of gender in a variety of languages, including Hebrew, show that children master the formal morphological parts of this system relatively early (Berman & Armon-Lotem, 1996; Levy, 1983; Mulford, 1985; Smoczynska, 1985). Thus, even before age 3, errors of linguistic gender on inanimate nouns, which mark gender morphologically, are infrequent. In cases of animate nouns in which linguistic gender is determined by the semantic notion of gender, errors are common and learning is a more protracted process. These findings hold across all languages studied so far, among them Hebrew (Levy, 1983, 1988b).

In a cross-sectional survey of productive syntax in Israeli children from ages 1;0 to 5;6, Dromi and Berman (1986) found an increase in the use of

---

[2]See Vainikka and Levy (1999) for an account of subject omission in mixed languages.

polyclause utterances and a decrease in the use of one-clause utterances, documented up to age 4. A decrease was observed in the production of nominal and copular clauses as well, along with an increase in the use of clauses with finite verbs. This is in line with the accepted view that an increase in the use of sentences with finite verbs characterizes more advanced grammatical stages (Berman, 1994; Berman & Armon-Lotem, 1996; Sano & Hyams, 1994).

The development of the mixed null subject system was studied by Berman (1990) and more recently by Elisha (1997) and by Levy and Vainikka (2001). Findings suggest a very early convergence on the basic facts of the mixed system, namely, preservation of overt subject in third person past and future and in all persons in the present tense with optional omission of overt subjects in first and second persons in the past and the future tense. By age 3, children are essentially adultlike in their performance.

Previous studies have shown that at or around MLU 3, children control agreement. Production of direct object marker -et- is likewise almost error free at this stage. This is the developmental phase during which children acquire crucial parts of the morphology and their errors become minimal (Berman, 1985; Levy, 1983, 1988a). However, from a quantitative point of view, the child continues to make a similar amount of errors of syntax and meaning, yet at the same time the child is also using longer sentences, more complex syntactic structures, and richer vocabulary (Levy et al., 2000). In other words, the child's linguistic repertoire is growing but it is still not error free.

STUDY I: LINGUISTIC PROFILES OF CHILDREN WITH NEURODEVELOPMENTAL DISORDERS[3]

Participants, Procedures, and Analysis

Eight Hebrew-speaking children, 5 boys and 3 girls, with a variety of neurological abnormalities (ND) were studied. Two of the children had fragile X syndrome (FX), one child had Sotos syndrome, two children had congenital hydrocephalus grade 4 with shunts, one child had a congenital LH infarct affecting the middle cerebral artery, one child had left hemiatrophy, and another had enlarged ventricles. Table 14.1 presents the diagnosed syndromes, ages, MLU, and number of analyzable utterances for each child (excluding imitations and repetitions).

The children and their families were monolingual. They lived at home and their parents had at least a high school education. The children's

---

[3]This section is a summary of Levy, Tennenbaum, and Ornoy (2000).

TABLE 14.1
Characterization of the Subjects

Child[a]	Syndrome	IQ	MLU	Age	Total Utterances
A	FX	[b]GCI = 48 verbal = 23	2.2	4;8	383
Mi	Sotos	GCI = 50 verbal = 24	2.5	6;10	376
M	Hydroc	GCI = 63 verbal = 35	2.5	3;3	587
B	FX	IQ = 70 verbal = 70	2.9	3;5	365
E	Hydroc	Leiter = 58	2.8	3;5	739
Av	LH Infarct	Leiter = 60	2.3	4;4	530
T	Left Hemiatroph	IQ = 69 verbal = 75	2.8	3;6	536
S	Enlarge V	Bayley = 74	2.4	3;6	533

[a]A, Mi, and M were tested on the McCarthy (1972). B and T were tested on the Stanford–Binet (1960). E and Av were tested on the Leiter (1969) and S was tested on the Bayley (1969).

[b]Note that verbal scores for the McCarthy (1972) have a mean of 50 ($SD = 10$), and the GCI has a mean of 100 ($SD = 15$).

speech was clear and intelligible and none had hearing impairment. As can be seen in Table 14.1, the children had mild to moderate retardation. It should be noted that these types of congenital conditions—chromosomal (FX), metabolic (Sotos), developmental (Hydrocephalus) and anatomical (infarct; hemiatrophy)—are representative of the most common *diagnosed* congenital causes of retardation in children.

Eight typically developing children, 5 boys and 3 girls from ages 2;0 to 2;4, served as controls. The groups were matched on two language measures: MLU and distribution of utterances of different length. The latter has been introduced in previous studies as a way of circumventing familiar problems with central measures such as MLU (Levy et al., 1992; see also Bol, chap. 10 in this volume).

The children were recorded two to three times in their homes with no more than 2 weeks interval between sessions. Each session lasted for an hour, during which the experimenter talked and played with the child, often in the presence of other members of the child's family. The experimenter was instructed to interact with the child in a natural way, focusing on activities that will encourage conversation such as joint play or joint personal activities. Specific manipulations were not attempted.

The study focused on 13 variables known to be diagnostic of a child's linguistic level. Three of the variables—correct syntactic agreement (coded as:

agr), correct use of direct object marker (coded as: **et**), and errors in gender marking on inanimate nouns (coded as: **gi**)—require grammatical knowledge that is inherently nonsemantic. The next list of variables reflects grammatical knowledge that involves semantic-pragmatic knowledge as well: use of nominal or copular sentences (coded as: **hc**), errors in marking gender on animate nouns (coded as: **ga**), proportion of verb roots to verb forms (coded as: **roots:vf**), use of past tense verbs (coded as: **past**), percentage of complex sentences (coded as: **coj + rel**), percentage of errors of morphology (coded as: **mor**), and percentage of errors of syntax (coded as: **syn**). Errors were always calculated out of the total numbers of errors committed by the child. The third group of variables concerns specifically semantic-pragmatic knowledge: pragmatic errors (coded as: **prg**), errors of word choice (coded as: **wc**), and percent of errors of meaning (coded as: **mean**). Note that the count of meaning errors includes **prg**, **wc**, and **ga**, as well as other types of meaning errors. **Coj + rel**, **agr**, and **et** are counted among the syntactic errors and **gi** is counted among the errors of morphology.[4]

Whereas many languages share some of the variables studied, others are specific to Hebrew. For example, production of subordinate and coordinate clauses, increased use of finite predicates, and control of morphology are among the defining characteristics of language development crosslinguistically. Measures such as proportion of verb roots to verb forms, use of verbless clauses, and use of direct object marker *et* are specific to Hebrew.

The mean and standard deviation (*SD*) of the control group provide measures of the performance and the variance seen in that group. Children with ND are considered similar to the controls with respect to a given variable if their achievements are within 1 *SD* from the normal mean. (See Conti-Ramsden, 1998, for a similar approach to the comparison between children with disorders and their normal controls.) Note that this criterion is rather stringent because, by definition, for each variable there also will be normally developing children who will be below or above 1 *SD* from the mean. Furthermore, the acceptable practice in previous research, borrowed from clinical practice, was to take between 1.5 and 2 *SD*s as marking deviation from the normal.

Findings

Table 14.2 presents percents of errors and of correct usage, in accordance with the previous coding system, for each child individually. Mean perform-

---

[4]Pragmatic errors include problems with extra sentential reference, inappropriate discourse behavior and wrong register. Meaning errors concern the types of errors referred to in the text as well as problems with logical form, e.g. asserting and negating the same attribute in the same sentence.

TABLE 14.2
Performance of Children with ND Relative to the Mean
Performance (+/– SD) of Typically Developing Controls

Variables	Controls M %	Subjects							
		A	Mi	M	B	E	Av	T	S
syn	29.5	^	^	^	^	^	^	^	^
	SD = 9.56	24	20	20	37	25	23	39	25
mor	13.6	^	^	—	^	^	^	^	^
	SD = 8.64	7	19	24	8	15	17	15	14
mean	58.2	^	^	^	^	^	^	^	^
	SD = 11.2	69	60	56	55	59	60	47	61
hc	12.3	—	^	^	^	^	^	^	—
	SD = 6.8	23.4	12	18.8	15	5.4	13	16.2	33.2
coj + rel	5.5	^	^	^	^	^	^	+	^
	SD = 4.9	1.4	3.1	2.3	7.6	2.1	3.7	14	3.4
et	93.4	^	^	^	^	^	^	^	^
	SD = 12.2	100	100	92.3	85.7	90	86.7	100	85.7
gi	3.1	^	^	—	^	^	^	^	^
	SD = 2.3	4.7	0	5.6	0	0	0	2	3.6
past	21.4	^	^	^	^	—	—	^	^
	SD = 7.65	19	17	20	21	11	8	21	38
root:vf	1:1.55	^	^	^	+	^	—	^	^
	SD = 0.27	1:1.5	1:1.8	1:1.8	1:2	1:1.8	1:1	1:1.8	1:1.5
agr	91.5	+	+	^	+	+	+	^	—
	SD = 4.04	100	100	88.2	100	100	100	93	82.4
ga	10.6	—	^	^	^	+	^	—	—
	SD = 5.4	28.6	10	5.6	6.7	0.8	15.4	21.6	17.8
wc	3.7	+	^	^	—	+	^	^	^
	SD = 1.2	1.5	3.4	3.7	7.4	1.2	3.5	2.6	4.5
prg	8.9	—	—	—	—	^	+	+	^
	SD = 3.1	24	16	13	17.2	8.5	4	3.3	8.3

Note: ^ = within 1 *SD* from the mean, - = below 1 *SD* from the mean, + = above 1 *SD* from the
mean. **syn** = % of syntactic errors, **agr** = % of correct agreement, **ga** = % of errors of gender in an
mate nouns, **mor** = % of errors of morphology, **mean** = % of meaning errors, **wc** = % of errors
word choice, **hc** = % of verbless clauses, **prg** = % of errors of pragmatics, **coj + rel** = % of comple
clauses, **past** = % of past tense verbs, **et** = % correct use of direct object marker, **gi** = % of errors
gender in inanimate nouns, **root:vf** = proportion of verb roots to verb forms.

ance on each of the variables for the typically developing children is pre
sented as well. When the child's performance in a given variable is withi
one *SD* of the mean seen in the typically developing group, it is marked a
^. The child's performance is marked – if it is below 1 *SD* and + if it is abov
1 *SD*.

As can be seen in Table 14.2, the children with ND score at or around th
mean achieved by the controls in the first nine variables. The difference

seen between the groups are distributed among different children. This is particularly clear in the first nine variables where differences are, in general, rather minimal. Thus, the only children who differ from the controls on two variables are M and Av, and all the others are either similar to the controls or different on just one variable. Notice that M is worse than the controls in **gi**, which is coded as a morphological error. It comes as no surprise that she is below normal on **mor**, which is the proportion of error of morphology as well. As for Av, he does not use many past tense verbs, which could have affected the ratio **root:vf**. This correlation, however, is not always critical, as can be seen in E, who does not do well with past tense forms but has a ratio of **root:vf** similar to that of the controls. In other words, growth in verb forms for E results from increase in use of forms other than past tense.

A larger variability is seen in the last four variables in Table 14.2. The children with ND differ most clearly from the controls with respect to errors of word choice (**wc**), errors of gender marking on animate nouns (**ga**), and pragmatic errors (**prg**). With respect to **agr**, although the children with ND make fewer errors than the controls, it can be seen from the mean and the *SD* that both groups are close to ceiling.

The findings from the children served to compare profiles through the use of Partial Order Scalogram Analysis by Base Coordinates (POSAC; Shye, 1985; Shye, Elizur, & Hoffman, 1994). Multiple scaling by POSAC is a technique for measuring individuals with respect to a multivariate attribute.[5] Profiles are plotted over multidimensional space according to overall proximity of their composite features (i.e., similar profiles are grouped together and profiles that differ are further apart). If the profiles of children with ND are different from those of the controls, then the space will divide between the groups.

Figure 14.1 gives the space diagram for the profiles of the children with ND and the controls. There was no separation on the POSAC multidimensional space between the linguistic profiles of the children with ND and the controls. That is, it was not possible to divide the POSAC space in such a way that children with ND will cluster in different areas than the controls. Rather, children were spread in space and the groups were indistinguishable.

So, at the basic level, the clinically observed language disorders seen in children with neurological deficits could not be explained in reference to disorders of grammar, because at this phase grammatical development as reflected in the children's linguistic profile, although delayed, did not differ from the observed pattern in typically developing children.

---

[5]For more details concerning the use of POSAC in the current study see Levy et al. (2000).

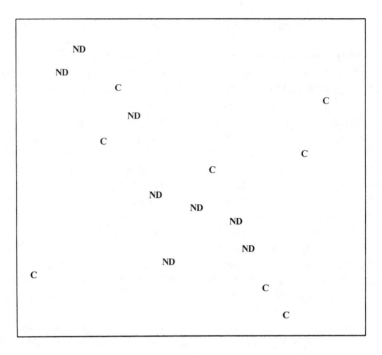

FIG. 14.1. General POSAC space diagram for children with neurological syndromes (ND) and for the controls (C).

STUDY 2: SPEECH MONITORING AS A REFLECTION
OF GRAMMATICAL KNOWLEDGE

Requests for Clarification

A different analysis performed on the linguistic products of children with
ND concerned their compliance with requests for clarifications during conversations. Consider the nature of conversational requests for clarification.
Earlier studies have drawn attention to the fact that there are two distinct
ways in which listeners may overtly express, in language, the fact that they
have not understood what has been said (Spilton, 1977). The listener may
pose contingent queries that are focused, guiding the speaker to the source
of the difficulty encountered by the hearer (e.g., "Where did he go?"). Following Garvey (1977), we term such a specific request **SR**. In response to
SR, speakers may either attempt to repair their previous utterance, repeat
it, or change the topic altogether.

Alternatively, difficulties of understanding may be conveyed through the
use of a nonspecific, neutral contingent query like "What?" We term such a
neutral request **NR** (Garvey, 1977). Because **NR** is a general query that does

not inform the speaker of the specific source of the difficulty, it requires the speaker to locate the problem and then do something about it, e.g., repair it, repeat it, or change the topic altogether. Note that ability to locate an error and ability to repair once the source of the difficulty has been identified are separate behaviors. Yet both are revelatory with respect to children's linguistic knowledge. In response to such requests, children can locate the error and attempt repair only in cases in which their grammar tells them that an error has been committed. Other behaviors, such as repeating the utterance, raising the voice, or changing the topic of the discourse, although often pragmatically appropriate in the context of requests for clarification, are not linguistically specific and hence are of no concern here.

Models of speech production and monitoring can provide a potential theoretical framework which will account for the kind of linguistic behavior that is the focus of the current investigation. Assuming Levelt's model (1989), speech monitoring is inseparable from speech comprehension. Ability to work on the products of the monitor for the sake of repair, a meta-operation, is part of speakers' knowledge of language. The prediction therefore is that even young children with basic linguistic knowledge will show speech monitoring. Furthermore, such monitoring will be at a level commensurate with the children's grammatical knowledge (Levy, 1999). Examining the products of monitoring and repair is therefore yet another way of gaining insights into children's grammatical knowledge. The current study asked whether children with neurodevelopmental disorders perform similar to their language matched controls when they encounter **NRs**.

Participants, Procedure, and Method of Analysis

Unfortunately, adults pose rather few **NRs** to young children and thus, of the 8 children in Study 1, only 4 participants with ND had enough instances of **NRs** in the recorded conversations. These were Mi, A, M, and E. Details concerning these children are given in Table 14.1.

All four children had achieved basic linguistic skills that they were readily using to communicate with people around them. Four typically developing children, age 2;2 to 2;6, with no reported health problems, matched individually on sex and socioeconomic status with the participants served as controls (**LC**). The children were matched on MLU and on distribution of sentences of different length. The typically developing children were part of the group reported in Levy (1999) in which repair behavior in typically developing children was investigated.

The following questions were investigated: (a) Do the children understand the conversational import of neutral requests for clarification? Evidence for such an understanding is prerequisite for the questions that follow. (b) Can the children access the representation of their utterance? (c) Can the children locate linguistic problems that may be the cause of the

NRs? Note that children may be able to access the representation of their spoken utterances, and thus Question (b) will receive a positive reply, and yet fail to locate the *specific error* that provoked the adult request for clarification, and thus Question (c) may be answered in the negative. (d) Can the children repair the problems that they have successfully located? Here again, it is quite possible that the children will be able to locate the problem while still unable to provide an appropriate repair.

The data consist of naturalistic adult–child conversations in which exchanges of the following type occurred: the child said something, the adult expressed lack of understanding of what had been said through an explicit request for clarification of either an **SR** or an **NR** type, and the child responded. The adult's difficulties in understanding were authentic and no manipulations were attempted.

Only exchanges in which the adult query could be related to some linguistic aspect of the child's utterance were analyzed. Similar to Levelt (1989) and to Marshall and Morton (1978), the current work adopts a definition of language broad enough to encompass grammar as well as lexical, semantic, and pragmatic aspects of language. Instances in which difficulties of understanding might have been caused by external circumstances (e.g., an unexpected noise or an event that required sudden attention or cases in which the adult did not hear what the child said, were excluded from the analysis). Altogether there were only a few such cases. Details of the procedure for data collection are similar to Study 1. A single experimenter collected the data from all four children and later transcribed the tapes. This person was unaware of the fact that repair constituted the topic of investigation.

The following steps were involved in coding an adult–child exchange: (a) The child's utterance was coded for the error it contained. (b) A decision was made concerning whether a request for clarification was of an **NR** or an **SR** type. (c) The child's response was coded.

Note the decision to relate the adult's requests for clarification to the errors that the children were committing. Of course, it may be argued that the adult was in need of clarification not because of the errors but for other reasons that were not obvious from the transcripts. Clearly, this possibility cannot be rejected altogether. However, with respect to the topic of the current investigation, namely, children's monitoring abilities, all that matters is that there was an error that the child could monitor for, even if the possibility exists that this error was not the actual trigger for the adult query. In line with this approach, if a request for clarification was issued yet, no aspect of the child's utterance was inappropriate or erroneous, that exchange was considered irrelevant to the current analysis.

As for the notion of an "error," whereas morphological or syntactic errors are relatively straightforward, semantic and pragmatic errors are less clearly defined within spontaneous, naturalistic conversations. Here and throughout the chapter, *error* is used in a broad sense to refer to an explicitly expressed linguistic aspect of the utterance that could be the cause for its infelicity.

Errors in children's productions and the corresponding requests for clarification were divided into three main categories: syntactic, morphological, and meaning. The *syntactic* category included errors in diverse syntactic phenomena such as subordinate constructions, agreement, use of direct object marker, use of prepositions, and ungrammatical subject omission. Recall that with respect to subject omission, Hebrew is "mixed." Omission of NP subject is typically grammatical in the first and second persons in the future and past tense. It is ungrammatical in the third person and in the present tense. However, as is the case in many languages, ungrammatical omission is allowed given specific contexts. Thus, errors of subject omission in the third person and in the present tense may be of two types: omissions that are ungrammatical in all contexts and thus constitute a syntactic error and omissions that would have been acceptable had the context been different. The latter cases were counted among the pragmatic errors.

Errors coded as morphological related to inflectional as well as derivational morphology. *Morphological* errors include errors of form involving root consonants, word patterns, or inflections. As for nonce words, these probably represent a confluence of factors including articulatory, morphological, and lexical. In the present work, they are counted among the morphological errors.

Errors of *meaning* and the corresponding clarification requests related to lexical, semantic, and pragmatic aspects. The following were considered as tapping lexicosemantic problems: errors in the choice of words, use of incompatible terms, and problems of reference. For example, utterances in which the child used a negative term and immediately contradicted it by using a positive term that reversed the meaning of the clause, or instances in which reference could not be determined from what was actually said, were coded as meaning problems (see footnote 4). Errors of gender marking on animate nouns, inappropriate marking of tense, person, and number, and lack of definite marker when definiteness is required were likewise counted among the meaning errors. Note that in Hebrew, tense, number, person, and gender are morphologically marked, thus knowledge of morphology is implicated in the linguistic encoding of these notions. These cases were coded as meaning errors whenever the focus was neither on agreement nor on problems of morphological form, but on the correct marking of the semantic concept.

Meaning errors also included pragmatic infelicity. These were cases in which the child's choice of words or construction was such that, had the general context been different, the same word or construction would have been appropriate. Examples concern omissions of sentence elements—subjects or objects—that are pragmatically constrained. Discourse conditions likewise permit omission of other sentence elements, for example, verbs or main clauses. Such omissions can therefore be well formed or can be pragmatically inappropriate, if the context is not right.

Note that whereas interesting insights may be gained from consideration of children's errors and adult queries as they divide between these separate categories, with respect to the main topic under investigation (viz. speech monitoring and repair), nothing really hinges on the accuracy of this categorization. What was crucial was that there be an identifiable linguistic problem in the child's utterance that might reasonably be assumed as the cause for the adult's request for clarification.

Apart from coding the child's errors, adult–child exchanges involving requests for clarification were coded for success of locating the errors as well as success of producing repair. Request for clarification of the **SR** type require only the former. Thus, those were coded in the following way: **SR + y** was chosen if the child successfully repaired the utterance. Unsuccessful repair included cases in which the child ignored the adult's request or changed the topic of the conversation or repeated the entire utterance.

With respect to **NR**, both questions were relevant, namely, did the children locate the error and did they repair it? **NR + y** was chosen if the children correctly identified the source of the problem. This was most clearly evident if they attempted a specific change in their utterance, for example, changing the morphology or substituting a lexical item. Repetition of part of the utterance that contained the error, but not the rest of the utterance, likewise indicated that the children had identified the locus of the problem. When locating the error was successful and appropriate repair was produced, the utterance was further coded as **NR + y + s**. Thus, the category **NR + y** subsumes correct as well as incorrect repairs, whereas **NR + y + s** refers exclusively to successful repairs.

Findings

Table 14.3 presents sample sizes, percentage of utterances with errors of different types calculated out of the total number of analyzable utterances for each child, and percentage of utterances with errors that were queried by the adult (**SRs + NRs**) calculated out of the total number of errors in each category. For example, of the 892 utterances that were analyzed for Mi, 6.5% had syntactic errors. The adult queried only 7% of these errors. The last row gives the means and ranges for the language-matched control group (**LC**).

As can be gleaned from Table 14.3, although the children make many errors, requests for clarification are rather infrequent, particularly in relation to syntax and to morphology. Errors of meaning are the most disruptive to the conversation and most requests for clarification relate to those aspects

TABLE 14.3

Sample Size, Percentage of Error Types, and Percentage of Requests
for Clarification for Mi, A, M, and E and for Typically Developing Children

		Syntax		Morphology		Meaning	
Subject	*Sample Size*	*Errors %*	*SR + NR %*	*Errors %*	*SR + NR %*	*Errors %*	*SR + NR %*
Mi	892	6.5	7	6.2	26.8	19.6	40.5
	882	12.5	5.4	3.4	23.3	27.7	35.1
M	958	10.7	2	11.4	16.5	26.8	29.5
	752	10.3	12.8	6.2	17	24.3	30.6
C	4075	7.4	12.6	4.9	55	21	41
		(4.8–9.4)	(6.4–20.5)	(2.5–7.2)	(51–63.2)	(17.2–23.5)	(27.2–50)

Note: Numbers in parentheses indicate ranges for the findings in the **LC**. **Syn** = syntactic, **Mor** = morphological, **NR** = neutral requests for clarification, **SR** = specific requests for clarification.

(Fisher Exact Test; Mi, $p < .04$; A, $p < .01$; M, $p < .005$; E, $p < .043$). Reluctance to pose requests for clarification to children was evident in conversations with typically developing children as well. However, unlike the children with **ND**, they were mostly required to clarify utterances with morphological errors (Levy, 1999). This was the case despite the fact that the percent of meaning errors was similar in both groups, as seen in Table 14.3. This point is taken up in the discussion.

The next paragraphs focus on the analysis of children's responses to **NR**s. Table 14.4 addresses the following questions: do the children understand the conversational import of **NR**s, and can they access the representation of their spoken utterances? The percentage of changes of topics (**CT**) following **NR**s offers a way of estimating the children's understanding of what is required of them. Although changes of topic do occur every now and then in conversation (if, e.g., a person thinks that the listener did not hear what was said), a systematic change of topic in response to **NR** is indication that the child does not understand the conversational force of **NR**. Repetition of the full utterance likewise may indicate a lack of understanding of the intent of **NR**. It suggests a default behavior when an individual does not know what, specifically, needs to be done. On the other hand, attending to part of the utterance, repeating it, or changing a certain aspect of it is prima facie indication that the child hypothesized that there was a specific problem in the expressed utterance.

Table 14.4 gives the number of **NR**s asked of each child, the percentage of changes of topic following such requests (**CT**), the percentage of repetition of whole utterances (**Rep**), and the percentage of **SP**. **SP** refers to cases in which the child attended to a specific part of the utterance. The figures given in Table 14.4 are similar for the children with **ND** and for the controls. The relatively small number of **CT**s suggests that all four children under-

TABLE 14.4
Neutral Requests for Clarification (NR), Percentage of Responses
Involving a Change of Topic (CT), Full Utterance Repetition (REP),
and Repetition of Part of the Utterance (SP) in Mi, A, M, and E

	Child				
	Mi	A	M	E	LC
NR	32	45	49	28	147
CT(%)	18.7	26.6	18.4	25	22
REP(%)	10.4	8.4	9.3	8	8.6
SP(%)	70.9	65	72.3	67	69.4

Note: **NR** = neutral request for clarification, **CT** = change of topic, **Rep** = whole utterance repetition, **SP** = repetition or change of specific parts of the utterance.

stood that by posing **NR**, the listener requests clarification of the previous utterance. The percentage of **SP** is close to or above 70% for all the children.

Table 14.5 presents findings that are relevant to several other questions, namely, are the children able to locate errors in their utterances, and can they provide repair? Table 14.5 gives the numbers of **NR**s, the percentage of

TABLE 14.5
Mi, A, M, and E: Neutral Requests for Clarification (NR), Percentage
of Successful Identification of Errors (NR + y), and Percentage
of Successful Repair Out of the Total Identified Errors (NR + y + s)

Subject	Syntax NR / NR + y(%) / NR + y + s(%)	Morphology NR / NR + y(%) / NR + y + s(%)	Meaning NR / NR + y(%) / NR + y + s(%)	Total NR + y(%) / NR + y + s(%)
Mi	— / — / —	5 / 1(20) / —	27 / 3(11) / 3(100)	4(12.5) / 3(75)
A	1 / — / —	4 / 3(75) / 2(66.6)	40 / 17(42.5) / 5(29.4)	20(44.4) / 7(35)
M	1 / — / —	10 / 6(60) / 4(66.6)	38 / 16(42.1) / 3(18.7)	22(44.8) / 7(31.8)
E	6 / 4(66.6) / 1(25)	4 / 1(25) / 1(100)	18 / 7(38.8) / 1(14.3)	12(42.8) / 3(25)
LC	20 / 18% / — / (33%–40%)	48 / 40.6% / 38% / (30.7%–46%) (16.6%–60%)	118 / 55.4% / 58.7% / (38.7%–70%) (41.6%–79%)	186 / 47% / 55% / (40.8%–55%) (40%–66.6%)

success in locating errors in specific parts of the utterances (**NR + y**), and the percentage of success in providing repair (**NR + y + s**).

The data in Table 14.5 highlight the difference between Mi and the other children. A, M, and E succeed in locating errors in more than 40% of the total number of **NR**s addressed to them, which is quite similar to the percent seen in the controls. Mi locates 12.5% of the errors in response to **NR**s and thus he is clearly outside the norm seen in typically developing children. The exceptionally small number of errors that Mi locates (**NR + y**) is striking in view of the fact that he seems to have understood the conversational import of **NR**s as seen in the relatively few cases of changes of topic and of whole-utterance repetitions in his data (see Table 14.4).

Although A and M are doing quite well in locating errors of morphology, E does rather poorly in morphology yet he does well in locating errors of syntax. All three children are within lower end of the norm in locating errors of meaning (**NR + y**), and are doing very poorly in providing repairs. (The fact that Mi succeeds in providing repair for 100% of the meaning errors that he locates is not very telling because he locates so few of them.) In general, the children's repairs (**NR + y + s**) are considerably fewer than those provided by the controls.

SUMMARY AND DISCUSSION OF THE FINDINGS

This study analyzed conversational repair in naturalistic settings in four children with intellectual impairments. These are case studies in which averaging over participants has not been attempted. The naturalistic setup had two drawbacks from the point of view of the investigation. The first concerned the fact that, under natural circumstances, adults tend not to pose too many requests for clarification to young children. In fact, although typically developing children are asked to clarify their speech slightly more often than the participants in the study, most of the errors they commit are left unqueried (Levy, 1999). Thus, despite the fact that large corpora have been analyzed, in some cases firm conclusions could not be reached because there were too few instances. The second drawback concerned the fact that the only errors that children had to react to were those that the adult considered disruptive to the conversation, whereas other errors were ignored.[6]

All four children seemed to grasp the conversational import of a neutral "What?" as evident in the fact that in 75% to 80% of the cases the children attempted to do something to their utterances when **NR**s were posed—repair them, change some components, or repeat what they said. This suggests

---

[6]Bowey and deBahl (1994) suggest an ingenious experimental procedure that might counteract these difficulties.

that failure to repair that is so often seen in these children is not a consequence of a lack of understanding of what is required when **NRs** are posed.

Not surprisingly, adults prefer **SRs**, which seem intuitively simpler, to **NRs**, which are nonspecific and therefore potentially ambiguous. A similar prevalence of **SRs** over **NRs** was found in conversation with typically developing children. However, whereas in conversation with normal children, most requests for clarification were provoked by morphological errors (Levy, 1999), queries addressed to the children in the current study arose mostly out of errors concerning aspects of meaning including, more specifically, pragmatic problems.

This finding is reminiscent of Brown and Hanlon's (1970) seminal work in which it was found that adults tended to repair aspects of meaning in children's speech ignoring formal errors. It may be hypothesized that, in conversations with children with intellectual impairments, adults may tend to be less concerned about grammatical well-formedness as long as they can understand what the child is saying. On the other hand, because the children are cognitively impaired, lexical, semantic, and pragmatic errors of production may express considerable conceptual problems and thus become quite disruptive to the conversation.

The main findings concern the ability of three of the children to detect over 40% of the errors in their own productions, in response to nonspecific requests for clarification. This is close to the mean level of detection seen in typically developing children. This behavior is a reflection of the operation of a speech monitor that can detect and repair speech errors. The absolute necessity of such a monitor for a functional language faculty is discussed in Marshall and Morton (1978) and a schematic model for its operation is given in Levelt (1989). The data presented here suggest that ability to monitor speech and detect errors is yet another aspect of children's early language competence for which similar to the normal developmental pattern is seen in children with intellectual handicaps in the early stages of language development.

A caveat is in place, however. Note that the child for whom evidence for speech monitoring and error detection was not evident was also the child with the most severe intellectual impairment. This raises the possibility that ability to carry out speech monitoring and effectively apply it in responding to requests for conversational repair may be differentially affected depending on the level of cognitive functioning. Further research is needed to pursue this idea.

As shown in Table 14.5, for the participants as well as for the typically developing children, locating the errors in response to **NRs** did not necessarily result in correct repair. Importantly, however, the participants' ability to repair in response to **NRs** is significantly less than that of typically developing children. This, then, is one aspect of the children's behavior in which they differed from typically developing children.

BRAIN PLASTICITY REVISITED

Work presented in the previous sections suggests that across populations, there is a similar-to-the-normal course of grammatical development regardless of the nature of the neurological deficit. Put differently, grammatical development in the early phases, with MLU 3 or under, until basic linguistic competence has been achieved is not diagnostic of the kind of disorder a child might have. (See Crago & Paradis, chap. 3, Tager-Flusberg, chap. 12, and de Villiers, chap. 17 in the current volume for data that is relevant to this claim.) This does not preclude, however, the possibility that phenotypic differences between the syndromes may be seen at later developmental phases, when MLU will exceed 3 and there will be larger percentage of longer sentences in the child's repertoire.[7]

This is a classical case for which a notion akin to brain plasticity may provide an explanation, for these are cases in which congenitally deficient neurological systems adapt such that language acquisition proceeds normally. Brain plasticity has been defined as the capacity of the brain to diminish the impacts of lesions through structural functional changes (cf. Bach, 1990). Because specific functional deficits often occur after injury to certain neuroanatomical locations, it has been tempting to suggest that within the brain, structure equals function (Boyeson, Jones, & Harmon, 1994). Support for this idea comes from the claim that the clinical manifestations of neuronal plasticity are observed especially after prenatal, neonatal, or childhood focal cerebral damage. Thus, recent work on developmental brain plasticity continues to focus on localized brain injuries as the clinical arena in which plasticity operates and much of the discussion of brain plasticity has been restricted to cases of focal brain insults, excluding etiologies such as have been studied here (e.g., H. T. Chugani, Muller, & D. C. Chugani, 1996; Nass, 1997).

Notice that the claim that the effects of plasticity are seen especially after focal damage depends on empirical evidence concerning the ultimate level of linguistic competence that children with this type of damage can reach (Dennis, 1980; Dennis & Kohn, 1975; Woods, 1980, and the critique offered in Bishop, 1988a). However, plasticity should further be interpreted in relation to the normalcy or pathology seen in the developmental course traversed by the children (Levy et al., 1992). The clearest effects of plasticity

---

[7]Note that a larger proportion of long sentences may fail to affect MLU if concomitant with it there is a decrease in 2–3 word sentences and an increase in one word utterances.

may be seen when basic linguistic skills are concerned, whereas the final outcome is expected to vary among syndromes as well as among individuals within each syndrome as a function of the specific neurological condition and the individual's unique experiences.

The data presented in the current chapter suggest that the effects of brain plasticity are not restricted to cases of focal damage. Brain plasticity may likewise be seen in children with congenital syndromes that typically result in diffuse damage. Current conceptualization of cerebral cortex functions as basic processes under continual modification with emphasis on the role of brain plasticity in adaptive behavior in fact point in this direction (Hertz-Pannier, 1999). Furthermore, there exists a biological mechanism that suggests that this may not be a radical hypothesis.

Consider, for example, the well-documented fact of a transient phase of synaptic overabundance that is observed in the young normal brain. This period is followed by selective synaptic regression that occurs as a function of exposure to experience. This early synapse abundance is biologically driven and is considered to form the neurobiological correlates of both learning and individual variability of cortical anatomy and functional organization (Hertz-Pannier, 1999). Such systems have been observed in a number of developing sensory systems in animals as well as in the autonomic and in the musculature peripheral systems. It has been described in the human visual and frontal cortex too (Huttenlocher, de Courten, Garey, & Van der Loos, 1982).

Greenough, Black, & Wallace (1987) suggested a linking between the period of excess of synaptic structures and what they referred to as learning effects produced by experience-expectant information. By experience-expectant information, Greenough et al. (1987) meant the kind of experience that every member of the species is likely to encounter. The production of an excess of synapses, which are eventually selected by an experience-based process, seems to underlie what is being referred to as the sensitive period in young age. In later development and in adulthood, any observed growth of synapses appears to take place in response to events in the environment (Karni & Bertini, 1997; Karni et al., 1998). Greenough et al. (1987) referred to this kind of learning as experience-dependent. This kind of learning is based on the individual's unique experiences. Although later synapse formation is localized to regions where the type of information that the event presents is processed, early synapse formation has been observed in a number of areas in the brain. One may hypothesize that a similar mechanism—one not tied to specific brain areas—can compensate for diffuse deficits as well.

On the cognitive plain, plasticity is analogous to a mechanism of monitoring and repair that operates in parallel to learning during the sensitive period. Monitoring is contingent on acting in the environment, because it is through action that the system will find out that the behavior of the organism has failed.[8] Thus, the system "knows" that it is failing because its products fail to correspond to other products in the environment, because its goals are not achieved, because it gets requests for clarification, and because it fails to receive positive feedback. Under such circumstances and as a function of plasticity, the system will self-repair such that basic skills can be achieved.

Monitoring and repair in the sense used here are functionally determined. That is, it works to guarantee that the individual will achieve basic cognitive skills, in this case, basic linguistic communication. The result is the familiar linguistic profile that has been repeatedly observed in children with various disorders in the early phases, as reported in the previous sections.

But what defines "basic"? On a linguistic level, basic may be related to universal grammar, yet it will have to be functionally determined (i.e., that which enables the organism to function linguistically). On a neurological level, basic is what can be compensated for under a variety of neurological conditions. Behavioral achievements that are beyond such basic level will vary among individuals depending on the specific neurological condition as well as the person's unique environmental experiences.

In sum, consider the following hypothesis: In cases of neurological deficits that affect language, brain plasticity allows for learning that is guided by functionally determined priorities that guarantee the preservation of basic levels of performance in critical domains (see Tager-Flusberg, chap. 12 in this volume, for data that might support this claim). The prediction, therefore, is that children will show similar linguistic profiles at various points in development, reflecting the fact that basic linguistic competences are achieved by all children (normal as well as children with neurological deficits), following essentially similar acquisitional course.

Brain plasticity, however, does not come for free and the often-observed global delay in development may be the cost of the required reorganization. This is different from delay in a specific linguistic construction (e.g., Rice and Wexler's EOI, 1996, which is the hypothesis that children with SLI are delayed in acquiring the obligatoriness of tense on verbs). The claim is that delay in the onset of language is not a characteristic of the developing linguistic system. Rather, it signals the extra effort that brain mechanisms are called on to exert so as to enable the development of language to take its normal course.

Does plasticity operate in the case of SLI? Whereas many studies have grappled with the uniqueness of SLI, and quite a few of the chapters in the present volume attest to that, most are concerned with language phases that

---

[8]I would like to thank Avi Karni of the Wiezmann Institute, Rehovot, Israel, who was very helpful in turning my thoughts into words and sentences. Whether plausible or not, is of course, entirely my responsibility.

are beyond the basic level (MLU 3) considered in this chapter. Although the early phases of language development in young children with SLI have not been studied in depth, there are several accounts in the literature that suggest that the linguistic profile of children with SLI may not be unique (See, e.g., Crago & Pradis, chap. 3, and de Villiers, chap. 17 in this volume).

In a review of the literature and of his own work, Leonard (1991) argued that children with SLI fall within the lower end of the normal distribution. If this is indeed the case, then accounting for SLI is no different than accounting for individual differences within the general population. Bishop (1994) studied twins with language impairment with and without additional intellectual impairments. She reached the conclusion that there is no fundamental difference between children with language impairment who do and do not have a large discrepancy between IQ and verbal abilities. Bishop (1994) questioned the uniqueness of SLI vis-à-vis language impairments that occur in individuals with retardation.

Finally, Tomblin and Zhang (1999) conducted a large-scale study of kindergarten children with language impairments. The study did not uncover a qualitatively different profile for the children with SLI. A cluster analysis performed on these children did not display evidence of any special group of poor language learners except for one small group of children who did stand out as possibly very different from the rest of the children.

In sum, whether children with SLI indeed present with a unique grammatical profile in the early phases is still in need of empirical investigation. If the effects of plasticity on language development are as described here, then the prediction is that the early linguistic profiles of typically developing children who will eventually develop specific language impairment, will not differ from profiles seen in children whose development is normal throughout or from what has been observed in children with a variety of other neurological syndromes affecting language development.

ACKNOWLEDGMENTS

This work was done with the support of the National Institute for Psychobiology in Israel and the Israel Foundation Trustees, grant 13/92-94. I thank A. Tennebaum and A. Ornoy, MDs, of the Jerusalem Child and Family Development Center for allowing me access to their patients. I also thank the children and their families for participating in this research.

REFERENCES

Bach, R. P. (1990). Brain plasticity as a basis for recovery of function in humans. *Neuropsychologia, 28*, 547–554.

auman, M. L. (1999). Autism: Clinical features and neurobiological characteristics. In H. Tager-Flusberg (Ed.), *Neurodevelopmental disorders* (pp. 383–400). Boston: MIT Press.

ates, E., Vicari, S., & Trauner, D. (1999). Neural mediation of language development: Perspective from lesion studies of infants and children. In H. Tager-Flusberg (Ed.), *Neurodevelopmental disorders* (pp. 533–582). Boston: MIT Press.

ayley, N. (1969). *Bayley Scales of Infant Development.* New York: The Psychological Corporation.

erman, R. A. (1985). The acquisition of Hebrew. In D. I. Slobin (Ed.), *The cross-linguistic study of language acquisition* (pp. 255–372). Hillsdale, NJ: Lawrence Erlbaum Associates.

erman, R. A. (1990). On acquiring an (S)VO language: Subjectless sentences in children's Hebrew. *Linguistics, 28,* 1135–1166.

erman, R. A. (1994). Developmental perspectives on transitivity: A confluence of cues. In Y. Levy (Ed.), *Other children, other languages* (pp. 189–242). Hillsdale, NJ: Lawrence Erlbaum Associates.

erman, R. A., & Armon-Lotem, S. (1996). How grammatical are early verbs? In C. Martinot (Ed.), *Annals Littéraires de L'Université de Franche-Compté: Actes du Colloque International sur l'Acquisition de la Syntaxe* (pp. 125–137).

ishop, D. (1994). Grammatical errors in specific language impairment: Competence or performance limitations? *Applied Psycholinguistics, 15,* 507–550.

ishop, D. V. M. (1988a). Can the right hemisphere mediate language as well as the left? A critical review of recent research. *Cognitive Neuropsychology, 5*(3), 353–367.

ishop, D. V. M. (1988b). Language development after focal brain damage. In D. V. M. Bishop & K. Mogford (Eds.), *Language development in exceptional circumstances* (pp. 203–219). Hillsdale, NJ: Lawrence Erlbaum Associates.

owey, J. A., & deBhal, M. C. (1994). Selectively prompting speech repairs in stages I to V: A technique for investigation early meta-linguistic abilities. *Journal of Psycholinguistic Research, 23,* 267–275.

rown, R., & Hanlon, C. (1970). Derivational complexity and order of acquisition in child speech. In J. R. Hayes (Ed.), *Cognition and the development of language* (pp. 11–54). New York: Wiley.

oyeson, M. G., Jones, J. L., & Harmon, R. L. (1994). Sparing of motor function after cortical injury: A new perspective on underlying mechanisms. *Archives Neurology, 51,* 405–414.

apirci, O., Sabbadini, L., & Volterra, V. (1996). Language development in William's syndrome: A case study. *Cognitive Neuropsychology, 13*(7), 1017–1039.

ardoso, M. C., Mervis, C. B., & Mervis, C. A. (1985). Early vocabulary acquisition by children with Down syndrome. *American Journal of Mental Deficiency, 90,* 177–184.

hugani, H. T., Muller, R. A., & Chugani, D. C. (1996). Functional brain reorganization in children. *Brain Development, 18,* 347–356.

onti-Ramsden, G. (1998). What is the nature of specific language impairment? Is SLI really specific? *ASCLD, 6*(71), 47–64.

ennis, M. (1980). Capacity and strategy for syntactic comprehension after left and right hemidecortication. *Brain and Language, 7,* 153–169.

ennis, M., & Kohn, B. (1975). Comprehension of syntax in infantile hemiplegics after cerebral hemidecortication: Left hemisphere superiority. *Brain and Language, 2,* 472–482.

romi, E., & Berman, R. A. (1986). Language-general and language-specific in developing syntax. *Journal of Child Language, 14,* 371–387.

isha, I. (1997). *Functional categories and null subjects in Hebrew and child Hebrew.* Unpublished doctoral dissertation, CUNY Graduate Center.

eldman, H. M., Holland, A. L., & Keefe, K. (1989). Language abilities after left hemisphere brain injury: A case study of twins. *Topics in Early Childhood Special Education, 9,* 32–47.

errier, L. J., Bashir, A. S., Meryash, D. L., Johnson, J., & Wolff, P. (1991). Conversational skills of individuals with fragile X syndrome: A comparison with autism and Down syndrome. *Developmental Medicine and Child Neurology, 33,* 766–788.

Fowler, A. (1990). Language abilities in children with Down syndrome: Evidence of a specific syn
tactic delay. In D. Cicchetti & M. Beeghly (Eds.), *Children with Down syndrome: A developmen
tal perspective* (pp. 302–328). Cambridge, England: Cambridge University Press.

Garvey, C. (1977). The contingent query: A dependent act in conversation. In M. Lewis & L. /
Rosenblum (Eds.), *Interaction, conversation and the development of language* (pp. 63–93). Ne*
York: Wiley.

Greenough, W. T., Black, J. E., & Wallace, C. S. (1987). Experience and brain development. *Chi*
Development, 58, 539–559.

Hagerman, R. J. (1991). Physical and behavioral phenotype. In H. J. Hagerman & A. C. Croniste
(Eds.), *Fragile X syndrome* (pp. 3–68). Baltimore: Johns Hopkins University Press.

Hendrick, D. L., Prather, E. M., & Tobin, A. R. (1975). *Sequenced inventory of communicative deve
opment.* Seattle: University of Washington Press.

Hertz-Pannier, L. (1999). Brain plasticity during development: Physiological bases and function.
MRI approach. *Journal of Neuroradiology, 26*(1), 66–74.

Huttenlocher, P. R., de Courten, C., Garey, L. J., & Van der Loos, H. (1982). Synaptogenesis in h
man visual cortex—evidence for synapse elimination during normal development. *Neurosc
ence Letters, 33,* 247–252.

Karni, A., & Bertini, G. (1997). Learning perceptual skills: Behavioral probes into adult cortic
plasticity. *Current Opinions in Neurobiology, 7*(4), 530–535.

Karni, A., Meyer, G., Rey-Hipolito, C., Jezzard, P., Adams, M. M., Turner, R., & Ungerlieder, L. (
(1998). The acquisition of skilled motor performance: Fast and slow experience-drive
changes in primary motor cortex. *Proceedings of the National Academy of Science, 95*(3
861–868.

Leiter, R. (1969). *Leiter International Performance Scale.* Chicago: C. H. Stoelting.

Lenneberg, E. (1967). *Biological foundation of language.* New York: Wiley.

Leonard, L. (1991). Specific language impairment as a clinical category. *Language, Speech ar
Hearing Services in Schools, 22,* 66–68.

Levelt, W. J. M. (1989). *Speaking: From intention to articulation.* Cambridge, MA: MIT Press.

Levy, Y. (1983). It's frogs all the way down. *Cognition, 15,* 75–93.

Levy, Y. (1988a). The nature of early language: Evidence from the development of Hebrew mc
phology. In Y. Levy, I. M. Schlesinger, & M. D. S. Braine (Eds.), *Strategies and processes in la
guage acquisition* (pp. 73–98). Hillsdale, NJ: Lawrence Erlbaum Associates.

Levy, Y. (1988b). On the early learning of formal grammatical systems: Evidence from studies
the acquisition of gender and countability. *Journal of Child Language, 15,* 179–187.

Levy, Y. (1997). The development of morphology and syntax in a pair of DZ twin boys. *Europec
Journal of Disorders of Communication, 32,* 165–190.

Levy, Y. (1999). Early metalinguistic competence—Data from children's conversational repai*
Developmental Psychology, 35(3), 822–834.

Levy, Y. (in press). Longitudinal study of language acquisition in two children with Williams sy
drome. Proceedings of the 26th Boston University Conference on Language Developmen
MA: Cascadilla Press.

Levy, Y., Amir, N., & Shalev, R. (1992). Language development in a child with a congenital LH
sion. *Cognitive Neuropsychology, 9,* 1–32.

Levy, Y., Tennebaum, A., & Ornoy, A. (2000). Spontaneous language in children with congeni*
neurological deficits. *Journal of Speech, Language and Hearing Research, 43,* 351–365.

Levy, Y., & Vainikka, A. (2001). Development of the so-called 'empty' subjects: A cross-linguis*
perspective. *Language Acquisition, 8*(4), 363–384.

Marshall, J., & Morton, J. (1978). On the mechanics of EMMA. In A. Sinclair, R. J. Jarvella,
W. J. M. Levelt (Eds.), *The child's conception of language* (pp. 225–239). Berlin: Springer-Verla

McCarthy, D. (1972). *McCarthy Scales of Children's Abilities.* New York: Psychological Corporatic

Mulford, R. (1985). Comprehension of Icelandic pronouns gender: Semantic vs. formal factors. *Journal of Child Language, 12*, 443–454.

Nass, R. (1997). Language development in children with congenital strokes. *Seminars in Pediatric Neurology, 4*(2), 109–116.

Owens, R. E., & MacDonald, J. D. (1982). Communicative uses of the early speech of non-delayed and Down syndrome children. *American Journal of Mental Deficiency, 86*, 503–509.

Pruess, J. B., Vadasy, P. F., & Fewell, R. R. (1987). Language development in children with Down syndrome: An overview of current research. *Education and Training in Mental Retardation, 22*, 44–55.

Rice, M., & Wexler, K. (1996). Toward tense as a clinical marker of specific language impairment in English-speaking children. *Journal of Speech, Language and Hearing Research, 39*, 1236–1257.

Rondal, J. A. (1993). Down's syndrome. In D. Bishop & K. Mogford (Eds.), *Language development in exceptional circumstances* (pp. 165–176). Hillsdale, NJ: Lawrence Erlbaum Associates.

Rondal, J. A. (1995). *Exceptional language development in Down syndrome: Implications for the cognitive-language relationship.* Cambridge, England: Cambridge University Press.

Rondal, J. A., Ghiotto, M., Bredart, S., & Bachelet, J. F. (1988). Mean length of utterance in children with Down syndrome. *American Journal of Mental Retardation, 93*, 64–66.

Rousseau, F., Heitz, D., Biancalana, V., Blumenfeld, S. Kertz, C., Boue, J., Tommerup, N., Van der Hagen, C., DeLouzier-Blanchet, C., Croquette, M-F, Gilgenkrantz, S., Jalbert, P., Voelckel, M. A., Oberle, I., & Mandel, J. L. (1991). Direct diagnosis by DNA analysis of the fragile X syndrome of mental retardation. *New England Journal of Medicine, 325*, 1673–1681.

Sabsay, S., & Kernan, K. T. (1993). On the nature of language impairment in Down syndrome. *Topics in Language Disorders, 13*(3), 20–35.

Sano, T., & Hyams, N. (1994). Agreement, finiteness and the development of null arguments. *NELS, 24*, 543–555.

Scarborough, H. S., Rescorla, L., Tager-Flusberg, H., & Fowler, A. (1991). The relation of utterance length to grammatical complexity in normal and language-disordered groups. *Applied Psycholinguistics, 12*, 23–45.

Shye, S. (1985). *Multiple scaling: The theory and application of partial order scalogram analysis.* Amsterdam: North Holland.

Shye, S., Elizur, D., & Hoffman, M. (1994). *Introduction to facet theory* (Applied Social Research Methods Series, 35). Thousand Oaks, CA: Sage.

Smoczynska, M. (1985). Acquisition of Polish. In D. I. Slobin (Ed.), *The cross linguistic study of language acquisition* (Vol. 1, pp. 595–686). Hillsdale, NJ: Lawrence Erlbaum Associates.

Spilton, D. (1977). Some determinants of effective communication on four year olds. *Child Development, 48*, 968–977.

Sudhalter, V., Cohen, I. L., Silverman, W., & Wolf-Schein, E. G. (1990). Conversational analysis of makes with Fragile X, Down syndrome and autism. *American Journal on Mental Retardation, 94*(4), 431–441.

Sudhalter, V., Scarborough, H. S., & Cohen, I. (1991). Syntactic delays and pragmatic deviance in the language of fragile X males. *American Journal of Medical Genetics, 38*, 493–497.

Tager-Flusberg, H., Calkins, S. Nolin, T., & Baumberger, T. (1990). A longitudinal study of language acquisition in autistic and Down syndrome children. *Journal of Autism and Developmental Disorders, 20*(1), 1–21.

Thal, D. J., Marchman, V., Stiles, J., Aram, D., Trauner, D., Nass, R., & Bates, E. (1991). Early lexical development in children with focal brain injury. *Brain and Language, 40*, 491–527.

Tomblin, B. J., & Zhang, X. (1999). Language patterns and etiology in children with specific language impairment. In H. Tager-Flusberg (Ed.), *Neurodevelopmental disorders* (pp. 361–382). Boston: MIT Press.

Vainikka, A., & Levy, Y. (1999). Empty subjects in Finnish and Hebrew. *Natural Language and Linguistic Theory, 17,* 613–671.

Verkerk, A., Pieretti, M., Sutcliffe, J. Fu, Y., Kuhl, D. P., & Warren, S. T. (1991). Identification of a gene containing a CGG repeat coincident with a breakpoint cluster region exhibiting length variation in fragile X syndrome. *Cell, 65,* 905–914.

Walzer, S. (1985). X chromosome abnormalities and cognition: Implications for understanding normal human development. *Journal of Child Psychology and Psychiatry, 26*(2), 177–184.

Woods, B. T. (1980). Observations on the neurological basis for initial language acquisition. In D. Caplan (Ed.), *Biological studies of mental processes* (pp. 149–158). Cambridge, MA: MIT Press.

15

On the Complementarity
of Signed and Spoken Languages

Wendy Sandler
The University of Haifa

This chapter considers some implications of the relation between sign language and spoken language for a general theory of human language. Previous research revealing both similarities and differences between languages in the two modalities is taken into account here. In addition, the nature of gesture that accompanies language in each modality is explored in an attempt to better understand universal features of human communication. Whereas speakers gesture with their hands, the preliminary investigation described here suggests that signers gesture with their mouths. The picture that emerges is one in which the two natural language modalities converge in some areas, but diverge in others, and only together reveal the human language capacity in its entirety.

Sign languages are normal languages that arise when the channel for oral–aural communication is absent. Linguists study the very ordered system that emerges from this situation to gain insight into the nature of human language in general. Natural sign languages, then, represent a special instantiation of language, and as such, they provide an important means for determining the essential properties of human language and the contribution that the physical modality makes to language structure and organization. This chapter deals particularly with sign language competence, and with a perhaps surprising overlap between speakers and signers in the use of gestures specific to each modality. The discussion ends with suggestions as to how the particular whole human language approach presented here may also be relevant to the study of language disorders in general and to SLI in particular.

TWO COMPLEMENTARY MODALITIES
OF NATURAL LANGUAGE

Forty years of research on sign languages has demonstrated that the languages themselves are full natural languages with phonological, morphological, and syntactic systems (Emmorey, 2002, in press-b; Sandler & Lillo-Martin, 2000). They have such purely linguistic characteristics as phonological substructure (Stokoe, 1960) with sequential properties (Liddell, 1984); autosegmental and hierarchical relations among phonological elements (Sandler, 1989, 1993b); productive inflectional and derivational morphology (Aronoff, Meir, & Sandler, 2000; Padden, 1988; Supalla, 1986; Supalla & Newport, 1978); recursivity in syntax (Padden, 1988); and licensing of null arguments (Lillo-Martin, 1991). This research explains that the human brain spontaneously creates alternative full language systems when the auditory channel necessary for spoken language is not available. In order to understand what language is, then, it seems imperative to reach a profound understanding of the characteristics of these "other" languages.

A hypothesis is presented here that spoken and signed language manifest two parts of a single human language faculty. This hypothesis is different from others that assume sign languages are essentially the same as spoken languages, peacefully existing in a single language module, differing only trivially in the peripheral systems. The theory proposes that these two natural systems, spoken and signed, are similar in certain ways but different in others, and they complement each other within the realm of human cognition, together forming the whole human language.

Compare the whole human language theory with two other viewpoints. The first proposes that sign languages are not real languages, and the second is its opposite, saying that sign languages are just like spoken languages in all the important respects:

1. *The Speech Is Language Theory.* Humans are endowed by evolution for speech. Sign languages are not part of this endowment, are not natural languages, but instead are adaptive communication systems. The theory would predict that either (a) sign languages are entirely derivative of spoken languages, or (b) the grammatical organization of sign languages should be substantially different from that of spoken languages; there should be a different language–brain map, and sign languages should not have the same innate underpinnings as spoken languages. Proponents of this view would need evidence to support the claim that humans are not innately endowed with a pro-

pensity for sign language: The course of sign language acquisition should be different and longer, and should contain errors not predicted by general linguistic principles such as those embodied in a theory of universal grammar.

2. *The Modality-Independent Language Module Theory.* This is the mirror image of the first theory. It holds that signed and spoken languages are the same in all important respects and are mediated by a single language module, cognitively and neurologically. Only the peripheral systems, which make a trivial contribution to language structure, are different. It would predict that the grammatical systems of sign languages should conform to all principles of general linguistic theory. Within this overall constraint, sign language grammars should differ from one another as do the grammars of spoken languages; humans are endowed with an innate propensity for spoken and signed languages equally, and should show the same acquisition course; and sign languages should be controlled in the same areas of the brain as spoken languages.

3. *The Whole Human Language Theory.* Signed and spoken languages are two parts of one language faculty, partly overlapping, partly complementing each other, and together manifesting the full human endowment for language. The mind encompasses the potential for both systems, but each modality plays a nontrivial role in determining the linguistic structure of the resulting language. The theory would predict that there should be both significant grammatical similarities between spoken and signed languages, but also significant grammatical differences due to modality. Language in the two modalities should be innate to the same extent: There should be similar courses and timetables of acquisition. The language–brain map should reflect the influence of modality, and early experience with either modality could result in selective differences in brain organization.

Other theories are possible.[1] These three are presented here because the predictions of each theory are relatively coherent, and each theory is clearly distinguishable from the others. This chapter is devoted to providing evidence to support the whole human language theory. The discussion begins by demonstrating both grammatical similarities and differences be-

---

[1]The theories as presented here reflect ideas that have been in the air in one form or another, but do not necessarily conform strictly to specific proposals in the literature. The Speech is Language Theory follows from the Speech is Special theory proposed by Liberman and his colleagues at Haskins Laboratories (e.g., 1967), although these researchers did not take sign language into consideration at the time. The Modality-Independent Language Module theory is in the spirit of Fodor's (1983) modularity theory. It is this theory that explicitly or tacitly underlies much current sign language research (e.g., Poizner, Klima, & Bellugi, 1987; Kegl, Senghas, & Coppola, 1999). Theory III, The Whole Human Language Theory, is compatible with the views of McNeill and his colleagues (e.g., McNeill, 1992), here somewhat expanded in scope and extended to include sign language.

tween spoken and signed languages. There is an overview of recent work on prosody and on verb agreement in Israeli Sign Language. Then some results in acquisition and brain research are briefly summarized. The chapter concludes by highlighting complementary traces of each system within the other—in manual and oral gestures.

GRAMMATICAL OVERLAP

Much of the past 40 years has been spent demonstrating that there are similarities in the grammars of spoken and signed languages. Stokoe's discovery that American Sign Language exhibits duality of patterning started the ball rolling. He showed that signs are not holistic gestures, but are comprised of a finite list of discrete, meaningless, contrastive units that combine to produce a potentially large vocabulary (Stokoe, 1960). A substantial body of linguistic research on the phonology of sign language followed, demonstrating that there are constraints on the combination of these units (e.g., Battison, 1978; Sandler, 1989), that despite significant simultaneous structure there is also sequential structure in sign language words (Liddell, 1984; Sandler, 1989), that there are autosegmental relations among phonological elements as well (Sandler, 1986, 1989), and that the sign language syllable has a visual equivalent of sonority (Brentari, 1990, 1998; Corina, 1990; Perlmutter, 1992; Sandler, 1993c).[2]

Others investigated morphology in American Sign Language, finding systems of verb agreement (Padden, 1988), verbal aspect inflection (Klima & Bellugi, 1979), and a rich system of classifier complexes (Supalla, 1982, 1986). Although most of these discoveries were made in studies of American Sign Language (ASL), research on other sign languages reported similar findings. Among the earliest studies of a sign language were those conducted by Schlesinger and his colleagues on Israeli Sign Language (ISL), which described certain grammatical regularities (Cohen, Namir, & Schlesinger, 1977; Schlesinger & Namir, 1978). Fundamental similarities in the syntactic structures of ASL and many spoken languages have also been shown to exist. For example, ASL has embedded sentences that can be formally distinguished from coordinated sentences (Padden, 1981, 1988); it has null arguments (Lillo-Martin, 1986, 1991), and wh-movement in questions (Neidle, Kegl, McLaughlin, Bahan, & Lee, 2000; Petronio & Lillo-Martin, 1997).

Recent research on prosody in Israeli Sign Language serves as one example of the many grammatical similarities that have been found between languages in the two modalities. Prosody is potentially of special interest for

---

[2]See Corina and Sandler (1993), Brentari (1995) for overviews of sign language phonology research.

two reasons. First, prosody is at the crossroads of all the components of language, systematically tying together phonology, syntax, and semantics. To be more specific, the syntactic structure and semantic intent of utterances are interpreted by manipulating rhythm, stress, and pitch of the voice (intonation) to create complex and multifaceted prosodic systems. Second, the physical expression of prosody seems to be frankly rooted in the physical modality. The primitives of prosody—rhythm, stress, and pitch—are the substantive material of phonology in the oral medium. If it can be shown that languages in two such different physical modalities both have prosody, and the prosodic systems have significant similarities to one another, then this would be strong evidence that there is essentially one system.

Similarity between the prosody of spoken and signed languages is shown in a recent study of two prosodic constituents in Israeli Sign Language (Nespor & Sandler, 1999; Sandler, 1999b): the phonological phrase[3] and the intonational phrase. For brevity, only the latter is described here.

The ISL prosody study demonstrates the existence of the intonational phrase in ISL—a significant similarity with spoken language, because the intonational phrase is the primary domain for the organization of intonational tunes, a strongly modality-dependent phenomenon. As is the case in spoken language, syntactically independent constituents such as topicalized elements, parentheticals, and nonrestrictive relative clauses tend to form independent intonational phrases in ISL. The study indicates that the intonational phrase is the primary domain of the sign language equivalent of intonational tunes as well.

Spoken language intonational tunes consist of sequences of tones that typically fall on prominent words and cluster at the boundary of the intonational phrase. Although a range of tones are perceived, it is now generally accepted that all contrasts can be expressed phonologically by a simple distinction between high (H) and low (L) tones, which are either accented (*) or not (Pierrehumbert, 1980). Example 1 shows a sentence from a study of Bengali by Hayes and Lahiri (1991), with a focus contour consisting of the tune L^* H_p L_I, plus continuation rise, H_I. The whole sequence occurs on *harlo*, the last word of the intonational phrase, *jodio ram harlo*.

(1) [jodio ram [harlo,] $_P$] $_I$ (o k^{h}ub b^{h}alo k^{h}elec^{h}ilo)
              L^* H_P L_I H_I

   Although Ram lost,   *(he very well played)*

The final sequence, L_I H_I is componential. The L is the boundary tone at the end of the focused constituent. It enters into a contour with a following H, signaling continuation.

---

[3]The present summary deals only with the intonational phrase. For findings on the phonological phrase, see Nespor and Sandler (1999), and Sandler (1999b).

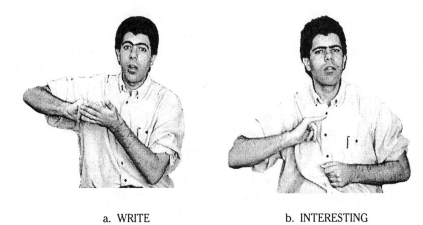

a. WRITE   b. INTERESTING

FIG. 15.1.   Change in body and face across Intonational Phrases.

In sign language, several researchers have claimed that facial expression corresponds to intonation in spoken language (e.g., Nespor & Sandler, 1999; Reilly, McIntire, & Bellugi, 1990; Wilbur, 1996).[4] The sign language correlate of intonation has been called *superarticulation*, and the combination of superarticulations *superarticulatory arrays* (Sandler, 1999b). Like intonational tunes of spoken language, the superarticulatory arrays of sign language also have the intonational phrase as their primary domain. For example, each of the intonational phrases in the sentence glossed in Example 2 is characterized by a completely different set of nonmanual markers, pictured in Fig. 15.1: a change of head position at the intonational phrase boundary, and differences in all aspects of facial expression (e.g., eyebrows, upper and lower eyelids, and mouth) in each intonational phrase.

(2) [[book-there]$_P$ [he write]$_P$]$_I$ [[interesting]$_P$]$_I$
'The book he wrote is interesting.'

As in vocal intonation, sign language superarticulation is also componential. For example, the superarticulatory array of a wh-question can be combined with the superarticulation that has the meaning, 'shared information'. The wh-question array in ISL is typically characterized by furrowed eyebrows, as shown in Fig. 15.2a. A different superarticulation—a squint of the eyelids, shown in Fig. 15.2b—signals information that is to be considered shared by both interlocutors. These two can be combined. For example, in the following wh-question, the underlined part is established as shared in-

---

[4]This view contrasts with the position of some researchers that grammatical facial expressions of sign languages reflect syntax directly (Liddell, 1980; Neidle et al., 2000).

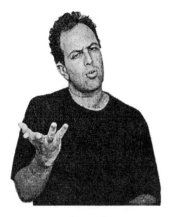

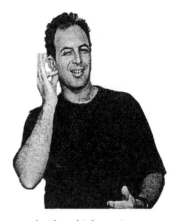

a. wh-question   b. shared information

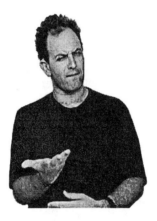

c. wh-question and shared information

FIG. 15.2. (a) Superarticulation for a wh-question in ISL. (b) Superarticulation for shared information in ISL. (c) Compotential superarticulation: Wh-question and shared information.

formation: 'Who is the woman you met last week?'. As Fig. 15.2c shows, the facial expression for the that part of the sentence combines the wh- furrowed brows with the shared information squint.

These examples show that sign language superarticulation, like spoken language intonation, is componential. But there is a difference, which is due to the modality. Each superarticulation can be superimposed simultaneously with the others, and with the whole stretch of the utterance that they characterize. As the facial articulators responsible for superarticulation are independent of each other and of the manual channel that transmits the words of the language, all articulations are free to combine simultaneously. This effect of the modality will be discussed further in the next section, in which other differences in the grammars of signed in spoken languages are presented.

GRAMMATICAL DIFFERENCES

The videotaped series, "The Human Language," presents an excellent and engaging introduction to the leading modern approach to linguistics conceived of primarily by Chomsky. One installment of the three-part series,[5] revealed that language is very good at some things—like expressing the relation of people and things to some activity or event (through agreement, case marking, word order, etc.). But it is also explained that language is bad at other things—like describing a map (how to get somewhere) or shapes and dimensions of objects (like "spiral shape"). Well, this statement as it stands is wrong. Spoken languages are bad at these things, but sign languages are great at them. Not only are sign languages extremely good at expressing things related to visuospatial cognition, but more than that, they all seem to do it pretty much the same way, and to encode visuospatial concepts in their grammars. Here is where the grammatical systems of spoken and signed languages part ways.

A typical example of a grammatical process in sign language that exploits visuospatial cognition is verb agreement. Although many spoken languages have verb agreement, the verb agreement of sign languages is different. First described and analyzed in detail for American Sign Language (ASL) by Padden (1988), the system indicates the referents of arguments of the verb by moving the hands among points in space that correspond to these referents. For example, the signs meaning 'I give you' and 'S/he gives me' are represented in Fig. 15.3.

In a discourse, there can be many referents (physically present or not), each with its own locus in space. The way in which this system exploits spatial relations is immediately obvious. But it might still be claimed, as many people have, that it is nevertheless just verb agreement—a system that grammatically marks on the verb certain properties of its arguments, much as Hebrew or Italian do. This claim is not accurate, however, because there are several other ways in which the sign language system differs from spoken language verb agreement. For example, not all verbs agree. There is a class of plain verbs that do not take any agreement. In addition, there is a class of verbs like TAKE that seem to move backward; instead of the hands articulating a movement that goes from the subject locus to the object locus as in GIVE (Fig. 15.3), the direction of movement in backward verbs is

---

[5]*The Human Language: Colorless Green Ideas*. 1993. Gene Searchinger, Producer. Equinox Films.

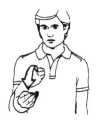   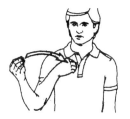

I GIVE YOU   S/HE GIVES ME

FIG. 15.3. Example of verb agreement in ASL. Reprinted with permission from A Basic Course in American Sign Language, T. Humphries, C. Padden, and T. J. O'Rourke. 1980. Silver Spring, MD: TJ Publishers.

from object to subject.[6] Meir (1998b, 2002) showed that these and other properties of the verb agreement system of Israeli Sign Language can be explained by a few simple principles that reveal how ISL reflects visuospatial cognition in its grammar.

VERB AGREEMENT PRINCIPLES

Meir (1998a) proposed the following verb agreement principles:

1. Agreement verbs are verbs involving *transfer*, physical or metaphorical.
2. Movement of the hand follows a path from *source to goal*.[7]
3. Facing of the hand is toward the *syntactic object*.

This analysis explains why some verbs are agreement verbs and others are not: Only verbs of transfer agree. For example, the verbs HOLD and THINK are not agreement verbs as there is no transfer involved, whereas the verbs GIVE and TEACH are both agreement verbs, involving transfer of goods and of information, respectively. In addition to explaining which are and are not agreement verbs, the principles also explain which agreement verbs are regular and which are backward. The regular agreement verb GIVE and the backward verb TAKE are both verbs of transfer. In both signs, the hand moves from source to goal as the second principle requires. This

---

[6]An additional difference, also first described by Padden (1988), is the existence of a third class, called spatial verbs, whose movement paths are interpreted literally, i.e., from specified point a to specified point b.

[7]Other researchers working within different theoretical frameworks have also claimed that the sign language agreement system refers to source and goal rather than subject and object, e.g., Friedman (1976), Kegl (1985), and Bos (1998).

explains why, in a sentence meaning 'I give you', the hand moves from the signer (subject) to the addressee (object), whereas in 'I take from you', the hand moves from the addressee (indirect object) to the signer (subject)—backward from a syntactic point of view. In both verbs, the signing hand faces the addressee, the syntactic object. What is backward about TAKE type verbs is their inherent lexical semantics, and not their agreement properties: The source corresponds to the object and the goal to the subject, unlike regular agreement verbs in which the source corresponds to the subject and the goal to the object (Meir, 1998a, 1998b). But as far as agreement is concerned, backward verbs are like other agreement verbs, moving from source to goal.

The verb agreement system is linguistic: It involves specific semantic and syntactic categories, and it is rule governed. However, it clearly exploits spatial locations and relations. In fact, the system may exploit essentially any visible and comfortably reachable spatial location within the signing area, and the grammar does not limit the number of locations that can be employed within a discourse. These aspects of agreement have been argued to rely on general cognition and not on a linguistic system (e.g., Liddell, 1995, 2000).

Another unusual property of sign language agreement is that the agreement morphology is superimposed on the sign in a way that is more simultaneous than is the case with the typically sequential affixal morphology of spoken languages. And yet another fact about sign language agreement makes it different from grammatical systems in spoken languages: All established sign languages have essentially the same system.[8] They all have a class of agreement verbs with the same spatial organization, a subclass of backward verbs, and a class of plain verbs that do not agree. It is clear that this system, although grammatical, reflects universal aspects of visuospatial cognition.

In addition to verb agreement, sign languages in general have other morphological systems in common, such as verbal aspect morphology and classifier complexes. Aronoff, Meir, and Sandler (2000) and Aronoff, Meir, Padden, and Sandler (in press) proposed that sign languages reflect this kind of cognitive system directly because they are visual. Spoken languages would if they could, but they can't, so they don't. Rather, the grammatical systems of spoken languages are for the most part not directly determined by visuospatial cognition, and they differ from one another much more widely. Under the whole human language theory, it is expected that some significant gram-

---

[8]Though strikingly similar in overall structure, some differences have been found among sign languages in verb agreement. For example, some sign languages have auxiliary verbs for marking agreement where the main verb does not inflect for agreement (Smith, 1990; Bos, 1994). Fischer and Osugi (2000), have found that in Nihon Syuwa (the Sign Language of Japan), an 'indexical classifier', articulated in neutral space by the nondominant hand, marks the locus of agreement.

matical differences between spoken and signed languages will result from the physical modality. Visually motivated, sign language universal morphological processes, such as verb agreement, are examples of such differences.

Lest the reader form the mistaken impression that sign language morphology has little in common with that of spoken language, it should be noted that there are also sequential affixes grammaticalized from independent words in ASL and ISL, the two sign languages studied in Aronoff et al. (2000, in press). These show the same kind of arbitrariness, language specificity, and idiosyncrasy that derivational affixes manifest in spoken languages. From a comparison of the two types of morphology, it may be concluded that sign languages do draw from the pool of grammatical possibilities available to all languages regardless of modality, but they also have some properties unique to them and predictable on the basis of visuospatial cognition (Aronoff et al., 2000, in press). It has also been argued that even the more typical simultaneous sign language morphology bears structural similarities to that of some spoken languages, in particular, to the templatic type of morphology found in Semitic languages (Sandler, 1990).

The superarticulation system described earlier, although bearing certain important similarities to intonation in spoken language, also manifests a nontrivial difference resulting from the modality, as explained. In particular, the primitives of the system and their distribution within a prosodic constituent are quite different from those of spoken intonation. Spoken language intonation consists of H and L tones that are lined up in a sequence, especially at phrase boundaries, but sign language superarticulation consists of configurations of the brows, upper and lower eyelids, cheeks, and mouth, which co-occur with each other simultaneously in different combinations as exemplified in Figs. 15.2a–c. In addition, the whole array cooccurs simultaneously across entire prosodic constituents, not just at their boundaries.

Spoken language intonational contrasts are produced by the frequency of vibration of a single articulator, the vocal cords, which is involved in the transmission of speech apart from intonation. Different frequencies or tones can only be produced and perceived in a sequence. The sign language modality recruits many more articulators (i.e., the brows, eyelids, cheeks, mouth, etc.) and none are involved in producing signs. This results in an intonational system in sign language that has more primitives than the H and L tones of spoken language. The primitives of sign language intonation co-occur simultaneously with each other instead of following one another in a sequence, and also co-occur simultaneously with the entire prosodic constituent that they characterize, rather than clustering at the boundary. It appears then that when sign language is considered alongside spoken language, the modality-determined differences between them cannot be considered trivial. Rather, in each case, the modality imposes significant aspects of linguistic structure on language (Sandler, 1999c).

THE COURSE OF ACQUISITION

There is quite an extensive literature on the acquisition of American Sign Language by deaf children of deaf signing parents. (For overviews, see Newport & Meier, 1985, and Peperkamp & Mehler, 1999; for syntheses, see Meier, 1991, and Sandler & Lillo-Martin, 2001.) Researchers concur that language is acquired by children along a comparable time course in the two modalities. Early milestones are reached at comparable ages.[9] Difficult parts of the grammar are acquired later than simpler parts in both modalities. For example, despite the fact that verb agreement is motivated by general properties of visuospatial cognition, the system is formally complex, and is only acquired in ASL between ages 3 and 4 (Meier, 1982). The error pattern of deaf children confirms that they are acquiring language as a formal, componential system, and not as an iconic gestural system. For example, small children can confuse the pronouns 'I' and 'you' in sign language as in spoken language, despite the fact that the ASL pronouns have the seemingly transparent form of pointing gestures toward oneself and one's addressee, respectively (Pettito, 1987).

THE LOCALIZATION OF LANGUAGE IN THE BRAIN

A range of different research methods has been applied in attempts to map various cognitive functions to specific areas of the brain. Traditionally, the field was based on the study of aphasics, and relied on comparing CAT scans picturing the brain lesions with language performance. Real-time studies on normal brains have been made possible by using the event-related potential (ERP) method, and more recent methods of positron emission tomography (PET) and functional magnetic resonance imaging (fMRI), and these studies have challenged some of the earlier assumptions. Overall, the most significant generalization is also the broadest: "In about 98 per cent of strong right-handers from right-handed families, the left perisylvian association cortex accomplishes most ... language processing functions" (Caplan, 2000, p. 594).

Sign languages rely on visuospatial abilities, as the discussion of verb agreement indicates. Visuospatial cognition is understood to be primarily controlled by the right hemisphere. If sign language is an adaptive system as the Speech is Language Theory proposes, then it might be expected that its organization in the brain is determined primarily by general cognitive abilities and not by operations specific to language. For example, sign lan-

---

[9]Some researchers have found an early advantage for the acquisition of first signs over first spoken words (see Newport and Meier 1990 for a theoretical discussion of these results). However these findings are based on studies of a small number of children, and other researcher have refuted them because of conflicting evidence (Volterra and Iverson, 1995).

guage might be expected to be controlled primarily in the right hemisphere like any other function relying on visuospatial cognition. However, if the linguistic organization of spoken and sign language are independent of the physical modality in which they are transmitted, as the modality-independent language module theory would have it, then sign language should be controlled by the left hemisphere to the same extent as spoken language. The predictions of the whole human language theory are less clear-cut at this stage, but ultimately may prove more interesting. If spoken and signed languages belong to the same system, then significant overlap in brain organization should be found. But differences in brain organization should also be found. These differences in brain organization should go beyond peripheral motor activity. They should also correspond directly to the ways in which each physical modality influences linguistic structure. The following paragraph summarizes some of what is known about sign language and the brain.

Poizner, Klima and Bellugi (1987) studied six deaf signing patients, three with right hemisphere lesions, and three with left hemisphere lesions. They found that the LH patients all exhibited aphasia in sign language production, whereas the RH patients did not, even though they did exhibit visuospatial deficits such as left neglect. These results are striking, but cannot be considered conclusive. First, although the sign language production of Poizner et al.'s RH patients was intact, they did have difficulties in comprehension of spatial syntax. Second, recent studies on normal brains, surveyed in Peperkamp and Mehler (1999), reveal a more mixed picture. For example, they described an fMRI study showing bilateral representation of both spoken and signed language in hearing native signers (i.e., hearing people with deaf parents; Soderfeldt, Risberg, & Ronnberg, 1994). They also reported on an ERP study by Neville et al. (1997) showing bilateral representation of visually presented written English and signed ASL in deaf and hearing native signers. Taken together, it appears that early acquisition of sign may lead to bilateral representation in the brain of any language, spoken or signed, whereas the acquisition of spoken language alone results in representation mostly in the left hemisphere.[10]

EVIDENCE FOR COMPLEMENTARITY: GESTURE IN BOTH MODALITIES

The primary channel for spoken language is the oral–aural channel. Largely as a result of this modality, speech is segmented and sequential, and the words of spoken language are mostly arbitrary. However, the spoken me-

---

[10]See Corina (1998, 1999) and Emmorey (2002) for overviews of research on sign language and the brain.

dium with its inherent arbitrariness and sequentiality of structure are apparently insufficient for human communication. Studying descriptive narratives from vastly different cultures, McNeill (1992) and his team found that people invariably gesture when they speak. Together with Kendon (1988) and others,[11] McNeill argued that gesture is part of language, and not extraneous to it:

> My own hypothesis is that speech and gesture are elements of a single integrated process of utterance formation." p 35 "The utterance has both an imagistic side and a linguistic side. The image arises first and is transformed into a complex structure in which both the gesture and the linguistic structure are integral parts. (pp. 29–30)

McNeill (1992) distinguished gestures from the linguistic units of language along the following five parameters:

1. Gestures are global (in the sense of having no subunits like the phonemes of words for example).
2. They are noncombinatoric: Each gesture is an idea unit with no ordered or hierarchical organization between it and other gestures.
3. Their interpretation is context dependent: The same entity can prompt different gestures in different contexts.
4. They are idiosyncratic; there are no standards of form.
5. They either anticipate or cooccur with speech. They neither follow speech nor occur independently.

Gesture is thus distinct from the linguistic elements of speech. But according to McNeill, gesture is part of language, as attested by the fact that gestures and speech do not always manifest the same information, often complementing each other instead. Speech and gesture are interwoven to form a rich communicative amalgam. The gestural component of this amalgam is divided into four categories: Gestures may be iconic, metaphoric, beat, or deictic. Anticipating a comparison with sign language, the focus here is only on iconic gestures. These are "gestures that bear a close formal relationship to the semantic content of speech . . . (and) display aspects of the same scene that speech also presents" (p. 78). An example from the McNeill corpus is a gesture that accompanies the words, *and he bends it way back*, in describing a scene in a cartoon in which a character bends back a tree. The hand appears to grip something anchored from below and to bend it toward the speaker. This iconic gesture is semantically related to the spoken utterance, and also adds information that is not present in the

---

[11]See Kendon (1994) for a recent overview of research on gesture in communication.

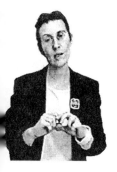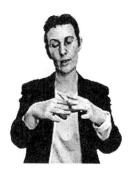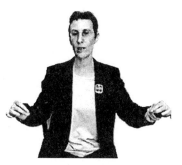

a. 'braid them'   b. 'slightly higher in the middle'   c. 'tapered at the ends'

FIG. 15.4. Iconic gestures accompanying speech.

utterance, information about shape, dimension, anchoring, and the spatial relation between the character and the object.

Even the most articulate speakers enhance their speech with gesture. A professor of English literature describes how she makes her favorite *hallah*, a traditional bread for Sabbath and holidays. The relevant part of the narrative is shown in Example 3, in which words that were accompanied by gestures are underlined. The specific gestures accompanying the words that are in boldface are shown in Fig. 15.4.

> (3) "I like to make . . . a traditional braided <u>*hallah*</u>, made with <u>three long</u> <u>segments</u> that are <u>narrower</u> at the ends than at the <u>middle</u>. Then when you **<u>braid them</u>** it'll be **<u>slightly higher in the middle</u>** and **<u>tapered at the ends.</u>**"

Whereas this speaker is especially articulate, describing objects and activities in clear detail verbally, she nevertheless enhances these verbal descriptions with simultaneous gestures.

It is clear that gestures are a natural part of linguistic communication, just as the basic organizing properties of language are natural for humans. People even gesture when they cannot be seen, for example, on the telephone. Iverson and Goldin-Meadow (1997, 1998) reported more impressive findings—that congenitally blind people use similar gestures to those of sighted people when they talk. Volterra and Iverson (1995) reported that small children (hearing and deaf alike) typically use a good deal of gesture in the early stages of language acquisition. One study (Iverson, Capirci, & Casell, 1994) showed that many small hearing children (16 months old) with no exposure to sign language use gesture more frequently than words, even when their verbal vocabulary is larger. Gesture, then, is natural.

The ability to organize and convey thoughts through a linguistic system that has a broad foundation of universal properties is, of course, also natural.

The naturalness both of gesture and of linguistic organizing principles explains why sign languages arise spontaneously wherever a group of deaf people has an opportunity to congregate and interact: Sign languages originate as gesture systems and quickly become grammaticized (Kegl et al., 1999).

It is extremely important to underscore the fact that the signs of established sign language are not gestures. Evaluated according to all of the criteria used by McNeill to define gestures, the lexical signs of real, grammatically organized sign languages are distinct from gestures, exactly as spoken words are distinct from gestures. Sign language signs are componential rather than global; they are combinatoric, entering into hierarchical phonological, morphological, and syntactic structures; they have meaning independent of context; and they are standardized (i.e., signs are like spoken words and unlike gestures).

However, signs do use the manual/visual channel that gestures use. Does the fact that the hands are busy "talking" preempt the possibility of gesture in sign language? Preliminary research indicates that it does not. Instead, signers may gesture with the other articulatory mechanism with which humans are endowed for linguistic communication: the mouth.

The mouth is very active in sign language communication, performing an eclectic variety of tasks. A small number of lexical signs in Israeli Sign Language require a mouth shape or movement of some kind as part of their lexical representation. Like any sign, such signs are lexically specified for hand configuration and for the location and movement articulated by the hand. But these signs are also lexically specified for a particular mouth shape or movement. Whether the mouth movements have internal structure is not yet clear; however, it is clear that they themselves are contrastive subunits like phonemes, entering into the higher word structure. These lexical mouth specifications are completely standard and required by the grammar.[12]

Other mouth movements function as grammatical morphemes. Certain mouth shapes, co-occurring with verbs or verb phrases, have an adverbial meaning (Liddell, 1980; Anderson & Reilly, 1998). For example, a laxly open mouth with the tongue visible but not protruding, co-occurring with an ISL verb, means 'for a long time'. Other mouth shapes add other adverbial modifications, such as 'carelessly' or 'with effort'. These two functions—as part of a lexical representation and as an adverbial morpheme on verb phrases—are part of the linguistic system of the language. They are standard subunits in the language, entering combinatorially into the grammatical system.

In addition to these native mouth shapes and movements, selective and sometimes partial mouthing of words from Hebrew is fairly common in ISL, as in many other sign languages (Boyes-Braem & Sutton-Spence, 2001). Although clearly borrowed from the spoken language, this mouthing has inher-

---

[12]See Woll (2001) and Bergman and Wallin (2001) for suggestions about internal structure to mouth movements in lexical signs.

ent patterns that are determined in large part by language-internal criteria. An example of such a pattern is found in ISL constructions of a content-word host plus a pronominal clitic. In these forms, if the Hebrew word corresponding to the sign that hosts the clitic is mouthed, the mouthing stretches over the whole host plus clitic construction (Sandler, 1999a, 1999b).

In sum, the investigation of Israeli Sign Language is showing that there is a stream of linguistic mouth shapes and movements with different functions accompanying the manual signing (Sandler, in preparation).[13]

Apart from this plethora of linguistic roles, the mouth is also used for gestures in ISL. These mouth gestures are all iconic, representing some physical aspect of an object or event.[14] For example, they may represent a tactile effect, either of an object (e.g., soft or lightweight) or of a motion event (e.g., friction or vibration); or a physical state, such as being filled to capacity. In the corpus studied, three native signers signed the same 20 sentences, which were elicited for a study on an unrelated topic and happened to be especially rich in mouth gestures. A detailed treatment of these phenomena is beyond the scope of this discussion. What follows demonstrates briefly what is meant by mouth gestures, so that the bearing they have on the more general topic under discussion may then be examined.

The mouth shapes that express physical properties in ISL indeed appear to be gestures. Unlike the linguistic mouth units already described, the mouth gestures are independent of the grammatical system. They have no internal structure, and they are also noncombinatoric in McNeill's sense that each gesture is an idea unit, and that no ordered or hierarchical organization exists among gestures (McNeill, 1992). Further distinguishing these gestures from linguistic mouth units is the fact that the gestures have no ordered or hierarchical relation with the linguistic content. The gestures are context dependent: The same gesture may have different interpretations, depending on the sentence with which it occurs. The three signers sometimes used the gestures idiosyncratically. In some cases, one or two signers used mouth gestures and the other(s) did not. In other cases, the same signer either used different gestures to describe the physical situation in-

---

[13]Linguistic functions for the mouth have been reported in other sign languages as well. Liddell (1980), Anderson and Reilly (1998), and others have described adverbial mouth positions in ASL. For example, Bergman and Wallin (2001) examine mouth 'segments' in Swedish Sign Language, and Woll (2001) describes the behavior of lexical mouth movements in British Sign Language. The reader is referred to Boyes-Braem and Sutton-Spence (in press) for a collection of interesting papers on the behavior of the mouth in a variety of sign languages. An additional role for the mouth is reported by Obando et al. (2000), who describe an elaborate system of lip pointing in Nicaraguan Sign Language that was apparently modeled on simpler lip pointing gestures of hearing Nicaraguans.

[14]The term 'mouth gestures' as used here refers only to a particular subset of what are labeled with the same term in Boyes-Braem and Sutton-Spence (2000).

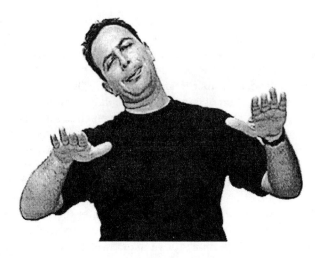

FIG. 15.5. *Friction* gesture.

volved, or gradient degrees of intensity to iconically reflect different degrees of intensity involved.

Consider three examples here. The first gesture accompanied the ISL translation of the sentence, 'He emptied the water out of the pool." The gesture, pictured in Fig. 15.5, creates friction as the air passes through the constricted lips, and represents the draining of water through a small opening. Like manual gesture accompanying spoken language, this mouth gesture complements the signed message, adding information about the way in which the water was emptied from the pool: creating friction (by forcing it through a small opening).

Goldin-Meadow and McNeill (2000) independently suggested that "the mouth movements associated with particular sounds might assume the mimetic function for signers," and cited an observation to this effect in Padden (1990). By putting such gestures to the tests listed earlier, the present investigation suggests that their speculation is correct, that mouth movements corresponding to sounds such as one created by friction are among the mouth gestures of ISL. Figure 15.5 is one of several examples in the corpus.

Another example focuses on the physical state of an object, specifically, the state of being filled to overflowing. The gesture is one or two puffed cheeks. In addition to conforming to other gesture criteria, this gesture is nonlinguistic in an additional respect: It is gradient rather than discrete. In the example shown in Figs. 15.6 and 15.7, as the wagon gets fuller, the puffing spreads from one cheek to two. These gestures occurred in sequence, with a signed utterance, meaning "He loaded the wagon with grass." The cheek-puff cannot be considered part of a lexical word, FULL. Rather, its interpretation is context dependent, another criterion of gesturehood. In a dif-

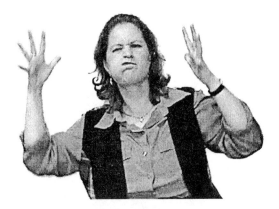

FIG. 15.6. Gradient mouth gesture—*full* gesture.

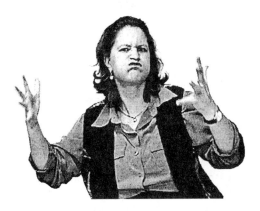

FIG. 15.7. Gradient mouth gesture—*stuffed* gesture.

ferent utterance in the corpus, the cheek-puff coincided with 'carried a suit-case', in which the suitcase had previously been described as heavy. In the utterance from which Fig. 15.8 was extracted, the gesture complements the words, adding the information that the suitcase was heavy. This sort of complementary function is analogous to McNeill's tree bending example described earlier.

It seems clear that these mouth gestures are qualitatively different from signs: They conform to McNeill's gesture criteria, whereas lexical signs do not.

At this stage of research, it is already becoming apparent that mouth gestures are also different from intonational use of the face. The mouth gestures in the corpus are iconic, representing either the appearance of something (e.g., stuffed-full, large, etc.) or another physical property, like vibration (e.g., to spray bullets vs. to pop bullets; spray or drain water, etc.). The

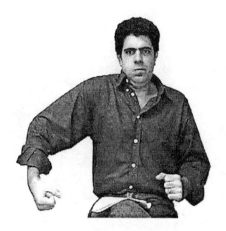

FIG. 15.8. *Heavy* gesture.

superarticulatory facial expressions of sign language intonation are not iconic in this way. The raising of eyebrows does not correspond in form to any external object or event, for example. In addition, the elements of intonational facial expression are componentially structured, and mouth gestures appear to be independent of each other and of the elements of superarticulation.

A good deal remains to be learned about mouth gestures and their place in sign language communication. Readers familiar with sign language may be interested to know that mouth gestures often accompany classifier constructions. Such constructions are arguably standardized and combinatorial and thus linguistic (e.g., Supalla, 1982, 1986), but they also differ in significant ways from lexical signs (see Emmorey, in press, for current views and analyses). The various functions of classifier complexes all involve visual aspects of some event. They describe size and shape of referents, spatial relations and interactions among them, and the path shapes and manners of movements that they enact. Current investigations concentrate on whether the tendency for mouth gestures to co-occur with classifier constructions is coincidental, because such constructions also tend to be used when describing physical shapes, states, and relations, or whether there is a more principled relation and interaction between the two.

Another area currently under investigation is the degree of idiosyncracy in sign language mouth gestures. Whereas idiosyncracy has been found in the ISL mouth gestures, it may turn out that McNeill's criterion—that gestures are idiosyncratic, having no standards of form—will have to be relaxed somewhat for the mouth gestures of sign language. The mouth gestures may be somewhat less free in form than are the manual gestures that accompany spoken language. In fact, it may turn out that there is a continuum from true mouth gestures to more conventionalized mouth shapes of the adverbial system, for example. There are two good reasons for a tendency from gesture toward conventionalization in this modality. First, the mouth has far fewer configurational options than the hands, especially the two hands together. This means that each mouth gesture is relatively simple and easy to process. The fact that the sign language addressee looks smack at the face of the signer, rather than at the hands (Siple, 1978), may make this processing even more immediate. Second, mouth gestures are transmitted visually, like the rest of sign language. The pressure to conventionalize simple and salient gestures that are transmitted in the same perceptual modality as the words of the language might in some cases overwhelm the idiosyncrasy that mouth gestures have at their origin.

To summarize the investigation thus far, natural sign language utterances are often accompanied by gestures. These gestures are made with the mouth and have much in common with the iconic gestures made by the hands of speakers of spoken language. The most obvious difference between the two is that the gestures accompanying spoken language are transmitted in a different modality from that of the language itself, whereas the gestures accompanying sign language are transmitted in the same modality.

THE WHOLE HUMAN LANGUAGE

If the preliminary results reported in the previous section are correct, then all human language requires augmentation with gesture. That is, both modalities require a holistic, idiosyncratic, iconic, and simultaneous means of complementing the linguistic signal. How can these new findings be integrated with the selective survey of sign language research contained in previous sections, and within the context of the theories of language introduced earlier? And what are some possible implications for the study of SLI?

An example in the literature showing that sign languages and spoken languages share certain key properties was presented earlier. The particular system described there was the prosodic system. Similarities to spoken language in the prosodic system are added to significant similarities at the phonological, morphological, and syntactic levels reported here and elsewhere in the sign language literature. In addition, both spoken and signed languages are acquired without instruction along the same time course. These two shared characteristics, specific structural and organizational features and the timetable for acquisition, are defining properties of natural language. It follows that a theory the Speech is Language Theory, predicting that only the spoken modality will have these features, should be rejected as an explanatory theory of language. This leaves the modality-independent language module theory and the whole human language theory for consideration.

The modality-independent theory predicts that, phonetics aside, the modality will have no important effect on grammatical organization. It also predicts that the organization of language in the brain should be the same in any modality. How do these predictions fare in the light of the sign language facts reported here?

As discussed earlier, intonational sequences of units that differ from each other in binary fashion (H or L), that fall on stressed words and cluster at prosodic constituent boundaries, characterize spoken languages but not sign languages. Rather, sign language superarticulation, which seems to have the same function as intonation, is comprised of a larger pool of primitives that combine simultaneously rather than sequentially and characterize whole constituents instead of occurring mainly at boundaries.

A previous section showed clear differences in the morphology of spoken and signed languages. The modality-independent theory predicts both that sign languages should draw from the same pool of morphological possibilities as spoken languages, and that individual sign languages should differ from each other to the same extent that spoken languages do. However, it was shown that significant blocks of sign language morphology have a predictable and nonarbitrary relation to visuospatial cognition that is lacking in spoken languages, and that all sign languages studied so far are very similar with respect to these morphological systems. The expected variation across sign languages has not emerged. More arbitrary morphology, like the sequential affixes in ASL and ISL, as well as more cross sign language variation will emerge and increase, to the extent that sign languages are able to accrue diachronic depth at a rate comparable to that of spoken language (Aronoff et al., 2000, in press). Because typically only fewer than 10% of deaf people are native signers, this diachronic depth is always confounded by the fact that interaction takes place in a community in which 90% are not native users of the language. Although the kinds of morphology more commonly found in spoken language are still predicted to increase over time, it is also expected that the sign language typical morphology will persevere in all sign languages, simply because of the modality. Such differences in grammatical organization between the two modalities are not expected under the modality-independent theory.

The results of brain research also challenge that theory. The use of language in both modalities involves extensive left hemisphere involvement, but the right hemisphere is also activated by sign language, quite possibly because of the interaction between visuospatial cognition and language. Interestingly, early acquisition of sign language by hearing people results in right hemisphere involvement for spoken language as well. Evidence of this kind argues against a language module like that proposed by Fodor (1983) and also predicted by the modality-independent theory, which requires fixed neural architecture for the language module.[15]

---

[15]See also Sandler (1993a) for several arguments from sign language against Fodor's (1983) modularity model.

However, if signed and spoken languages are complementary aspects of the whole human language faculty, such differences would be expected. The whole human language view holds that, within the human mind, the propensity for language in both modalities exists. This seems to be true despite the apparent evolutionary predominance of speech. Such predominance seems indisputable, as no known hearing community just happens to use sign language as its primary means of communication. But, regardless of the conditions under which one modality emerged as dominant, the potential for sign language is as much a part of the human language capacity as is the potential for spoken language. Whereas similarities abound between languages in the two modalities, there are important differences as well. The Whole Human Language is the combination of the two.

GESTURES ARE INTEGRAL TO LINGUISTIC COMMUNICATION

The gesture studies are especially intriguing in the pursuit of the defining characteristics of human language. The claim that natural gestures are integral to linguistic communication has four solid pieces of evidence to support it.

1. Speaking people apparently must gesture when they speak, whether or not these gestures are even perceived by the speakers or their interlocutors.
2. The gestures are often not redundant; they complement the message being conveyed.
3. In the absence of the auditory channel, human communities create bona fide languages from gesture spontaneously and in a short time.
4. Gesture accompanies any natural language, whether spoken or signed.

The language–gesture amalgam may hint at a more primal bimodal foundation for linguistic communication: Both modalities use oral and manual channels simultaneously in the service of language. If the oral channel is used for the purely linguistic signal, then the hands supply the gestural complement. If the manual channel is the medium for language, then the mouth provides the complementary gestures. Both modalities are natural; traces of each are found in the other, and together they comprise the whole human language.

One implication of this theory is clear. In order to study language, whether in linguistically normal populations such as speakers or signers, or in populations with language impairments such as those seen in aphasia, autism, or SLI, it is not possible to rely on the structure of spoken language alone, sign language alone, or gesture alone. Rather, serious consideration must be given to the organization of language in both spoken and signed modalities, as well as to the interaction of each with gesture.

ACKNOWLEDGMENTS

This study was supported by Israel Science Foundation grant number 750/ 99-1.

I am grateful to the participants of the Workshop on Communication Disorders, Jerusalem, 1999 for discussion of this work, an earlier version of which was presented there. I also thank Irit Meir for helpful comments on this paper, and Marina Nespor for useful discussion of prosodic constituents and examples. Finally, my thanks to Yonata Levy for her insightful comments on this chapter.

REFERENCES

Anderson, D. E., & Reilly, J. S. (1998). PAH! The acquisition of adverbials in ASL. *Sign Language and Linguistics, 1*(2), 117–142.

Aronoff, M., Meir, I., Padden, C., & Sandler, W. (in press). Classifier complexes and morphology in two sign languages. In K. Emmorey (in press-b).

Aronoff, M., Meir, I., & Sandler, W. (2000). *Universal and particular aspects of sign language morphology.* Unpublished manuscript, SUNY Stony Brook and University of Haifa.

Aronoff, M., & Rees-Miller, J. (Eds.). *Handbook of linguistics.* Oxford, England: Blackwell.

Battison, R. (1978). *Lexical borrowing in American Sign Language.* Silver Spring: Linstok Press.

Bergman, B., & Wallin, L. (2001). A preliminary analysis of visual mouth segments in Swedish Sign Language. In Boyes Braem & Sutton-Spence (Eds.), (pp. 51–68).

Bos, H. (1994). An auxiliary verb in sign language of the Netherlands. In I. Ahlgren, B. Bergman, & M. Brennan (Eds.), *Perspectives on sign language structure: Papers from the fifth internationa symposium on sign language research* (Vol. 1, pp. 37–53). Durham, England: International Sigr Linguistics Association.

Bos, H. (1998, December). *An analysis of main verb agreement and auxiliary agreement in sign lan guage of the Netherlands with the theory of conceptual semantics.* Paper presented at the 6th conference on Theoretical Issues in Sign Language Research, Washington, DC.

Boyes Braem, P., & Sutton-Spence, R. (Eds.). (2001). *The hands are the head of the mouth. The mouth as articulator in sign languages.* Hamburg: Signum Verlag.

Brentari, D. (1990a). *Theoretical foundations of American Sign Language phonology.* PhD dissertation, University of Chicago, Chicago, Ill. [Published 1993 by University of Chicago Occasiona Papers in Linguistics, Chicago, Ill.]

Brentari, D. (1995). Sign language phonology: ASL. In J. Goldsmith (Ed.), *A handbook of phonolog cal theory* (pp. 615–639). Oxford, England: Blackwell.

Brentari, D. (1998). *A prosodic model of sign language phonology.* Cambridge, MA: MIT Press.

Caplan, D. (2000). Neurolinguistics. In M. Aronoff & J. Rees-Miller (Eds.), (pp. 582–607).

Corina, D. (1990). Reassessing the role of sonority in syllable structure: Evidence from a visua gestural language. *Papers from the Chicago Linguistic Society, 26*(2), 33–44.

Corina, D. P. (1999). On the nature of left-hemisphere specialization for signed language. *Brain and Language, 69,* 230–240.

Corina, D., & Sandler, W. (1993). On the nature of phonological structure in sign language. *Phonology, 10*(2), 165–208.

Emmorey, K. (2002). *Language, cognition, and the brain: Insights from sign language research.* Mahwah, NJ: Lawrence Erlbaum Associates.

Emmorey, K. (2002). *Sign language: A window into human language, cognition and the brain.* Mahwah, NJ: Lawrence Erlbaum Associates.

Emmorey, K. (Ed.). (in press). *Perspectives on classifier constructions in sign languages.* Mahwah, NJ: Lawrence Erlbaum Associates.

Fischer, S., & Osugi, Y. (2000, July). *Thumbs up vs. giving the finger: Indexical classifiers in NS and ASL.* Paper presented at the 7th International Conference on Theoretical Issues in Sign Language Research, Amsterdam.

Fischer, S., & Siple, P. (Eds.). (1990). *Theoretical issues in sign language research* (Vol. 1). Chicago: University of Chicago Press.

Fodor, J. (1983). *The modularity of mind.* Cambridge, MA: MIT Press.

Friedman, (1977). Formational properties of American Sign Language. In L. Friedman (Ed.), *On the other hand: New perspectives in American Sign Language* (pp. 13–56). New York: Academic Press.

Goldin-Meadow, S., & McNeill, D. (1999). The role of gesture and mimetic representation in making language the province of speech. In M. C. Corballis & S. Lea (Eds.), *The descent of mind* (pp. 155–172). Oxford: Oxford University Press.

Hayes, B., & Lahiri, A. (1991). Bengali intonational phonology. *Natural Language and Linguistic Theory, 9,* 47–96.

Iverson, J. M., Capirci, O., & Caselli, M. C. (1994). From communication to language in two modalities. *Cognitive Development, 9,* 23–43.

Iverson, J., & Goldin-Meadow, S. (1997). What's communication got to do with it? Gesture in children blind from birth. *Developmental Psychology, 33*(3), 453–467.

Iverson, J., & Goldin-Meadow, S. (1998). Why people gesture when they speak. *Nature, 396,* 228.

Kegl, J. (1985). *Locative relations in American Sign Language word formation.* Doctoral dissertation. MIT, Cambridge, Mass.

Kegl, J., Senghas, A., & Coppola, M. (1999). Creation through contact: Sign language emergence and sign language change in Nicaragua. In M. DeGraff (Ed.), *Language creation and language change: Creolization, diachrony, and development* (pp. 179–237). Cambridge, MA: MIT Press.

Kendon, A. (1988). How gestures can become like words. In F. Poyatos (Ed.), *Cross-cultural perspectives in nonverbal communication* (pp. 131–141). Lewiston, NJ: C. J. Hofgrefe.

Kendon, A. (1994). Do gestures communicate?: A review. *Research on Language and Social Interaction, 27*(3), 175–200.

Klima, E., & Bellugi, U. (1979). *The signs of language.* Cambridge, MA: Harvard University Press.

Liberman, A. M., Cooper, F. S., Shankweiler, D. S., & Studdert-Kennedy, M. (1967). Perception of the speech code. *Psychological Review, 74,* 431–461.

Liddell, S. (1980). *American Sign Language syntax.* The Hague: Mouton.

Liddell, S. (1984). THINK and BELIEVE: Sequentiality in American Sign Language. *Language, 60,* 372–392.

Liddell, S. (1995). Real, surrogate, and token space: Grammatical consequences in ASL. In K. Emmorey & J. Reilly (Eds.), *Language, gesture, and space* (pp. 19–41). Hillsdale, NJ: Lawrence Erlbaum Associates.

Liddell, S. (2000). Indicating verbs and pronouns: Pointing away from agreement. In K. Emmorey & H. Lane (Eds.), *The signs of language revisited* (pp. 303–320). Mahwah, NJ: Lawrence Erlbaum Associates.

Lillo-Martin, D. (1986). Two kinds of null arguments in American Sign Language. *Natural Language and Linguistic Theory, 4,* 415–444.

Lillo-Martin, D. (1991). *Universal Grammar and American Sign Language: Setting the null argument parameter.* Dordrecht: Kluwer Academic Publishers.

McNeill, D. (1992). *Hand and mind: What gesture reveals about thought.* Chicago: University of Chicago Press.

Meier, R. (1982). *Icons, analogues, and morphemes: The acquisition of verb agreement in American Sign Language.* Unpublished doctoral dissertation, University of California, San Diego.

Meier, R. (1991). Language acquisition by deaf children. *American Scientist, Jan–Feb.,* 60–70.

Meir, I. (1998a). *Thematic structure and verb agreement in Israeli Sign Language.* Unpublished doctoral dissertation, the Hebrew University of Jerusalem.

Meir, I. (1998b). Syntactic-semantic interaction of Israeli Sign Language verbs: The case of backwards verbs. *Sign Language and Linguistics, 1*(1), 3–38.

Meir, I. (2002). A cross-modality perspective on verb agreement. *Natural Language and Linguistic Theory, 20,* 413–450.

Namir, L., & Schlesinger, I. M. (1978). The grammar of sign language. In I. M. Schlesinger (Ed.), *Sign languages of the deaf* (pp. 97–140). New York: Academic Press.

Neidle, C., Kegl, J., McLaughlin, D., Bahan, B., & Lee, R. G. (2000). *The syntax of American Sign Language: Functional categories and hierarchical structure.* Cambridge, MA: MIT Press.

Nespor, M., & Sandler, W. (1999). Prosody in Israeli Sign Language. *Language and Speech, 42*(2&3), 143–176.

Nespor, M., & Vogel, I. (1986). *Prosodic phonology.* Dordrecht: Foris.

Nevile, H., & Lawson, D. (1987). Attention to central and peripheral visual space in a movement detection task: An event-related potential and behavioral study: II. Congenitally deaf adults. *Brain Research, 405,* 263–283.

Neville, H., Coffey, S., Lawson, D., Fischer, A., Emmorey, K., & Bellugi, U. (1997). Neural systems mediating American Sign Language: Effects of sensory experience and age of acquisition. *Brain and Language, 47,* 285–308.

Newport, E., & Meier, R. (1985). The acquisition of American Sign Language. In D. Slobin (Ed.), *The cross-linguistic study of language acquisition* (Vol. 1, pp. 881–938). Mahwah, NJ: Lawrence Erlbaum Associates.

Newport, E., & Meier, R. (1990). Out of the hands of babes: On a possible sign advantage in language acquisition. *Language, 66,* 1–23.

Obando, I., Vega, E., Javier, E., Ellis, M., & Kegl, J. (2000, July). *Lip pointing in Idioma de Senas de Nicaragua.* Paper presented at 7th International Conference on Theoretical Issues in Sign Language Research, Amsterdam.

Padden, C. (1981). Some arguments for syntactic patterning in American Sign Language. *Sign Language Studies, 32,* 237–259.

Padden, C. (1988). *Interaction of morphology and syntax in American Sign Language.* New York: Garland. [1983: Doctoral dissertation, University of California, San Diego]

Peperkamp, S., & Mehler, J. (1999). Signed and spoken language: A unique underlying system? *Language and Speech, 42*(2&3), 333–346.

Perlmutter, D. (1992). Sonority and syllable structure in American Sign Language. *Linguistic Inquiry, 23,* 407–442.

Petronio, K., & Lillo-Martin, D. (1997). WH-movement and the position of SPEC-CP: Evidence from American Sign Language. *Language, 73,* 18–57.

Pettito, L. (1987). On the autonomy of language and gesture: Evidence from the acquisition of personal pronouns in American Sign Language. *Cognition, 27,* 1–52.

Pierrehumbert, J. (1980). *The phonology and phonetics of English intonation.* PhD Dissertation, MIT. Published 1988 by Indiana University Linguistics Club.

Poizner, H., Klima, E., & Bellugi, U. (1987). *What the hands reveal about the brain.* Cambridge, MA: MIT Press.

Reilly, J., McIntire, M., & Bellugi, U. (1990). The acquisition of conditionals in American Sign Language: Grammaticalized facial expressions. *Applied Psycholinguistics, 11,* 369–392.

Sandler, W. (1986). The spreading hand autosegment of American Sign Language. *Sign Language Studies, 50,* 1–28.

Sandler, W. (1989). *Phonological representation of the sign: Linearity and nonlinearity in American Sign Language.* Dordrecht: Foris.

Sandler, W. (1990). Temporal aspects and ASL phonology. In S. Fischer & P. Siple (Eds.), (pp. 7–35).

Sandler, W. (1993a). Sign language and modularity. *Lingua, 89*(4), 315–351.

Sandler, W. (1993b). A sonority cycle in ASL. *Phonology, 10*(2), 243–280.

Sandler, W. (1993c). Hand in hand: The roles of the nondominant hand in ASL phonology. *The Linguistic Review, 10,* 337–390.

Sandler, W. (1999a). The medium is the message: Prosodic interpretation of linguistic content in sign language. *Sign Language and Linguistics, 2*(2), 187–216.

Sandler, W. (1999b). Cliticization and prosodic words in a sign language. In T. Hall & U. Kleinhenz (Eds.), *Studies on the phonological word* (pp. 223–254). Amsterdam: Benjamins.

Sandler, W. (1999c). Prosody in two natural language modalities. *Language and Speech, 42*(2&3), 127–142.

Sandler, W. (in preparation). *Gestures and other roles of the mouth in sign language.*

Sandler, W., & Lillo-Martin, D. (2000). Natural sign languages. 533–562.

Sandler, W., & Lillo-Martin, D. (in preparation). *Sign language and linguistic universals.* Cambridge University Press.

Selkirk, E. (1986). On derived domains in sentence phonology. *Phonology Yearbook, 3,* 371–405.

Siple, P. (1978). Visual constraints for sign language communication. *Sign Language Studies, 19,* 95–110.

Stokoe, W. (1960). Sign language structure: An outline of the visual communication systems of the American deaf. In G. Trager (Ed.), *Studies in linguistics, occasional papers* 8. University of Buffalo. [1978. Silver Spring: Linstok Press.]

Supalla, T. (1982). *Structure and acquisition of verbs of motion and location in American Sign Language.* PhD Dissertation. University of California, San Diego.

Supalla, T. (1986). The classifier system in American Sign Language. In C. Craig (Ed.), *Noun classification and categorization* (pp. 181–214). Amsterdam: John Benjamins.

Supalla, T., & Newport, E. (1978). How many seats in a chair? The derivation of nouns and verbs in American Sign Language. In P. Siple (Ed.), *Understanding language through sign language research* (pp. 91–132). New York: Academic Press.

Volterra, V., & Iverson, J. M. (1995). When do modality factors affect the course of language acquisition? In K. Emmorey & J. Reilly (Eds.), *Language, gesture, and space* (pp. 371–390). Hillsdale, NJ: Lawrence Erlbaum Associates.

Wilbur, R. (1996). *Prosodic structure of American Sign Language.* Unpublished manuscript, Purdue University.

Woll, B. (2001). The sign that dared to speak its name: Echo phonology in British Sign Language (BSL). In P. Boyes-Braem & R. Sutton-Spence (Eds.), (pp. 87–98).

410 - Blank

TOWARD A DEFINITION
OF SLI?

16

Understanding SLI:
A Neuropsychological Perspective

Dorit Ben Shalom
Ben-Gurion University of the Negev

This chapter considers some of the basic themes in this book—exclusionary criteria as part of the definition of SLI (specific language impairment), the nature of the linguistic deficits found in SLI—in light of other types of cognitive disorders. It is argued that the study of SLI can benefit from the ways in which similar fundamental issues have been dealt with in the study of other disorders. The approach is neuropsychological, that is, it is concerned with brain–behavior relations as they are revealed through the study of SLI.

The first part of this chapter studies SLI from the point of view of brain research. It starts out with current beliefs about the specificity of brain mechanisms subserving grammatical processing, and asks what these views may entail with respect to SLI. It is suggested that such beliefs predict the existence of selective deficits in grammatical processing in some children, but do not require that SLI is defined by exclusionary criteria. To illustrate his position, SLI is compared with prosopagnosia (impaired face recognition), since face recognition, like grammatical processing, is often described as being subserved by a specific brain mechanism.

The second part takes the opposite approach, namely, it looks at brain research from the viewpoint of the linguistic behavior of people with SLI. It asks what current clinical markers of SLI mean with regard to the brain basis of grammatical processing. Three general similarities between clinical markers of SLI and acquired grammatical impairment (agrammatism) are noted: deficits in the production of tense morphology, in the comprehension of reversible passives, and in nonword repetition. Based on this discussion, it is suggested that the question of separate syntactic and phonological subtypes of SLI may have implications for the understanding of grammatical processing in the brain.

FROM BRAIN RESEARCH TO SLI

Many definitions of SLI contain exclusionary criteria, excluding children with intellectual, sensory, physical, or neurological impairments that co-occur with grammatical impairments (see Rice, chap. 2; Leonard, chap. 8; van der Lely, chap. 4; Schaeffer, chap. 5; & de Villiers, chap. 17, in this volume). The need for exclusionary criteria is motivated by the belief that the specificity of brain mechanisms subserving grammatical processing predicts "pure" impairments, as well as by the importance of such individuals for genetic research.

Certain empirical considerations, however, challenge this approach. Consider the case of autism. Autism spectrum disorders are characterized by impairments in three domains: social interaction, communication, and a restricted repertoire of activities and interests (APA, 1994). A diagnosis of "classical autism" requires, in addition to impairments in the aforementioned domains, a history of significant language delay. As already noted, many definitions of SLI characterize it as a selective impairment in the development of language, which is not accompanied by other intellectual, sensory, physical, or neurological impairments. These definitions in fact mean that a child cannot receive both a diagnosis of autism spectrum disorders and of SLI.

Recent work by Tager-Flusberg (see chap. 12 in this volume), however, has demonstrated that a group of children with autism spectrum disorders exhibit two widely accepted clinical markers of SLI: deficits in tense production and in nonword repetition. She argues that general considerations of language development in autism make it desirable to characterize this group of individuals as exhibiting both autism spectrum disorders and SLI. First, other individuals with autism spectrum disorders do not show these clinical markers, so grammatical impairment of this specific type does not seem to be a necessary component of autism spectrum disorders. Second, there is some genetic evidence that children with autism spectrum disorders and language impairment share genetic characteristics with some children with SLI (Warburton et al., 2000; see discussion in Tager-Flusberg, chap. 12 in this volume). In order to allow for a double diagnosis of autism and SLI, it seems necessary to redefine SLI in such a way that it does not include exclusionary criteria. This requires addressing the two arguments for exclusionary criteria already mentioned: the belief that the specificity of the brain mechanisms subserving grammatical processing predicts specific impairments, and the need for individuals with "pure" impairments for genetic research on SLI.

First consider the former argument. Suppose the brain mechanisms subserving grammatical processing are specific (Chomsky, 2000). Then it is predicted that there are some individuals with impairments that uniquely involve this mechanism. In other words, if developmental grammar impairment is consistently paired with another specific developmental impairment, then this would make it harder to maintain that the brain mechanisms subserving grammatical processing are specific (cf. van der Lely, chap. 12 in this volume). However, this belief does not imply that there are no individuals with SLI who exhibit additional impairments.

Neuropsychology offers an alternative way of dealing with issues of specificity, through the use of "double dissociations" (A. W. Ellis & Young, 1986). When there are individuals who perform well on measures of a given cognitive process A, but poorly on measures of another cognitive process B, and other individuals exhibit an opposite pattern of cognitive impairment—namely, they perform well on measures of process B but poorly on measures of process A—there is talk of *double dissociations*. Note that it is crucial to find both types of individuals. If only one type is found, say individuals who perform well on measures of process A but not B, then it is possible that processes A and B involve the same cognitive process, but that A is for some reason easier than B. This assumption makes the prediction that individuals doing well on measures of process B but not A will not be found.

Double dissociations can be applied in the case of grammatical processing. Let grammatical processing be Process A and any other cognitive process of interest be Process B. To argue that grammatical processing and Process B are distinct, it is necessary to find at least one individual who is impaired on measures of Process B but not on measures of Process A (i.e., grammatical processing) and one with impairment on measures of grammatical processing but not Process B.

A concrete example of the application of double dissociations is Schaeffer's (chap. 5 in this volume) work on pragmatic processing. She shows that some children with SLI perform poorly on measures of grammatical processing, but do well on measures of pragmatic processing. The opposite pattern has long been associated with a subgroup of individuals with autism spectrum disorders (e.g., Tager-Flusberg, 1996). Together these dissociations support the claim that pragmatic processing and grammatical processing are distinct cognitive processes.

The use of double dissociations as a tool for dealing with specificity can be further illustrated in the case of face recognition, another cognitive process often argued to be subserved by a specific brain mechanism (Nachson, 1995). Grammatical processing and face recognition are similar in important ways. For example, both grammatical processing and face recognition take sensory inputs (auditory in the case of oral languages, visual in the case of face recognition) and perform a specific computation on specific aspects of the input (grammatical structure in the case of grammatical processing, face identity in the case of face processing). Moreover, it has been argued that both these cognitive processes are subserved by specific brain mechanisms (e.g., Fodor, 1983; see van der Lely, chap. 4; Schaeffer, chap. 5; and Wexler, chap. 1, in this volume, for arguments that grammatical processing is a specific brain mechanism).

Tzavaras, Hecaen, and Le Bras (1970) suggested that some strategies for the analysis and integration of facial details have innate specificity. This position has been supported by various indirect arguments: Attraction to faces but not to other visual stimuli is evident very early on in life; appreciation of differences among faces is earlier than that of differences among other visual objects, and face recognition has a different developmental course than the recognition of other visual objects (Yin, 1978). One of the more convincing pieces of evidence for innateness of face recognition comes from Goren, Sarty, and Wu's (1975) study, in which 9-minute-old babies preferred a moving schematic face to other visual stimuli. More recent studies have shown neonatal imitation of lip movements a minute or two after birth when the model face was the first facial stimulus to which the neonate was exposed. This is interpreted as further evidence for the innateness of face recognition (see Johnson & Morton, 1991).

Fried, Mateer, Ojemann, Wohns, and Fedio (1982) found that electrical stimulation to specific areas in the brain disrupts face recognition in humans. Allison et al. (1994) reported event-related brain potentials that are specific to face recognition. Recent functional imaging studies help pinpoint the location of specific areas in the brain that are activated during face recognition (Sergent, Ohta, & MacDonald, 1992). These areas are by and large compatible with the brain areas implicated in face recognition through electrical stimulation and event-related potentials.

Face recognition can exhibit selective impairment as a result of either development or acquired brain lesions. A deficit in recognizing familiar faces is known as prosopagnosia, and is a recognized neuropsychological syndrome (Bodamer, 1947). It is usually linked to specific brain areas (for a review, see Benton, 1990). Double dissociations have been demonstrated between face recognition and many other related processes. Some people cannot recognize familiar faces but can recognize facial expressions, whereas others show the opposite pattern of impairment (Hecaen & Angelergues, 1962). Some people do not recognize familiar faces but can recognize unfamiliar faces. Others can recognize familiar faces but not unfamiliar ones (Warrington & James, 1967). In experiments conducted with farmers, one farmer could not recognize familiar faces, but could recognize his individual animals (Bruyer et al., 1983). Other farmers could recognize familiar faces but not their animals (McCarthy & Warrington, 1986). Interestingly, for the present purposes, the definition of face recognition impairment does not include exclusionary criteria, rather, the issue of specificity is assessed through double dissociations. "Pure" cases of prosopagnosia are in fact very rare (H. D. Ellis & Young, 1989). This fact is not used to argue that face recognition is not specific, but rather as evidence for the multiple anatomical and functional connections between the brain areas involved in face processing and other brain areas.

Turning now to the second argument in favor of using exclusionary criteria to define SLI, namely, genetic research, it has been argued that investigations into the genetic basis of SLI require the use of individuals with selective impairments. This assumption is, however, unwarranted.

Many clinical syndromes are defined behaviorally, resulting in heterogeneous clinical populations. This heterogeneity makes genetic research more difficult because different genetic deficits can result in partly overlapping clusters of behavioral symptoms. One way to reduce heterogeneity in a clinical population is to focus on "nonpure" subpopulations who share more than the core symptoms of the "pure" disorder. One recent example concerns individuals with both autism spectrum disorders and SLI. Bradford et al. (2001) pointed out the involvement of chromosome 7 in some cases of autism spectrum disorders, but only when analysis was restricted to the subgroup of children with both autism spectrum disorders and severe language impairment. The genetic generalization was no longer evident when all available children with autism spectrum disorders were considered. Thus, the study of nonpure subpopulations may help the discovery of genetic generalizations that are not true for the whole population.

Thus, it seems that the use of exclusionary criteria to define SLI cannot rely on either the specificity of brain mechanisms subserving grammatical processing or on arguments from genetic research. This provides support for definitions of SLI without exclusionary criteria, and for treatment of the specificity of grammatical impairment through the use of double dissociations rather than that of exclusionary criteria.

FROM SLI TO BRAIN RESEARCH

Thus far this chapter has discussed SLI from the perspective of brain research, but as already noted in the introduction, the connections between brain research and SLI run both ways. This section examines what might be learned about brain research from the study of SLI.

Acquired and developmental deficits of the same cognitive process often result in somewhat different patterns of impairment. Comparing these patterns may help isolate the essential properties of the process in question. In the case of grammatical processing, it is natural to compare SLI and *agrammatism*, which is probably the purest form of acquired grammatical impairment.

Agrammatism is caused by brain injury to the left hemisphere, usually in Broca's area or its vicinity (cf. Zurif, 1995). There are some general similarities between currently accepted clinical markers of agrammatism and SLI. They come from three core domains of language performance: production, comprehension, and repetition.

A widely accepted syntactic marker for SLI in many languages is the extended use of infinitives in syntactic contexts where finiteness is obligatory (Rice & Wexler, 1996; Wexler, chap. 1, and Rice, chap. 2, in this volume). When English-speaking children with SLI are matched on mean length of utterance with typically developing younger children (around 3 years old), the children with SLI make significantly more errors in tense production, even when performance on other inflections does not differ significantly between the two groups. Similarly, omitted or incorrect grammatical morphemes are a clinical hallmark of agrammatism (Goodglass, 1976). Interestingly, in both SLI and agrammatism, the structure of the relevant language seems to play a role in determining the type of errors produced: More omissions are seen in languages that allow bare roots as verbs, and more incorrect inflected forms are seen in languages that do not allow bare stems (but see Crago & Paradis, chap. 3 in this volume; Friedmann, 2001). Deficits in question formation might be part of this group of symptoms as well (van der Lely, chap. 4 in this volume, for SLI; Friedmann, 2001, for agrammatism).

A second reliable syntactic finding in SLI is errors in the comprehension of reversible passives (van der Lely & Dewart, 1986; van der Lely, chap. 4 in this volume). Children with SLI typically interpret sentences such as "The man is eaten by the fish" as "The man is eating the fish." Similar deficits have been documented in agrammatism. Grodzinsky, Pinango, Zurif, and Drai (1999) surveyed comprehension scores of people with agrammatism on active versus reversible passive sentences. Active sentences were comprehended correctly in almost 100% of the cases. Reversible passives distributed binomially with a mean comprehension score of 55%, and the two distributions differed significantly from one another.

A third widely accepted marker for SLI is phonological in nature, consisting of a deficit in nonword repetition (i.e., the ability to repeat pseudowords presented auditorily; Bishop, North, & Donlan, 1996; cf. its use in Tager-Flusberg, chap. 12 in this volume). The score on such a test is considered an index of phonological short-term memory (Gathercole & Baddeley, 1989). Impairment in word repetition is known to be a core clinical symptom of Broca's aphasia, the more general type of aphasia to which almost all agrammatisms belong (e.g., Victor, Ropper, & Adams, 2000). Whereas lit-

tle is known about nonword repetition in agrammatism, there is no reason
to expect it to be better than word repetition.

Now consider some potential explanations of these phenomena in the
language of agrammatic aphasics and children with SLI. Some hypotheses
compatible with deficits in tense production and passive comprehension
rely on properties of syntactic processing. For example, in the Chomskian
paradigm, sentences are assumed to have syntactic structures resembling
the tree in Example 1, whose top part is presented here:

(1)

CP
(wh-question)   C'
        C⁰   TP
(complementizer)
                T'
            T⁰   AgrP
          (tense)
                    Agr'
                Agr⁰   VP
            (agreement)
                        V'
                    V
                  (verb)

The tree in Example 1 contains three grammatical projections corresponding to grammatical morphemes: a CP (complementizer projection), motivated by grammatical morphemes introducing complement clauses, such
as "that" or "whether," or by question words like "who" or "how"; a TP
(tense projection), motivated by various tense morphemes; and an AgrP
(agreement projection) motivated by agreement morphemes like the third
person s in English (e.g., in the sentence "The man eats the fish."). In a sentence like "Why did the man eat the fish?", the question word "why" is assumed to be under CP, the grammatical subject "the man" is assumed to be
under TP, and the grammatical object "the fish" is assumed to be inside the
VP (verb projection). A fourth projection, NegP (negation projection), is
added for sentences with sentential negation such as "The man didn't eat
the fish."

It is well-known that Broca's area in the brain plays a crucial role in the
processing of syntactic structure. Friedmann (2001) argued, more specifi-

cally, that in production, people with agrammatism cannot process the higher nodes of syntactic trees, such as CP, TP, and AgrP (see Example 1). As these higher nodes tend to be grammatical projections, the result is impaired processing of grammatical projections in agrammatics. For example, an agrammatic might produce a sentence with a bare verb, such as "The man eat the fish," without any tense or agreement. One way to think of Friedmann's (2001) hypothesis is in terms of a syntactic buffer that contains only grammatical projections, starting with the lower grammatical projections in the syntactic tree. This syntactic buffer can be assumed to be implemented in Broca's area. A healthy adult would have a syntactic buffer that can stack at least four grammatical projections (AgrP, NegP, TP, and CP). An agrammatic would have a smaller syntactic buffer. Extending the hypothesis to SLI, children with SLI are predicted to have syntactic buffers that are smaller than those of younger controls matched for mean length of utterance. Deficits in tense production in SLI and agrammatism are interpreted as supporting an impaired processing of the tense projection in Example 1.

Impaired processing of grammatical projections can also be linked to the deficits in reversible passives comprehension in SLI and agrammatism. This prediction relies on another core assumption of the Chomskian paradigm, concerning passive sentences like the one in Example 2:

(2) The man was eaten by the fish.

The assumption talks about the syntactic status of grammatical subjects of passive sentences ("the man" in Example 2). In general, grammatical subjects are assumed to be in the tense projection in Example 1, but subjects of passive sentences are assumed to be additionally linked to a position after the passive verb ("eaten" in Example 2). This link is assumed to be crucial for correct syntactic processing of the subject ("the man" in Example 2). These links fall under the heading of "syntactic movement."

According to the syntactic buffer hypothesis, a grammatical subject of a passive sentence would be, in general, misprocessed in SLI and agrammatism, as the connection between TP and the postverbal position would be lost as a result of impaired processing of the tense projection (cf. Grodzinsky, 2000). Consequently, reliance on nonsyntactic interpretation would result in the observed contrast between reversible and irreversible passives: Only in the irreversible passives is there enough semantic information to determine the role of the grammatical subject, despite the failure of syntactic processing. This account is consistent with the optional syntactic movement part of van der Lely's RDDR (representational deficit for dependent relations, chap. 4 in this volume), according to which syntactic movements to both TP and CP are disrupted in SLI.

Syntactic hypotheses like the syntactic buffer hypothesis tell little about phonological deficits like nonword repetition, thus requiring separate accounts for the syntactic and phonological clinical markers in SLI. Whether or not this separation is desirable depends to a large extent on the existence of separate syntactic and phonological subtypes of SLI.

The question of possible subtypes of SLI is discussed extensively in other chapters of this volume (e.g., see van der Lely, chap. 4, and de Villiers, chap. 17, in this volume). It is reasonably accepted at this point that there are cases of phonological SLI without syntactic impairment, putting one at risk for later phonological dyslexia (Snowling & Hulme, 1994), but it is less clear at present whether there are pure cases of syntactic SLI. A priori, two options are possible: One is that pure cases of syntactic SLI exist, even if they are extremely rare. In this case, there would be a double dissociation between syntactic and phonological subtypes of SLI, and separate accounts of syntactic and phonological deficits in SLI would be desirable. A second option is that pure cases of syntactic SLI do not exist. In this case, there would be no double dissociations between syntactic and phonological subtypes of SLI, and separate accounts of syntactic and phonological deficits in SLI would be undesirable. To date, the empirical evidence is insufficient to decide between these two options.[1]

Not surprisingly, given the general similarities between clinical markers in agrammatism and in SLI, the questions that arise concerning agrammatism are parallel to those arising in the case of SLI: What is the precise extent of phonological deficits in the purest cases of syntactic agrammatism? Are there any cases of agrammatism unaccompanied by phonological deficits? Is there a double dissociation between syntactic and phonological subtypes of acquired disorders of grammatical processing? As is the case for SLI, these questions are largely unanswered at present.

Finally, the question of syntactic and phonological subtypes of grammatical impairment is intimately connected to the question of syntactic and phonological types of grammatical processing. It is widely accepted that in the unimpaired brain, Broca's area has a pivotal role in both syntactic and phonological processing, but parallel to the options regarding grammatical impairment, two options exist with regard to the relation between syntactic and phonological types of processing in the unimpaired brain. Are there separate mechanisms in the brain responsible for syntactic and phonological processing or is there one set of mechanisms responsible for both? If there are separate brain mechanisms subserving syntactic and phonological processing, then double dissociations would be expected in the case of impairment. If, on the other hand, there is only one brain mechanism for grammatical processing, then separate syntactic and phonological process-

---

[1]A different approach to phonological deficits in SLI was suggested by Tallal and her colleagues (Tallal, Stark, & Mellits, 1985), who saw these deficits as reflecting a general auditory difficulty in processing rapid transient stimuli.

ing, or double dissociations between respective impairments, would not be expected. Thus, the existence of separate syntactic and phonological subtypes of SLI may have implications for general models of grammatical processing.

To summarize, examining brain research from the point of view of SLI, it was argued that the study of grammatical behavior in SLI populations may shed light on the underlying process of grammatical processing in the brain. A concrete example concerns the separation between syntactic and phonological types of grammatical processing, where the existence of separate syntactic and phonological subtypes of SLI may provide important clues for resolution of a general grammatical processing question.

CONCLUSIONS

This chapter has explored connections between SLI and brain research. Looking at SLI from the viewpoint of brain research, it has been argued that even if brain mechanisms subserving grammatical processing are specific, it does not require that SLI should be defined by the use of exclusionary criteria. Instead, a technique often used in neuropsychology, double dissociation, could serve to evaluate the specificity of grammatical impairment. Examining brain research from the point of view of SLI, it has been argued that the study of grammatical impairment in SLI may shed light on underlying processes of grammatical processing. Specifically, the possible existence of syntactic and phonological subtypes of SLI may have wider implications for theoretical models of grammatical processing, giving clues about the general question of separate mechanisms for syntactic and phonological types of grammatical processing in the human brain.

REFERENCES

Allison, T., Ginter, H., McCarthy, G., Nobre, A. C., Puce, A., Luby, M., & Spencer D. D. (1994). Face recognition in human extrastriate cortex. *Journal of Neurophysiology, 71,* 821–825.

American Psychiatric Association. (1994). *Diagnostic and statistical manual of mental disorder* (4th ed.). Washington, DC: American Psychiatric Association.

Benton, A. (1990). Facial recognition. *Cortex, 26,* 491–499.

Bishop, D. V. M, North, T., & Donlan, C. (1996). Nonword repetition as a behavioral marker for inherited language impairment: Evidence from a twin study. *Journal of Child Psychology and Psychiatry, 37,* 391–403.

Bodamer, J. (1947). Die Prosop-Agnosia [The propos-agnosia]. *Archiv fur Psychiatrie und Nerver krankheiten, 179,* 6–53.

Bradford, Y., Haines, J., Hutcheson, H., Gardine, M., Braun, T., Sheffield, V., Cassavant, T., Huang W., Wang, K., Vieland, V., Folstein, S., Santangelo, S., & Piven, J. (2001). Incorporating lar guage phenotypes strengthens evidence of linkage to autism. *American Journal of Medical Genetics, 105*, 539–547.

Bruyer, R., Laterre, C., Seron, X., Feyereisen, P., Strypstein, E., Pierrard, E., & Rectem, D. (1983). A case of prosopagnosia with some preserved covert remembrance of familiar faces. *Brain and Cognition, 2*, 257–284.

Chomsky, N. (2000). *New horizons in the study of language and mind.* New York: Cambridge University Press.

Ellis, A. W., & Young, A. W. (1986). *Human cognitive neuropsychology.* Hove: Psychology Press.

Ellis, H. D., & Young, A. W. (1989). Are faces special? In A. W. Young & H. D. Ellis (Eds.), *Handbook of research on face processing* (pp. 1–26). Amsterdam: North-Holland.

Fodor, J. (1983). *Modularity of mind.* Cambridge, MA: MIT Press.

Fried, I., Mateer, C., Ojemann, G., Wohns, R., & Fedio, P. (1982). Organization of visuospatial functions in human cortex. Evidence from electrical stimulation. *Brain, 105*, 349–371.

Friedmann, N. (2001). Agrammatism and the psychological reality of the syntactic tree. *Journal of Psycholinguistic Research, 30*, 71–90.

Gathercole, S. E., & Baddeley, A. D. (1989). Evaluation of the role of phonological STM in the development of vocabulary in children: A longitudinal study. *Journal of Memory and Language, 28*, 200–213.

Goodglass, H. (1976). Agrammatism. In H. Whitaker & H. A. Whitaker (Eds.), *Studies in neurolinguistics* (pp. 237–260). New York: Academic Press.

Goren, C. C., Sarty, M., & Wu, P. Y. (1975). Visual following and pattern discrimination of face-like stimuli by newborn infants. *Pediatrics, 56*, 544–549.

Grodzinsky, Y. (2000). The neurology of syntax: Language use without Broca's area. *Behavioral and Brain Sciences, 23*, 1–21.

Grodzinsky, Y., Pinango, M. M., Zurif, E., & Drai, D. (1999). The critical role of group studies in neuropsychology: Comprehension regularities in Broca's aphasia. *Brain and Language, 67*, 134–147.

Hecaen, H., & Angelergues, R. (1962). Agnosia for faces. *Archives of Neurology, 7*, 92–100.

Johnson, M. H., & Morton, J. (1991). *Biology and cognitive development: The case of face recognition.* Oxford, England: Blackwell.

McCarthy, R. A., & Warrington, E. K. (1986). Visual associative agnosia: A clinico-anatomical study of a single case. *Journal of Neurology, Neurosurgery, and Psychiatry, 49*, 1233–1240.

Nachson, I. (1995). On the modularity of face recognition: The riddle of domain specificity. *Journal of Clinical and Experimental Neuropsychology, 17*, 256–275.

Rice, M. L., & Wexler, K. (1996). Toward tense as a clinical marker of specific language impairment in English-speaking children. *Journal of Speech and Hearing Research, 39*, 1239–1257.

Sergent, J., Ohta, S., & MacDonald, B. (1992). Functional neuroanatomy of face and object processing. *Brain, 115*, 15–36.

Snowling, M., & Hulme, C. (1994). The development of phonological skills. *Philosophical Transactions of the Royal Society B, 346*, 21–27.

Tager-Flusberg, H. (1996). Brief report: Current theory and research on language and communication in autism. *Journal of Autism and Developmental Disorders, 26*, 169–172.

Tallal, P., Stark, R. E., & Mellits, E. D. (1985). Identification of language-impaired children on the basis of rapid perception and production skills. *Brain and Language, 5*, 314–322.

Tzavaras, A., Hecaen, H., & Le Bras, H. (1970). Le probleme de la specificte du deficit de la recconoissance du visage humain lors des lesions hemispheriques unilaterales [The problem of specificity of deficit of human face recognition in unilateral hemispheric lesions]. *Neuropsychologia, 8*, 403–416.

van der Lely H. K. J., & Dewart M. H. (1986). Sentence comprehension strategies in specifically language impaired children. *British Journal of Disorders of Communication, 21*, 291–306.

Victor, M., Ropper, A. H., & Adams, R. D. (2000). *Principles of neurology* (7th ed.). New York: McGraw-Hill.

Warburton, P., Baird, G., Chen, W., Morris, K., Jacobs, B. W., Hodgson, S., & Docherty, Z. (2000). Support of linkage of autism and specific language impairment to 7q3 from two chromosome rearrangements involving band 7q31. *American Journal of Medical Genetics, 96,* 228–234.

Warrington, E. K., & James, M. (1967). An experimental investigation of facial recognition in patients with unilateral cerebral lesions. *Cortex, 3,* 317–326.

Yin, R. K. (1978). Face perception: A review of experiments with infants, normal adults, and brain-injured persons. In R. Held, H. W. Leibovitz, & H. L. Teuber (Eds.), *Handbook of sensory physiology* (Vol. 3, pp. 147–172). New York: Springer Verlag.

Zurif, E. B. (1995). Brain regions of relevance to syntactic processing. In L. R. Gleitman & M. Liberman (Eds.), *An invitation to cognitive science: Language* (pp. 381–397). Cambridge, MA: MIT Press.

17

Defining SLI:
A Linguistic Perspective

Jill G. de Villiers
Smith College

This is an exciting time to be working on language disorders. Several contemporary trends converge to make the prospect of a breakthrough in understanding the nature of specific language impairment (SLI) more likely then it has been in the past:

1. The success of the human genome project, and the possibility that with a sufficiently clear description of the phenotype, the genetic basis of language disorders, long suspected, may be clarified or even located.
2. The rapid progress in contemporary linguistic theory, with some real convergence on an articulated and deep description of human language.
3. The cross-training of clinicians and linguists who are beginning to speak the same theoretical language.
4. The influx of evidence beyond the usual languages, making for fertile crosslinguistic tests of hypotheses.

Each of these is reflected in the work reported in this volume. This chapter reviews some of the various linguistic proposals concerning the fundamental nature of SLI. Linguistic theory and work on language development pathology can work together in several important ways. Linguistics promises the best current analysis of the categories and principles of importance in language, which shift every decade or so to reflect the newest insights, and, we can only hope, retain the old ones. Work on child language pathology must keep abreast of these discoveries because they hold the prospect of illuminating puzzling co-occurrences of symptoms, or dissociations among parts of language that may seem superficially connected. These patterns, and the path and course of development over time, can in turn feed linguistic theory with significant empirical data to allow choice among competing theoretical analyses. Several chapters in this volume reflect this symbiosis, and serve as points of reflection in this chapter.

But there is a lot of ground clearing ahead if the promising strands are going to converge and bring a new understanding. Replication and comparison of research results require clearly defined populations, as does the search for a common genetic profile. Large-scale empirical efforts must choose a population to study: who these children are and how they are selected can interact in complicated ways with the goals mentioned previously. But, if the tools for defining the populations are insufficiently refined, then the whole theoretical endeavor is in peril. Herein lies the dilemma.

As Crago and Paradis (chap. 3 in this volume) point out, the notion of "specific" in specific language impairment is at the heart of the matter. Consider what it has meant, and what it could mean. The original term was coined to capture the fact that researchers meant to include in this category children who only have a problem with language, that is, the problems they exhibit are not because of other sensory, cognitive, or social developments that might impact indirectly on language. So, deaf children had to be excluded, or children with attentional problems or retardation, or children with autism or severe emotional difficulties. All of these problems, it was argued, could result in a child who scored poorly on a standardized language test, but not for reasons that would interest linguists. Furthermore, the difficulty portrayed by children with specific language impairment was supposed to be "soft" neurologically, that is, there should not be clear evidence of brain injury, abnormal EEG, epilepsy, or other physical impairments that might explain the deficit on other grounds. Nevertheless, it is a common assumption that neurological signs specifically for SLI would be uncovered. So, specific language impairment has been traditionally defined by exclusion. The issue is taken up first and its ramifications are explored. This might be called the "specifically, language impairment" issue.

A second meaning of specific language impairment is a slight variant, namely, that children who fall into this category have a problem specific to language, with no other concomitant problems. That is, having defined by exclusion the class of children who fit the previous definition, is it the case that the only problem they have is in some aspect of their linguistic system? Or, is that secondary to some domain-general difficulty whose impact is primarily reflected in language? This second issue is discussed next as "specific-to-language impairment."

A third meaning of specific language impairment is also pertinent to the chapters in this volume, namely, is the language impairment highly specific? Children with SLI have been said to display many problems: Are these all manifestations of one basic linguistic problem, or might there be several subgroups each with distinct problems?

That is, not only is the impairment in the language system itself, and domain specific, but it is also highly circumscribed, say to the tense system. The ramifications of some highly specific omission within the linguistic system can be widespread, so it does not necessarily mean that such a child would have only a few things wrong in their speech. Crago and Paradis (chap. 3 in this volume) take up the further question of the specificity of the problems in SLI to particular languages, which is addressed here as well.

The final question concerns what is meant by impairment in specific language *impairment*: That is, is there a part of the grammar that has gone awry or is missing? Or, is the grammar intact, with all the principles, parameters, categories, and properties of universal grammar (UG), but delayed in maturation, with that delay having clearly demarcated consequences? This is an essential debate, and where the prospect of locating a gene becomes especially tantalizing. It is also where crosslinguistic work becomes essential.

The path through these varied concerns can be represented as a binary branching tree, as in Fig. 17.1. It is not really accurate as a decision tree, be-

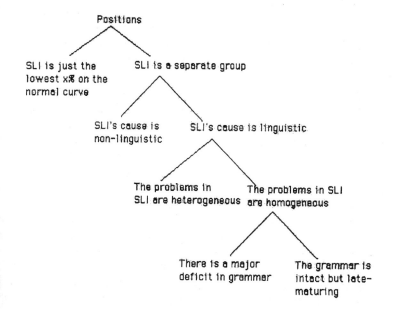

FIG. 17.1. A hierarchy of decisions about the nature of SLI.

cause there are theories of SLI that incorporate combinations of these positions that are not represented, but it does represent a path that has proved popular with those who adopt a more linguistic approach. Certain difficulties arise when researchers interested in decisions captured in the bottommost nodes retain assumptions reflected in the earlier decision points. In other words, embarking on the traditional path toward specificity of subject selection may risk obscuring linguistic questions about possible language disorders.

SPECIFICALLY, LANGUAGE IMPAIRMENT: IS SLI A DIFFERENT GROUP?

The first branching node reflects the decision about considering SLI to be a particular group defined by exclusion (Stark & Tallal, 1981; Stromswold, 1997). The exclusion of children with difficulties in areas other than language would seem to be an obvious decision. It is traditionally argued that researchers need to define the population of children who have a disorder that is specifically in the language area in order to discover what they have in common. The exclusionary criteria are under reexamination currently primarily for empirical reasons (Tager-Flusberg & Cooper, 1999; Plante 1998). But the discussion should also consider theoretical assumptions concerning modularity.

Fodor (1981) proposed that human cognition is comprised of special purpose systems designed for particular domains: face perception, three dimensional object recognition, speech perception, syntax processing. He argued that modules are designed for specialized kinds of input; the processing is fast, mandatory, not accessible to introspection, and most importantly, encapsulated (i.e., impervious to the influence of general knowledge or cognitive processes). In further refinements, the particular subparts of language are also modularized (syntax, phonology, semantics, pragmatics are separate modules), specialized, and perhaps encapsulated from general cognition, but not completely from each other. Chomsky (2000) and Crain and Wexler (1999) upheld the idea of modularity of language (J. G. de Villiers, 2001).

However, if syntax is a genuine module, then it should not be possible for a disorder in some other cognitive module—such as attention, memory, social, or sensory impairment—to manifest as a genuine syntax problem. Admittedly, children with a serious cognitive problem might never enter the right condition for testing their syntax: They may not look at the test, or fail to recognize that a question is being asked of them. The potential dangers here are of overinclusion for the wrong reasons. However, the danger is only possible if the test instrument is too gross: The profile of perform ance, not the score, should allow differentiation of the alternatives. Van der Lely (chap. 4 in this volume) points to growing evidence that within language impaired groups, IQ level seems to make little difference to the profile of language performance (e.g., Tomblin & Zhang, 1999).

What might be learned, and what might be lost, by casting the net wider to include subjects who show a deviant/delayed syntax profile but also have other problems, say, cognitive or social? This is an issue under renewed consideration.

One goal of research on SLI is to discover aspects of linguistic functioning that may uniquely define the phenotype of the disorder, if the syndrome is indeed unique. Therefore, it is necessary to compare the language of children defined by exclusion as having SLI with that of children with different identified syndromes. The chapters by Tager-Flusberg (chap. 12) and Levy (chap. 14) suggest there may be more overlap in language behavior across groups with different etiology than has been assumed. Levy argues that the very earliest stages of language acquisition take the same form regardless of specific etiology, and only later might distinct syndromes appear. Tager-Flusberg shows that there is considerable overlap among some groups of autistic subject and SLI subjects, even on the particular clinical markers: nonword repetition and tense marking, which have been held to be distinctive in SLI.

If Tager-Flusberg is correct in positing three distinct modules that can disassociate—one for theory of mind, one for syntax, and one for general cognition—then there is also no reason why they could not be jointly impaired in some varieties of disorder. A child might have impairment in both theory of mind and syntax, as in some autistic subjects, or even in syntax and general cognition, as in some syndromes of retardation. If the goal is to identify what is unique to the phenotype of SLI, then it would seem important to continue to search for linguistic properties or profiles that are not shared across syndromes, by comparing groups (see also Plante, 1998). If it should turn out that the linguistic properties are never unique, then SLI will have to be defined by exclusion of other difficulties.

If the goal is not necessarily to look for an associated genetic profile, but to understand the ways in which language can go wrong, then it can also be argued that exclusionary criteria will distort the picture. At the very least, close comparison groups should be part of the research endeavor (Mervis & Robinson, chap. 9 in this volume), and failures to find group differences should not languish unreported. More refined linguistic analyses might well reveal that different groups are more different than alike in their grammars. Alternatively, further research may suggest that all children who are delayed in the onset of syntax, no matter why, have grammars that exhibit certain common characteristics. To find the ways that grammar can go awry, it is necessary to take into account a broader range of subjects instead of a very narrow range, and continually to enrich the range of linguistic tests (Cooper & Tager-Flusberg, 1999).

SPECIFIC-TO-LANGUAGE IMPAIRMENT: IS SLI DOMAIN SPECIFIC?

The second issue is a refinement of the first issue: Is the difficulty in language exhibited by children who are defined as having SLI restricted to the language domain? In other words, is the language deficit primary or secondary to something else? Three alternatives occur. First, Tallal and her colleagues (Tallal, 2000; Tallal & Piercy, 1973) argued for many years that a central problem in SLI lies in the fast temporal resolution required by phoneme perception, and this is more general than speech. The hypothesis is that SLI subjects have capacity limitations for processing rapidly successive auditory verbal and nonverbal stimuli. In other words, language is where the problem is most obviously manifest, but it has a primary cause in auditory or even temporal resolution that is broader. Again, this represents a contradiction to the premise that the phonetic perception module is designed for specialized input and presumably does not draw on more general temporal processing skills. But the group with auditory deficits may also just be one subgroup of SLI. Van der Lely (chap. 4 in this volume) demonstrates that the auditory deficits are unrelated to the grammatical impairments in her group of grammatical-SLI subjects, and goes on to raise the possibility that there might be parts of phonology that are domain specific and parts that are domain general.

A second proposal of a general deficit is that by Bishop, North, and Donlan (1996), who argued that nonword repetition is an excellent task for detecting problems specific to language. This raises the possibility that short-term auditory memory deficits are fundamental to the language problems seen in typical SLI. If this is so, then modularity is again challenged. The language problems are secondary to a broader deficit lying beyond the bounds of language.

A third alternative is that children exhibiting language deficits are poor generalizers. In other words, they have trouble finding rules and patterns. Language demands more of this skill than other aspects of early cognition, so language is where the primary deficit appears. Note that this position is also strongly antimodular in that it assumes language acquisition involves general purpose learning processes that build up rules and patterns by induction. The case of Williams syndrome (Clahsen & Temple, chap. 13 in this volume) would seem to counter such a position in that children who are otherwise poor at finding patterns seem to be excellent (or even excessive) at extracting linguistic rules. However, this is far from uncontroversial, with some researchers on Williams syndrome finding language problems compatible with problems in general pattern making in nonverbal domains (Karmiloff-Smith, 1998).

If syndromes of this general sort exist, they constitute a challenge to models of language acquisition derived from the contemporary generative tradition. That is, how can something in general cognition have an impact on language competence, especially if it is reflected in performance across tasks? Or should the reverse be considered: Could more general difficulties be parasitic on the central language difficulty? Modularity is one way: Language may be encapsulated, but many aspects of general cognition are not, and can be influenced, scaffolded, or enabled by language. Plante (1998) discussed how children with language impairment may necessarily have depressed IQ scores if language is the tool by which certain aspects of cognition are mastered, so artificially setting an exclusionary IQ criterion can distort the picture of the disorder.

IS SLI A HETEROGENEOUS LANGUAGE DISORDER?

There are two related issues here. The first concerns the population and the second concerns the individual with SLI. The first asks: Is the population of children with SLI heterogeneous or homogeneous? That is, even when children who have other problems are excluded, and even if cases of articulation difficulty and verbal apraxia are excluded, is the result a group who exhibits the same language problems? Many researchers concur that there are still definable subgroups: Neville, Coffey, Holcombe, and Tallal (1993), van der Lely (chap. 4 in this volume; 1998), Stromswold (1997), Rapin and Allen (1983), and Leonard (chap. 8 in this volume) all reviewed evidence suggesting that there are even further subdivisions necessary in an already narrow definition.

The second issue concerns the problem in an individual with SLI: Do the difficulties and deficits form a single linguistic core problem, or are they several separate problems? This question is no doubt the most interesting for linguistics and language acquisition, and raises the greatest theoretical and methodological difficulties. The claim is that the impairments seen in SLI are not only domain specific but also narrowly definable (de Jong, chap. 6 in this volume). That is, it is not the case that a child with SLI exhibits a broad range of language impairments of great variety. Rather, the child has a well-defined deficit with several ramifications that are theoretically linked.

Before considering the varieties of answers to this question, it is useful to return to the issue of modularity within the language system. Consider the specific modules in language itself: phonology and syntax, semantics and pragmatics. Several chapters raise suggestions that there are influences between these linguistic submodules, and nonlinguistic cognition, that might or might not be symmetrical. For example, van der Lely suggested that children with vocabulary impairments might divide into at least two distinct groups. One group fails because of difficulties in joint attention and social scaffolding, and one group fails because they do not use syntactic bootstrapping to fast-map effectively. Imagine the many possibilities here in effects on lexical development. But complex grammar is also full of lexical effects, in the particularities of argument structure, complementation, factivity, and so forth, that a child with a difficulty acquiring vocabulary might then fail (Roeper & J. de Villiers, 1994).

Schaeffer (chap. 5 in this volume) has a fascinating discussion about how the pragmatics module might be structured, and the directionality of effects between interface pragmatics and morphology. She argues, along with Kasher (1991), that linguistic structure (morphosyntax) is the input for linguistic pragmatics—namely, speech acts, discourse regulation, conversational participation, and code switching. Surely then, a child with primary grammatical difficulties will also manifest problems in these areas of pragmatics (cf. Bishop, 2000). Yet, the first three of these aspects of discourse are traditionally the areas of pragmatics that autistic subjects have been found to be particularly weak at, even when they were claimed to have normal syntax and morphology (Tager-Flusberg, chap. 12 in this volume).

Schaeffer contends that interface pragmatics is a separate part of the module, dealing with understanding indexical expressions such as *he, she, there*. Interface pragmatics must "interface" between language and perception to achieve reference, coordination of knowledge with a hearer, as well as presupposition and article use. Interface pragmatics influences morphosyntax, and not vice versa. Schaeffer contends, with van der Lely (chap. 4 in this volume; van der Lely & Henessey, 1999), that children with grammatical forms of SLI have no problem with the concept of shared and nonshared knowledge, acquiring that on a normal timetable at around age 3. Hence she predicts and finds no apparent difficulty in SLI (or children older than age 3) with the distinction between determiners that depends on this understanding.

There are at least two difficulties with this picture. First, 3 years old is slightly too young an age for sophisticated understanding of the contents of others' minds, which most experts on theory of mind would put at nearer to 4 years (J. G. de Villiers, 1999; J. G. de Villiers & P. A. de Villiers, 2000; Perner, 1991; Wellman, 1990). Admittedly, however, the use of presupposition in language may be less demanding than false belief reasoning, which typically means predicting overtly what people know and therefore how they will act (Bartsch & Wellman, 1995; Wimmer & Perner, 1983). Some argue that the implicit understanding of false beliefs comes in around age 3 (Clements & Perner, 1994). On the other hand, not everyone finds that determiners are fully mastered in just these crucial respects, namely, sensitivity to what a listener could know at age 3. Using tasks such as elicited production or comprehension, rather than spontaneous speech, to assess whether children command the appropriate use of determiners, the age of mastery climbs nearer to 4 to 5 years (Cziko, 1986; Maratsos, 1976, Schafer & J. de Villiers, 2000).

Second, there is other work that also calls on interface pragmatics, again with the particular meaning that it calls for an assessment of what a listener can know with respect to what is being referred to. Consider the failure of children to obey Principle B of the binding conditions (Wexler, 1999; Wexler & Chien, 1986), in which children mistakenly think that *Ernie patted him* can mean 'Ernie patted himself'. Wexler argued that young children do in fact know Principle B, as shown by their behavior with bound pronouns. They get this case right: *Every boy patted him*. Wexler (1999) argued that, in addition, children know the "grounding principle"—namely, that a Noun Phrase must be grounded, either by a proper name, or deixis (pointing) or by being coindexed with another grounded Noun Phrase. Whereas coindexation is purely syntactic, deixis involves subtle coordination of the attention of hearer and speaker, hence lies outside the domain of syntax itself, and is therefore part of interface pragmatics. Arguing that the child lacks the "ability to make inferences about what speakers and listeners can infer in discourse situations" (p. 88), Wexler pointed out that the child might mistakenly assume that a Noun Phrase is successfully grounded when it is not. Hence a much older child, age 5 or 6, is said to be failing to obey binding Principle B because they have not yet mastered interface pragmatics. There is an inconsistency here that needs further investigation. It can presumably be refined so that interface pragmatics is not acquired all at once, but without that refinement the direction of effects among the modules is left in a tantalizing but questionable state.

SPECIFIC LANGUAGE IMPAIRMENT: DEFICIT OR DELAY?

If it is argued that SLI is a property of a distinct group, the language problem is domain specific, and homogeneous, then what specifically is the impairment? Several proposals exist in the current literature, and are divided by whether the problems in children with SLI can be described in terms of an essentially intact grammar subject to a maturational delay, or a grammar with a piece missing, a deficit.

The archetype of the first kind is that proposed by Rice and Wexler (1995, 1996, chaps. 1 and 2 in this volume). They put forward an elegant and intriguing possibility about the nature of the deficit in SLI—the extended optional infinitive hypothesis—that has received an enormous amount of attention, testing, and attempts at crosslinguistic replication. It has also received perhaps the largest test on a national sample of children in the United States identified as meeting the criteria for SLI described earlier. Rice (chap. 2 in this volume) reports that the sensitivity and selection scores of the tense composite index are very high (85%–90%), a goal only dreamed of by other investigators and test-makers seeking a clinical marker. So, on many grounds, it deserves a very serious look.

Quite apart from the empirical data on its behalf, the proposal may have attracted attention for theoretical reasons. Unlike most other proposals suggesting a particular deficit in the grammar of SLI, the extended optional infinitive hypothesis maintains one of the pillars of the paradigm of generative grammar in the Chomskyan framework, namely, continuity of principles and structures between adult and child grammar (J. G. de Villiers, 2001). In normally developing children, Wexler (1994, 1996, 1998) argued that tense (say past, third person) is completely represented in the child's grammar, complete with a full functional node from the earliest stages. This maintains a full clause hypothesis from the very beginning, that is, there is no need to grow categories or add nodes to the tree (see also Poeppel & Wexler, 1993). Yet, tense inflections are variably supplied, sometimes present and sometimes not (Brown, 1973). Wexler pointed out that when the verb is finite, it invariably preserves the other grammatical properties: For example, negation is in the right place with respect to it (at least in French; Pierce, 1992). So, tense is optional for the young child: The child does not know that tense is obligatory in matrix clauses. But Wexler argued that, in all other respects, the grammar is preserved. Just as in the adult grammar, if the verb is finite, it moves from the VP node to the inflection node to check tense, creating the kinds of word order patterns seen with negation in French. In the early period, then, the child uses the (nonfinite) infinitival form (the bare verb, in English, e.g., 'walk', the infinitive in French, e.g., 'marcher'). The child moves (gradually, apparently) to a grammar in which tense is obligatory rather than optional, usually resolving this at around age 3. Hence, there is a model in which there is full continuity of structure and principle with the adult grammar, unless, there is doubt, and there is, about whether any adult grammar permits optionality of this kind. On Wexler's model, biological maturation alone resolves the difference in optionality between adult and child: No learning, no parameter setting, and no gradual assembly of functional nodes is required.

In the case of the child with SLI, the proposal is that there is a maturational delay in the change to obligatory tense. Hence the SLI child persists for a prolonged period in using the infinitival form instead of the tensed form, with the resolution happening as late as 7 years, and perhaps not as completely resolved as in normal children. However, Rice, Wexler, and Hershberger (1998) documented a similar growth curve in SLI that starts at a later point (age 5) as compared to normal children. The attractiveness of the possibility is again theoretical. The claim that genes could code for particular linguistic deficits, such as "missing tense" is disputed (Marcus, 1999; Tomblin & Pandich, 1999), but if maturation is linked to the timing of gene expression, then a maturational delay linked to a genetic disorder is easily imagined (Wexler, 1996).

The crosslinguistic investigation of the central idea has run into some problems, primarily because the basis for the difficulty in SLI (a delay in the normal pattern) requires knowing about the normal manifestation. And the optional infinitive stage does not occur in all languages: It has been attested in French, German, and Irish, for instance, but not in Italian or Catalan Spanish. So what should be expected in SLI in those languages? Oddly enough, Crago's data on Inuktitut, which is definitely not an optional infinitive language (Crago & Allen, 2001), suggests that children with language impairments in Inuktitut may show use of bare forms never attested in normal development. But as Crago and Paradis (chap. 3 in this volume) point out, the stage cannot be called "extended" anything, and is not characterizable as a delay. Furthermore, the infinitive form is not a choice in Inuktitut: The SLI child in the case study used the bare form despite it being a form that never appears as an isolated root in normal language. As for French, Crago and Paradis claim that the form used as the default is not in fact the infinitive, but the past participle, often homophonous with the infinitive. De Jong (chap. 6 in this volume) raises a less severe but still interesting problem for Dutch, in which the normal path is a three-stage one, and the difficulty is in knowing which stage is "extended" in SLI. In Dutch, evidently other forms are sometimes substituted in place of tense, so the errors are not just of omission as in English, so not easily called either the infinitive or the bare form. Dromi, Leonard, and Blass (chap. 11 in this volume) present data on Hebrew, in which it is not apparent that there is a problem with tense at all, or what the default form is. In general, Hebrew-speaking children with SLI do not differ from age matched controls in their percentage of supplied obligatory morphology, except for the most difficult morphemes that combine person, number, and gender, and perhaps causality. The infinitive in Hebrew is varied in form, and does not serve as a default. The only hint of a difference between SLI and normal controls is in the minor use of "stripped," or bare, verb forms. Is it possible that the affected morphemes will differ according to the special characteristics of the language, and may not even always encode tense?

To illuminate the nature of the default forms for French, Crago and Paradis (chap. 3 in this volume) ask whether second language learners pass through an optional infinitive or extended optional infinitive stage. They find that children with SLI and the second language learners (in immersion programs in Canadian schools) had significantly more difficulty inflecting verbs for tense than age or language matched normally developing mono-lingual children. The second language learners were in fact the worst with past (48%) and future tense (49%) inflections, lower than the children with SLI (past tense: 74%; future tense: 64%). But the error forms of these two groups of language learners did have some differences. Second language learners used many more commission errors (e.g., using present instead of past tense), whereas SLI children primarily used nonfinite forms (i.e., infini-tive for the future, past participles for the past). Thus, the second language learners seemed more often to recognize the necessity for a finite form of some sort. But Crago and Paradis find the error patterns have considerable overlap, and most importantly, the stage of problems with tense is persis-tent in both groups.

Crago's work raises a fascinating possibility, namely, that the profile of optional nonfinite forms is shared by second language learners. But second language learners cannot possibly share the delayed maturation gene with SLI. The logical possibility is that what the two groups have in common, for different reasons, is that they start on the process of fixing tense later than normal: in the case of SLI, possibly because of maturational delay, and in the case of second language learning, for experiential reasons. If Crago is correct in arguing that the result is a plateau of tense acquisition, that the late onset does not just delay obligatoriness but can permanently affect it, then it might be argued that the empirical data are in keeping with a critical period for fixing the obligatoriness of tense. Both groups have missed it for different reasons. Furthermore, data on oral deaf subjects who have de-layed language acquisition would support such a model. Bare verbs instead of tensed forms are used extensively in the English of the oral deaf (J. G. de Villiers, P. A. de Villiers, & Hoban, 1993).

Tager-Flusberg (chap. 12 in this volume) claims there is a shared profile in at least some autistic subjects, which overlaps with SLI. They too show the optional tense profile, at least on the surface. Tager-Flusberg raises the interesting possibility that there is comorbidity between the "gene" respon-sible for this in SLI, and autism itself. But there is an alternative now brought up indirectly by Crago's findings. From everything now known about autism, a delayed onset of language is a defining feature. So these children too have a slow start, if a start at all, in language learning. Yet the slow start could exist for radically different reasons in autism than in SLI. For example, the classic problems that autistic subjects show in shared attention, gaze following, reference, and intentionality has been directly linked to their problems in early communication and first words. These are not problems usually associated with SLI. So both groups have delayed onset, and not enough time before the "critical period"[1] runs out to fix the properties of tense. But it might be premature to assume there is a shared genetic explanation.

So the notion of the extended optional infinitive period as a universal explanation for SLI runs into the following list of problems to be resolved: (a) It is not necessarily extended from a normal stage (Crago & Paradis); (b) the infinitive is not always a default (Crago & Allen; De Jong; Dromi, Leonard, & Blass); (c) it is not necessarily restricted to SLI (Crago & Paradis; Tager-Flusberg); and (d) in some languages, tense morphology may not be particularly affected (Dromi, Leonard, & Blass).

What alternative conceptions exist of the linguistic deficit in SLI? Other theoretical suggestions call on the notion of a grammar with something missing or mis-set.

One option is Clahsen's (1991) argument based on the case of German, in which a basic problem in SLI centers on agreement between two heads in the syntactic tree, leading to difficulties in subject-verb agreement or determiner-noun agreement. As de Jong noted, the problem arose that English children with SLI apparently did not have problems with determiners (Rice, 1994). However, Ramos (1999) found using experimental tasks that English-speaking children with SLI have significant problems with appropriate use of determiners. Consequently, the solution Rice (1994) proposed, in which German and English differ in the position of their determiners, loses some of its force. Schaeffer's data on Dutch suggests that SLI children continue to produce bare nouns, called "determiner drop," as do normally developing young children learning Dutch. Crucially, however, she argues that when they do produce determiners, they recognize the rules of word order ("scrambling") that can apply. Dutch children with SLI thus do not scramble determinerless nouns, and do obligatorily scramble pronouns. But the evidence on nouns with definite determiners is equivocal because it is so minimal (3 examples, 1 wrong, from all 20 children). It is premature to conclude that this represents a stage of extended optional determiners similar to the extended optional infinitive stage. That is, the form is variably supplied, but exhibits the right grammatical placement rules vis-à-vis the rest of grammar. More evidence is needed, preferably using elicitation procedures to collect a reasonable sample from each child. It certainly remains a strong possibility that subjects with SLI in languages other than German exhibit problems with determiners (e.g., in Spanish; Restrepo & Gutierrez-Clellen, 2001).

Roeper, Ramos, Abdulkarim, and Seymour (2001) argued on the basis of a case study that a child with SLI could exhibit a problem with agreement

---

[1]It needs to be mentioned that the critical period here invoked might itself be subject to variation in different groups (Levy, personal communication). This is an empirical question still to be explored.

that had pervasive effects throughout the grammar. For example, their subject (at 4.5 years) produced numerous case errors in subject position—*Me like ketchup, Her can cook something, Them have a party*—and in possessives—*Me sister name Dawn, He lost he family,* and *Them Mom could let them play outside.*

Both are argued to be related to agreement conceived as an abstract formal feature or relation applying in head complement and spec head environments, that is, in subject-verb agreement and also in the determiner phrase, as in possessives and demonstratives ("these hats"). The child also exhibited problems with prepositional phrases, specifically relational prepositions that are predictable from the verb (e.g., *to, of, for*). Such prepositions have been found before to be selectively affected in young children (Brennan, 1991) compared to spatial prepositions (*into, on, around*). Here are some examples from Roeper et al.'s subject: *Then me no have to go bath What beach you going?, Some wake up middle of the night.*

Roeper et al. argued that the verb contains, for example, a locative feature with which the preposition must agree. Thus, these quite distinct seeming errors might all fall under a common abstract rubric of a failure of agreement.

An attractive proposal by van der Lely (1998; chap. 4 in this volume) argues that some children with grammatical-SLI exhibit a representational deficit for dependency relations. Her account provides a systematic account of difficulties in argument structure (passive, dative, questions) as well as inflection (tense), thus providing an account that embraces a much wider range of difficulties than the extended optional infinitive account. She argues that a basic difficulty in the grammars of these subjects lies in the obligatoriness of movement, not in movement itself. But counter to the claim from Rice and Wexler that maturation is just delayed in SLI subjects van der Lely argues that something is missing in grammatical-SLI (G-SLI). To account for the optionality of movement, van der Lely contends that the economy 2 ("Must-Move") principle of last resort is missing in G-SLI grammar. The particular problem is part of the computational module of syntax hence a fundamental deficit. The problems are predicted and found to be widespread with tense, agreement, and argument structure, even extending to binding relations (van der Lely & Stollwerk, 1997) and wh-questions (van der Lely & Hennessey, 1999), but not to processes that do not fall under movement such as negative placement (Davies & van der Lely, 2000). In addition, van der Lely contended that some of the more subtle phonological deficiencies in grammatical SLI may stem from the same computational deficit in dealing with hierarchical structures.

Van der Lely's G-SLI subjects constitute a very highly selected group of children with persistent language difficulties that have not resolved. The subject population studied by van der Lely is considerably older (9 to 18 years, in specialized schools) than those studied in much other work. De Jong (chap. 6 in this volume) also finds his older Dutch SLI subjects to exhibit difficulties extending beyond morphology into argument structure in causative and resultative structures. One criticism against working with older SLI subjects is the possibility that the production and comprehension of older children becomes affected over time by their failures, so that they find compensatory strategies, or their responses reflect the therapy, the special education they have received, or the cumulative effect of persistent testing. Van der Lely has, however, adopted tasks such as truth–value–judgment that are held to minimize extraneous performance variables (Crain & Thornton, 1998). It seems probable then that children with SLI even at an older age reveal problems in grammatical operations or structures beyond morphology. Ravid, Levie, and Ben-Zvi (chap. 7 in this volume) finds that the problems extend into derivational as well as inflectional morphology.

So van der Lely's theoretical account accommodates interesting empirical work, but the concern is that it may only apply to a very specialized subset of children with SLI who have persistent problems into adolescence. How can such children be identified earlier? Researchers in the field may need to pay more attention to subtle syntax in younger language impaired children to bring the disparate accounts into closer connection, and to ensure that the oddities of the older groups are not a product of their prolonged adaptation. It might turn out to be the case that inflectional problems say, on tense, achieve their prominence just because young children with SLI avoid using complex syntactic structures in which other deficits would be noticeable.

In addition to these claims of a problem with the computational module in syntax, Penner (personal communication) argued that there is a different problem in SLI children having to do with the nature of variable binding. He contended that a striking feature of their grammar is a lack of appropriate use of variables, such as in answering wh-questions with a singular instead of an exhaustive set. That is, when asked *Who came to school today?*, the children might answer "*Henry*" and stop, instead of at least trying to list the people who fit the description, "*Henry, Alicia, Fred, I think maybe James,*" etc.

In addition, children with SLI have been found to have prolonged difficulty with appropriate use of quantifiers like *every, all, some*. Van der Lely and Stollwerk (1997) found some hints of this in their study of binding with quantifiers (also learning quantifiers: van der Lely & Drozd, unpublished data, cited in van der Lely, chap. 4 in this volume). But SLI children also make the "spreading" error characteristic of younger children (Philip, 1995) in which they interpret a sentence, such as *Every boy sat on an elephant*, to require one-to-one matching of boys and elephants. If there is an extra elephant in the picture, a fact irrelevant to the truth for adults, then these children say the sentence does not match the picture because of the extra elephant (Finneran, 1993).

Of course, as Leonard points out (chap. 8 in this volume), the fundamental problem with these very interesting observations is that the case studies or the subgroups prove to be shifting ground, not replicable in new samples. But the new samples, of course, are defined by the very criteria that may need to be questioned: no other associated difficulties, high enough IQ, less than 1.5 standard deviations below the mean on some omnibus standardized test of questionable linguistic value, and scores below the mean on several subtests. To clarify the existence of subgroups defined by deep linguistic properties, maybe at least some of these selection criteria need to be suspended. Especially if possible linguistic deficits turn out to be rather narrowly circumscribed, it seems odd to require poor performance across a range of relatively crude subtests (e.g., vocabulary, morphology) for a child to enter the definition.

Furthermore, the standard of comparison shifts across studies, ranging from the weakest, "compared to children of the same age," in which case SLI children look worse on just about everything, and "compared to children of the same MLU," who are naturally much younger. This latter criterion seems to be the one that a new observation finds hard to survive, and maybe it should be examined more closely. The point of an MLU matched group as well as an age matched group is to ask whether the child with the suspected language difficulty has a different path or pattern of acquisition from a child who is acquiring language on a normal timetable. It is by this criterion that the tense-composite measure has achieved its victories over other candidates as the clinical marker for SLI. That is, when children with SLI are matched in MLU with normally developing (3-year-old) children, they differ significantly in their use of tense markers even when other indices (e.g., other inflections, vocabulary, argument structure, etc.) remain fairly equivalent in the two groups. Obviously, this does not mean SLI children are normal in these other regards, just that they are delayed rather than deviant. But their tense use is below what would be expected for that MLU level. To avoid artifact, given that tense adds morphemes to MLU, Rice has used MLW (i.e., measured in words) as the matching index, and apparently there is not a significant reduction in the separability of the two groups by tense. So the tense composite survives the strictest comparison.

Nevertheless, because not all of the competing linguistic descriptions have been involved in the massive empirical effort to test SLI subjects from the great prairie states (Rice, chap. 2 in this volume), it is too soon to conclude that any other indices would do worse. But the strong suspicion given the data so far is that they might not be as revealing, and may indeed be fragile, variable, and harder to predict in form. Should the tense-composite clinical marker be adopted, at least for English? Before drawing that conclusion, consider some social consequences. They may turn out to be serious enough to provoke reconsidering the alternatives, and questioning the foundation for the search for a single index.

As background, notice that a critical period for the acquisition of inflectional morphology has been suggested before, in particular for the acquisition of a full American Sign Language (ASL) by Newport (1990; Gleitman & Newport, 1995). This research showed that people who attempted to learn ASL later in life showed much more optional marking of inflectional morphology to do with agreement, compared to normal first language acquisition of ASL that occurs at a young age. In fact, the critical period in their study seemed to stop around age 6 to 8 years. These subjects included individuals for whom ASL was really their first language, in that they had failed to learn the oral language to which they were exposed as an educational choice.

The ASL comparison brings out another significant point. When late-learning ASL users expose children to the impoverished model they provide, the young children pick up full use rather than optional use of morphology. In other words, they clean up their parents' mistakes. Newport (1999) and Singleton (1989) studied this process of "creolization" in deaf children who are born to hearing parents who choose to learn ASL to teach their children (also Singleton & Newport, 2000). So even an impoverished and optional input cannot deter a young normal language learner from acquiring full morphology. The optionality in the parental speech is presumably compensated for on different occasions and by occasional support from more effective ASL users, so the child can distinguish competence and performance.

In contrast, some dialects differ from Standard English in exhibiting what some linguists have dubbed "variable rules." For example, there are dialects in which speakers do not supply the past tense, or the copula, in all the contexts that a standard speaker would consider obligatory. Belfast English is such a case, as studied by Henry (1995). Yet young children exposed to Belfast English do not "fix" it to become Standard English. They end up speaking the same dialect as the parents, with the same variable use of the past tense and copula across different contexts (Henry, Wilson, Harrington, & Finlay, 1999). The only possible conclusion is that imperfect ASL and dialects are two different species of variability. One is genuine deviation from a standard, and the other is a full-fledged language with systematic rules that have conditions on them. And young children can tell the difference even when linguists have sometimes failed.

So, why not use optional tense as a clinical marker? Consider the situation in the United States. Tomblin estimated that from 5% to 10% of 5-year-olds are language impaired and in need of testing and services. Some 10% of 5-year-olds are African American. A majority of those children speak a dia-

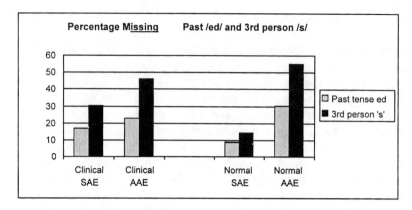

FIG. 17.2. Preliminary data on tense markers from AAE- and SAE-speaking children with and without language impairments.

lect, African American English, with properties resembling those of Belfast English: variable rules for copula, third person, and past tense. Figure 17.2 shows some preliminary data on spontaneous speech analysis of past tense -*ed* and third person -*s* from a much larger project investigating African American English (AAE) headed by Seymour (Seymour, J. G. de Villiers, & Roeper, 2000). Although these numbers are relatively small (< 30 per group), it is evident that the children speaking AAE who are healthy, talkative, normally developing 5-year-old children, score the lowest in their use of these two tense indices, even compared to children with SLI. The logic of the previous argument indicates that it is not the case that these children are being exposed to and are therefore learning an "impoverished" English. If it were performance variability, then they would fix it. Instead, African American English must contain subtle subrules governing the conditions of use of the morphology (Green, 1993; Labov, 1969; Wolfram, 1969) and to which children are sensitive (Abdulkarim, Benedicto, Garrett, Johnson, & Seymour, 1998; Benedicto, Abdulkarim, Garrett, Johnson, & Seymour, 1998; Jackson et al., 1996; Seymour, Bland-Stewart, & Green, 1998; Seymour & Roeper, 1999; Wyatt, 1991).

Notice that the very characteristics that distinguish these children's English use are those that have been identified as a clinical marker for SLI by Wexler and Rice. Unless the understanding of SLI is broadened to accommodate other possibilities for how it might be manifested, there is a serious risk of either grossly overdiagnosing or leaving out from services an already underserved population. This problem of relying on morphology in standardized tests and hence putting speakers of dialects at risk has been recognized for 25 years by the American Speech and Hearing Association. Thus, the tense-composite marker cannot be sufficient to the clinical task across dialect groups.

CONCLUSIONS

This chapter has come full circle back to the issues of definition of specific language impairment. Investigations of the linguistic basis for SLI are gaining momentum but are still in their infancy. There is a real risk in premature decisions about the likely common factor. It is also unlikely that linuistically based investigations can go forward under the methodological restrictions imposed by the broad definitions of the past. That is, although things have moved "down the tree" in Fig. 17.1 to arrive at the question of the nature of the specific language impairment, the debris of old branches are still dragging behind. It may be necessary to abandon some of the methodological strictures that go with the decisions about who to include and exclude, before there can be any progress on the questions of what constitutes a possible language disorder. Consider the requirements for inclusion that the child fail an omnibus language assessment:

The second consideration is performance on a comprehensive standardized language test (Tomblin, 1996; Tomblin et al., 1997). Ideally, such a test should include lexical, morphosyntactic, phonological, and pragmatic abilities in both comprehension and production. When such tests yield both an overall score and subtest scores, the overall score is required to fall below an established level X, usually −1.25 standard deviations below the mean for the child's age. In addition, the researcher may require that some minimum number of subtests also show low scores. The latter is essential if the standardized test yields subtest scores but no overall score. (Leonard, chap. 8 in this volume)

Omnibus language assessment was designed under many constraints, often having more to do with ease of use, ease of scoring, time limits, and differential diagnosis, than with systematic testing of deep linguistic knowledge. Clinicians are aware of their limitations in this latter regard. The gap from those scores to an appropriate characterization of the linguistic problem, and possible remediation procedures, is unimaginable. Even the submodules discussed strike many linguists as too broad: What about a "module" for agreement? Or for recursion? Or for binding? The chance is unfortunately slim that scores on a subtest of the average standardized test coincide with something that linguists OR biologists might consider worth measuring. Designing tests that test something BOTH linguists and biologists consider worth measuring may take a further revolution in education.

A new generation of tests needs to explore what the possible forms are that a language disorder might take from a linguistic perspective (e.g., Roeper et al., 2001). This might put researchers in a position to discover whether there are subgroups (as almost everyone suspects), whether the patterns they evidence ever occur in normal development, how the different modules of both language and cognition collaborate or dissociate, an whether children with these problems are distinct in any other way. But may be necessary to start at the bottom of the tree in Fig. 17.1, defining po. sible disorders in small groups, and work up. Although this may not be th way to find a gene in a hurry, it may be the only way to work out the the· retical puzzle of SLI, and it will also be a more direct way to help clinician diagnose and remedy the difficulties in children's grammars.

ACKNOWLEDGMENTS

Thanks to Yonata Levy and Jeannette Schaeffer for their invaluable help i stimulating and critiquing the writing of this chapter. Harry Seymour, To· Roeper, Barbara Pearson, and Peter de Villiers also gave very useful cor ments, for which I thank them. Preparation of the chapter was assisted b support from NIH Contract No. N01 DC8 2104.

REFERENCES

Abdulkarim, L., Benedicto, E. Garrett, D., Johnson, V., & Seymour, H. (1998). Syntactic-semant constraints on overt copulas in African American English. *ASHA Annual Convention Progra·* American Speech-Language-Hearing Association, San Antonio, TX.

Bartsch, K., & Wellman, H. M. (1995). *Children talk about the mind.* New York: Oxford Universi Press.

Benedicto, E., Abdulkarim, L., Garrett, D., Johnson, V., & Seymour, H. (1998). Overt Copulas in *l* rican American Children. In A. Greenhill, M. Hughes, H. Littlefield, & H. Walsh (Eds.), *Procee ings of the 23rd annual Boston University Conference on Language Development* (Vol. 1). Some ville, MA: Cascadilla Press.

Bishop, D. V. M. (2000). Pragmatic language impairment: A correlate of SLI, a distinct subgrou or part of the autistic continuum. In D. Bishop & L. Leonard (Eds.), *Speech and language i· pairments in children: Causes, characteristics, intervention and outcome* (pp.). Hove, Susse UK: Psychological Press.

Bishop, D. V. M., North, T., & Donlan, C. (1996). Nonword repetition as a behavioural marker f inherited language impairment: Evidence from a twin study. *Journal of Child Psychology a· Psychiatry, 37,* 391–403.

Brennan, V. (1991). Formal semantics of telegraphic speech. In B. Plunkett (Ed.), *Issues psycholinguistics* (pp.). Amherst, MA: University of Massachusetts Occasional Papers in L guistics.

Brown, R. (1973). *A first language: The early stages.* Cambridge, MA: Harvard University Pres

Chomsky, N. (2000). *New horizons in the study of language and mind.* New York: Cambridge Univ· sity Press.

Clahsen, H. (1991). *Child language and developmental dysphasia: Linguistic studies of the acquisiti· of German.* Amsterdam: Benjamins.

Clements, W. A., & Perner, J. (1994). Implicit understanding of belief. *Cognitive Development,* 377–395.

Crago, M., & Allen, S. (2001). Early finiteness in Inuktitut: The role of language structure and put. *Language Acquisition, 9*(1), 59–111.

Crain, S., & Thornton, R. (1998). *Investigations in universal grammar: A guide to experiments on the acquisition of syntax and semantics.* Cambridge, MA: MIT Press.

Crain, S., & Wexler, K. (1999). Methodology in the study of language acquisition: A modular approach. In W. C. Ritchie & T. K. Bhatia (Eds.), *Handbook of child language acquisition* (pp. 387–425). San Diego: Academic Press.

Cziko, G. (1986). Testing the language bioprogram hypothesis: A review of children's acquisition of articles. *Language, 62*(4), 878–898.

Davies, L., & van der Lely, H. (2000, November). *The representation of negative particles in children with SLI.* Paper presented at the 25th annual Boston University Conference on Language Development, Boston.

de Villiers, J. G. (1999). Language and theory of mind: What is the developmental relationship? In S. Baron-Cohen, H. Tager-Flusberg, & D. Cohen (Eds.), *Understanding other minds: Perspectives from autism and developmental cognitive neuroscience* (pp.). New York: Cambridge University Press.

de Villiers, J. G. (2001). Continuity and modularity in language acquisition and research. In F. Wijnen, M. Verrips, & L. Santelmann (Eds.), *Annual review of language acquisition* (Vol. 1, pp. 1–66). Amsterdam: John Benjamins.

de Villiers, J. G., & de Villiers, P. A. (2000). Linguistic determinism and false belief. In P. Mitchell & K. Riggs (Eds.), *Children's reasoning and the mind* (pp. 191–228). Hove, UK: Psychology Press.

de Villiers, J. G., de Villiers, P. A., & Hoban, E. (1994). The central problem of functional categories in the English syntax of oral deaf children. In H. Tager-Flusberg (Ed.), *Theoretical approaches to atypical language* (pp. 9–47). Hillsdale, NJ: Lawrence Erlbaum Associates.

Finneran, D. A. (1993). *Bound variable knowledge in language disordered children.* Unpublished master's thesis, University of Massachusetts, MA.

Fodor, J. A. (1981). *Modularity of mind.* Cambridge, MA: MIT Press.

Gleitman, L. R., & Newport, E. L. (1995). The invention of language by children: Environmental and biological influences on the acquisition of language. In L. R. Gleitman & M. Liberman (Eds.), *An invitation to cognitive science: Vol. 1. Language* (2nd ed.). Cambridge, MA: MIT Press.

Green, L. J. (1993). Topics in African American English: The verb system. Unpublished doctoral dissertation, University of Massachusetts, Amherst, MA.

Henry, A. (1995). *Belfast English and Standard English: Dialect variation and parameter setting.* Oxford, England: Oxford University Press.

Henry, A., Wilson, J., Harrington, S., & Finlay, C. (1999, November). *Language acquisition from variable input: Differences between parameter setting and lexical acquisition.* Paper presented at the 24th annual Boston University conference on language development, Boston.

Jackson, J., Ramos, E., Hall, F., Coles, D., Seymour, H., Dickey, M., Broderick, K., & Hollebrandse, B. (1996). They be taggin,' don't they?: The acquisition of invariant Be. In A. Stringfellow, D. Cahana-Amitay, E. Hughes, & A. Zukowski (Eds.), *Proceedings of the 20th annual Boston University Conference on Language Development* (Vol. 1, pp. 364–373). Somerville, MA: Cascadilla Press.

Karmiloff-Smith, A. (1998). Is atypical development necessarily a window on normal language development? In A. Greenhill, M. Hughes, H. Littlefield, & H. Walsh (Eds.), *Proceedings of the 22nd annual Boston University Conference on Language Development* (pp. 1–13). Somerville, MA: Cascadilla Press.

Kasher, A. (1991). On the pragmatic modules: A lecture. *Journal of Pragmatics, 16,* 381–397.

Labov, W. (1969). Contraction, deletion and inherent variability of the English copula. *Language, 45,* 715–762.

Maratsos, M. (1976). *The use of definite and indefinite reference in young children.* Cambridge, England: Cambridge University Press.

Marcus, G. (1999). Genes, proteins and domain-specificity. *Trends in Cognitive Sciences, 3,* 367.

Neville, H., Coffey, S., Holcombe, P., & Tallal, P. (1993). The neurobiology of sensory and language processing in language-impaired children. *Journal of Cognitive Neuroscience, 5,* 235–253.

Newport, E. L. (1990). Maturational constraints on language learning. *Cognitive Science, 14*, 11–28.

Newport, E. L. (1999). Reduced input in the acquisition of signed languages: Contributions to the study of Creolization. In M. DeGraff (Ed.), *Language creation and language change: Creolization, diachrony and development* (pp.). Cambridge, MA: MIT Press.

Perner, J. (1991). *Understanding the representational mind.* Cambridge, MA: MIT Press.

Phillip, W. (1995). *Event quantification in the acquisition of universal quantification.* Unpublished doctoral dissertation, University of Massachusetts, Amherst, MA.

Pierce, A. (1992). *Language acquisition and syntactic theory: A comparative analysis of French and English child grammars.* Dordrecht: Kluwer.

Plante, E. (1998). Criteria for SLI: The Stark and Tallal legacy and beyond. *Journal of Speech, Language and Hearing, 41*, 951–957.

Poeppel, D., & Wexler, K. (1993). The full competence hypothesis of clause structure in early German. *Language, 69*, 1–33.

Ramos, E. (1999). *Acquisition of noun-phrase structure in children with Specific Language Impairment (SLI).* Unpublished doctoral dissertation, University of Massachusetts, Amherst, MA.

Rapin, I., & Allen, D. (1983). Developmental language disorders: Nosologic considerations. In U. Kirk (Ed.), *Neuropsychology of language, reading, and spelling* (pp. 155–184). New York: Academic Press.

Restrepo, M. A., & Gutierrez-Clellen, V. F. (2001). Article use in Spanish-speaking children with specific language impairment. *Journal of Child Language, 28*(2), 433–452.

Rice, M. L. (1994). Grammatical categories of children with specific language impairment. In R. V. Watkins & M. L. Rice (Eds.), *Specific language impairments in children* (pp. 69–88). Baltimore: Brookes.

Rice, M., & Wexler, K. (1995). Extended optional infinitive (EIO) account of specific language impairment. In D. MacLaughlin & S. McEwen (Eds.), *Proceedings of the 19th annual Boston Conference on language Development* (pp. 451–462). Somerville, MA: Cascadilla Press.

Rice, M., & Wexler, K. (1996). Toward tense as a clinical marker of specific language impairment in English-speaking children. *Journal of Speech, Language and Hearing Research, 39*, 1236–1257.

Rice, M., Wexler, K., & Hershberger, S. (1998). Tense over time: The longitudinal course of tense acquisition in children with specific language impairment. *Journal of Speech, Language and Hearing Research, 41*, 1412–1431.

Roeper, T., & de Villiers, J. (1994). Lexical links in the WH-chain. In B. Lust, G. Hermon, & J. Kornfilt (Eds.), *Syntactic theory and first language acquisition: Cross-linguistic perspectives: Vol. 2. Binding, dependencies, and learnability* (pp. 357–390). Hillsdale, NJ: Lawrence Erlbaum Associates.

Roeper, T., Ramos, E., Abdulkarim, L., & Seymour, H. (2001). Language disorders as a window on universal grammar. *Brain and Language, 77*, 378–397.

Schafer, R., & de Villiers, J. (2000). Imagining articles: What *a* and *the* can tell us about the emergence of DP. In *Proceedings of the Boston University Language Development Conference* (pp. 609–620). Somerville, MA: Cascadilla Press.

Seymour, H., Bland-Stewart, L., & Green, L. J. (1998). Difference versus deficit in child African-American English. *Language, Speech, and Hearing Services in Schools, 29*, 96–108.

Seymour, H., de Villiers, J. G., & Roeper, T. (2000, November). *A dialect-sensitive language screener.* Paper presented at American Speech and Hearing Association, Washington, DC.

Seymour, H. N., & Roeper, T. (1999). Grammatical acquisition of African American English. In O. Taylor & L. Leonard (Eds.), *Language acquisition in North America: Crosscultural and cross-linguistic perspectives.* San Diego: Singular Press.

Singleton, J. (1989). *Restructuring of language from impoverished input: Evidence for linguistic compensation.* Unpublished doctoral dissertation, University of Illinois.

Singleton, J., & Newport, E. L. (in press). When learners surpass their models: The acquisition of American Sign Language from inconsistent input. *Cognitive Psychology.*

Stark, R. E., & Tallal, P. (1981). Selection of children with specific language deficits. *Journal of Speech and Language Disorders, 46*, 114–122.

Stromswold, K. (1997). Specific language impairments. In T. E. Steinberg & M. Farah (Eds.), *Behavioral neurology and neuropsychology* (pp. 755–772). New York: McGraw-Hill.

Tager-Flusberg, H., & Cooper, J. (1999). Present and future possibilities for defining a phenotype for specific language impairment. *Journal of Speech, Language, and Hearing Research, 42*, 1275–1278.

Tallal, P. (2000). Experimental studies of language learning impairments: From research to remediation. In D. Bishop & L. Leonard (Eds.), *Speech and language impairments in children: Causes, characteristics, intervention and outcome* (pp. 131–155). Hove: Psychological Press.

Tallal, P., & Piercy, M. (1973). Defects of non-verbal auditory perception in children with developmental aphasia. *Nature, 241*, 468–469.

Tomblin, J. B. (1996). Genetic and environmental contributions to the risk for specific language impairment. In M. Rice (Ed.), *Towards a genetics of language* (pp. 191–210). Hillsdale, NJ: Lawrence Erlbaum Associates.

Tomblin, J. B., & Pandich, J. (1999). Lessons from children with specific language impairment. *Trends in Cognitive Science, 3*, 283–285.

Tomblin, J. B., Records, N., Buckwalter, P., Zhang, X., Smith, E., & O'Brien, M. (1997). Prevalence of specific language impairment in kindergarten children. *Journal of Speech, Language, and Hearing Research, 40*, 1245–1260.

Tomblin, J. B., & Zhang, X. (1999). Are children with SLI a unique group of language learners? In H. Tager-Flusberg (Ed.), *Neurodevelopmental disorders* (pp. 361–382). Cambridge, MA: MIT Press.

van der Lely, H. K. J. (1998). SLI in children: Movement, economy and deficits in the computational-syntactic system. *Language Acquisition, 7*, 161–192.

van der Lely, H. K. J., & Hennessey, S. (1999, November). *Linguistic determinism and theory of mind: Insight from children with SLI.* Paper presented at the 24th Boston University Conference on Language Development, Boston.

van der Lely, H. K. J., & Stollwerck, L. (1997). Binding theory and specifically language impaired children. *Cognition, 62*, 245–290.

Wellman, H. M. (1990). *The child's theory of mind.* Cambridge, MA: MIT Press.

Wexler, K. (1994). Optional infinitives, head movement and the economy of derivations. In D. Lightfoot & N. Hornstein (Eds.), *Verb movement* (pp. 305–382). Cambridge, England: Cambridge University Press.

Wexler, K. (1996). The development of inflection in a biologically based theory of language acquisition. In M. Rice (Ed.), *Toward a genetics of language* (pp. 113–144). Hillsdale, NJ: Lawrence Erlbaum Associates.

Wexler, K. (1998). Very early parameter setting and the unique checking constraint: A new explanation of the optional infinitive stage. *Lingua, 106*(1–4), 23–79.

Wexler, K. (1999). Maturation and growth of grammar. In W. Ritchie & T. K. Bhatia (Eds.), *Handbook of child language acquisition* (pp. 55–109). San Diego, CA: Academic Press.

Wexler, K., & Chien, Y.-C. (1986). Development of lexical anaphors and pronouns. *Papers and Reports on Child Language Development*, Vol 24. Stanford University.

Wimmer, H., & Perner, J. (1983). Beliefs about beliefs: Representation and constraining function of wrong beliefs in young children's understanding of deception. *Cognition, 13*, 103–128.

Wolfram, W. (1969). *A sociolinguistic description of Detroit Negro speech.* Washington, DC: Center for Applied Linguistics.

Wyatt, T. (1991). *Linguistic constraints on copula production.* Unpublished Ph.D. dissertation, University of Massachusetts.

Author Index

Fox, M., 318
Frangiskakis, J. M., 323, 348
Frank, M., 324, 325, 349
Freese, P. R., 301, 320
Freyd, P., 175, 191
Frick, R. W., 237, 239, 242, 258
Fried, I., 416, 423
Friedman, D., 333, 348
Friedman, L. A., 391, 407
Friedmann, N., 278, 288, 418, 420, 423
Fristoe, M., 304, 307, 318
Frith, U., 120, 130
Fu, Y., 382

G

Galaburda, A., 312, 318
Gall, F., 210, 229
Gallagher, A., 120, 130
Ganger, J., 31, 45, 47 58, 59
Garcia, M., 316
Gardine, M., 422
Gardiner, M., 316
Garey, L. J., 376, 380
Garrett, D., 442, 444
Garvey, C., 366, 380
Gathercole, S., 120, 130, 213, 229, 308, 318, 418, 423
Gathercole, V. C. M., 171, 191
Gathercole, V. V., 326, 327, 342, 349
Gavin, W. J., 82, 94
Gavruseva, L., 105, 109
Gelman, S. A., 174, 178, 191, 193
Genessee, F., 101, 102, 105, 110
Gérard, C. L., 57, 59, 125, 131
Gerber, E., 211, 230
Gerla, B., 78, 94, 217, 230
German, M., 259, 271
Ghiotto, M., 354, 381
Gibson, E., 12, 23, 58, 59,
Gilbert, J. R., 316
Giles, L., 82, 94
Gilgenkrantz, S., 381
Gillis, S., 172, 175, 177, 191
Gilman, S., 316
Ginter, H., 422
Gleitman, H., 37, 60
Gleitman, L., 37, 60
Gleitman, L. R., 199, 207, 441, 445
Goad, H., 226, 229, 327, 349
Godzinsky, Y., 21, 59
Goellner, S., 121, 130, 348

Goldberg, A., 200, 207
Goldin-Meadow, S., 397, 400, 407
Goldman, R., 304, 307, 318
Gollner, S., 125, 130
Goode, S., 317, 319
Goodglass, H., 418, 423
Goodman, J., 118, 129, 235, 257
Goodman, W. K., 319
Gopnik, M., 114, 121, 130, 132, 214, 226, 229, 327, 345, 349, 350
Gordon, P., 121, 130, 342, 349
Goren, C. C., 416, 423
Gosch, A., 243, 254, 258
Gottesman, I., 316, 319
Grant, J., 350
Graziano-King, J., 325, 347, 349
Green, E. D., 318, 348
Green, L. J., 442, 445, 446
Greenberg, F., 323, 349
Greenbough, W. T., 376, 380
Greenfield, P., 147, 150
Grice, S., 350
Grimm, H., 110, 223, 230
Grodzinsky, Y., 278, 288, 418, 420 , 423
Grondin, N., 105, 106, 109
Gsödl, M., 350
Guasti, M., 37, 59
Guralnik, E., 282, 288
Gutierrez-Clellen, V. F., 437, 446
Gutowski, N. J., 348, 349

H

Hadley, P., 300, 318
Hafeman, L., 301, 318
Hagen, E. P., 350, 352
Hagerman, R. J., 355, 380
Hagstrom, 35
Haight, W., 43, 59
Haines, J. L., 316, 422
Håkansson, G., 104, 109
Häkkinen-Rhu, P., 213, 229
Hall, F., 445
Hall, S., 299, 319
Hamann, C., 57, 59, 125, 131, 154, 169
Hamburger, H., 12, 21, 23, 59, 60
Haney, K. R., 58, 60, 212, 215, 230, 308, 320
Hanlon, C., 374, 379
Hansen, D., 221, 222, 229
Hansson, K., 104, 109, 151, 169, 218, 219, 229
Happé, F., 120, 130
Harcum, E. R., 236, 258

Subject Index

A

Acquired grammatical impairment, *see*
    Agrammatism
Age matching confounds, 244–248, 256
Agrammatism, 413
    SLI, comparison with, 418–422
Approach bias, 6, 199–206
Auditory processing, 114–117, 430
Autism, 297–315, 355–356
    broader phenotype of, 301
    diagnosis of, 300
    genetics of, 301
    language, 297–315, 356
        age, relations with, 304–305, 310
        IQ, relations with, 304–305, 310
        profiles of, 305–308
        structural deficits, 299–300, 302
        variability, 305
    pragmatics, 299–300
    secondary symptoms of, 300
    SLI, comparison with, 91, 294, 298–302,
        414, 429, 436
    genetics, 311–312, 314
    neurobiology, 312–313
    tense marking, 90–91
Automaton view, 19–21, 23–25, 30

B

Brain plasticity, 293–294, 375–378
    and SLI, 377–378

C

Case, *see* Subject case
Case studies, 202
Clinical markers, 54–58, 63–69
    extended optional infinitive stage,
        54–58
    of SLI, 54–58, 63–66, 68–69, 93, 414,
        429–430
    tense, 54–58, 63–66, 68–69, 93, 440–442
Cognitive-functionalist approach, 199–206
Computational system of language, 4,
    11–14, 31–32
    parameters, 4, 7, 12, 13, 18–19, 29–31,
        34–36, 38, 53
    principles, 4, 7, 12, 13, 29–31, 38
Connectionism, 293, 339–347
Critical mass hypothesis, 203–206

D

Deixis, 433
Delay versus deviance, *see* Language
    delay versus deviance
Diagnosis of SLI, 300, 315
    exclusionary criteria, 3, 4, 9, 211–212,
        413–414, 417, 426, 428–429
    inclusionary criteria, 3, 4, 10, 210–211
Differential rates of development, 245–248,
    251–252
Distributional learning, 200, 205